COVID-19 AND GLOBAL INEQUALITIES

This timely and powerful autoethnography traces the spread of and responses to Covid-19: from the uncertainty surrounding its outbreak, to its devastating and continued aftermath. Following the virus in real time, it explores the fears, risks and responses to the global pandemic, and how it has shaped our everyday lives against the backdrop of social and political upheaval, and the looming climate crisis.

Social theorist and moral philosopher, Victor Jeleniewski Seidler, discusses fundamental questions of inequality and injustice regarding race, class and gender brought to the fore by the visibility of varying risk levels, vulnerabilities and protections provided by legislative measures against the virus. This interdisciplinary analysis scrutinises values, ethics, responsibilities and uncertain futures formed by the global health crisis, and evaluates media and communications strategies, government responses and political communications at domestic and international levels. Seidler shares critical insights into the cultural history of pandemics, highlighting lessons to be learned from anticipating, preparing for and enduring moments of crisis. Perceiving how the pandemic and climate emergency are interwoven, the book concludes with an urgent call to rebuild sustainable economic, political and ecological imaginations.

This wide-reaching volume will appeal to a broad academic readership in environmental studies, sociology, philosophy, health studies, cultural studies, gender studies, media and communication.

Victor Jeleniewski Seidler is Professor Emeritus in Social Theory at the Department of Sociology, Goldsmiths, University of London, UK. He has worked and published across the boundaries of social theory and philosophy, including works such as *Urban Fears and Global Terrors: Citizenship, Multiculture and Belongings after 7/7*; *Remembering Diana: Cultural Memory and the Reinvention of Authority*; *Remembering 9/11: Terror, Trauma and Social Theory*; *Making Sense of Brexit: Democracy, Europe and Uncertain Futures* and, most recently, *Ethical Humans: Life, Love, Labour, Learning and Loss*.

Routledge Studies in Environment and Health

The study of the impact of environmental change on human health has rapidly gained momentum in recent years, and an increasing number of scholars are now turning their attention to this issue. Reflecting the development of this emerging body of work, the *Routledge Studies in Environment and Health* series is dedicated to supporting this growing area with cutting edge interdisciplinary research targeted at a global audience. The books in this series cover key issues such as climate change, urbanisation, waste management, water quality, environmental degradation and pollution, and examine the ways in which these factors impact human health from a social, economic and political perspective.

Comprising edited collections, co-authored volumes and single author monographs, this innovative series provides an invaluable resource for advanced undergraduate and postgraduate students, scholars, policy makers and practitioners with an interest in this new and important field of study.

Research Ethics for Environmental Health
Edited by Friedo Zölzer and Gaston Meskens

More-than-One Health
Humans, Animals, and the Environment Post-COVID
Edited by Irus Braverman

Covid-19 and Global Inequalities
Vulnerable Humans
Victor Jeleniewski Seidler

For more information about this series, please visit: https://www.routledge.com/Routledge-Studies-in-Environment-and-Health/book-series/RSEH

COVID-19 AND GLOBAL INEQUALITIES

Vulnerable Humans

Victor Jeleniewski Seidler

Routledge
Taylor & Francis Group
LONDON AND NEW YORK

Designed cover image: © Daniel Ickowitz Seidler

First published 2024
by Routledge
4 Park Square, Milton Park, Abingdon, Oxon OX14 4RN

and by Routledge
605 Third Avenue, New York, NY 10158

Routledge is an imprint of the Taylor & Francis Group, an informa business

British Library Cataloguing-in-Publication Data
A catalogue record for this book is available from the British Library

ISBN: 978-1-032-28445-3 (hbk)
ISBN: 978-1-032-28447-7 (pbk)
ISBN: 978-1-003-29687-4 (ebk)

DOI: 10.4324/9781003296874

Typeset in Times New Roman
by codeMantra

In Memory of Tony
and all those who died from Covid-19 across the world.
And for all those in Covid-19 Bereaved Families for Justice seeking justice for those who died of Covid-19.

And in memory of Anna, whose love is always with us.

Days are scrolls: write on them what you want to be remembered.

Bachya

Just as the water reflects one's face, so does one's heart reflect other human hearts.

Proverbs 27:1

Teach your tongue to say, "I don't know."

Berachot 4a

From each according to his abilities, to each according to his needs.

Karl Marx

Every single person is required to say: For my sake the world was created.

Mishnah Sanhedrin

It is forbidden to harm any living creature. It is one's duty to save any living creature from pain.

Kitzur Shulchan Aruch

CONTENTS

PREFACE AND ACKNOWLEDGEMENTS

Fearful Times and Disrupting Worlds

Governments across Europe, the United States and Latin America were slow to react to the Coronavirus emerging from Wuhan in China and are still unsure whether the outbreak could have come from an animal market. With international flights across the world, the virus was just hours away, but this did not stop Donald Trump and Boris Johnson minimising the threats. They told their populations their health services were in good order, and it was only like a bad flu. We were to learn that in a globalised world we were vulnerable humans to a Covid-19 pandemic in ways that we had never anticipated and governments across the world had not effectively prepared for.

Their lack of transparency made it easy to distrust the severe warnings when they did come. Then, they assured people "we are all in this together." But it soon became evident that the middle class and the wealthy could work from home and escape the cities. They were not affected in the same way. Global inequalities were suddenly to be clearly exposed not only between the Global North and Global South but within nation states where issues of class, race, age, gender and sexual inequalities were to show that we were also differently vulnerable as human beings not only to a climate emergency but to a vast spreading Coronavirus.

At 1.38am on 31 December, a Chinese government website announced the detection of a "pneumonia of unknown cause". Over the next 100 days the world would be transformed. The virus would freeze international trade, extinguish economic activity and confine half of humanity to their homes.

The speed and severity of the lockdowns, first in Italy and then across Europe, left people shocked. Emergency workers were obliged to carry on working whatever the risks. People were inundated with contrasting information from a globalised media, which put out broadcasts 24/7, and social media.

The threat of a global pandemic had been anticipated for years by scientists but few of the preparations had been put in place. There was widespread anger in the UK when people realised that the years of austerity, since the 2008 global financial crisis, had left the National Health Service severely weakened and inadequately staffed. It was hard for people to evaluate the *risks* they faced in their everyday lives. British Prime Minister, Boris Johnson, at a press conference on 3 March 2020, cheerfully boasted that he was still shaking hands with people he met – including, he said, people infected with Coronavirus. This was a story of change so rapid that we can still, even years later, barely absorb it.

In February 2020, the future had suddenly been erased. It was hard to say how long the crisis would last, especially as it was evident that a second wave, probably worse than the first, was about to hit in the autumn of 2020. With our family stretched across different countries and the pandemic taking on a different rhythm and pace in different spaces, we were relieved to discover we could communicate through Zoom, a system most people in Britain had never heard of till then, even if it was often difficult to engage emotionally with what one was hearing.

You would hear different stories and different strategies of coping in different places. Often, they would make little sense in the context you found yourself in. People were living in radically *different* material worlds facing different threats, especially if they were obliged to continue working. Inequalities in risk, to do with class, race and gender quickly became visible. The middle class who could work from home because of new technologies found themselves living in a very different Covid world from those living in overcrowded housing and obliged to work as essential workers.

We were living through an unprecedented and fearful time of health and climate crises that fundamentally challenged our relationship with nature and our visions of the future. We pondered, *as* ethical humans, the need to decolonise the world as we shaped new democratic imaginations. Social theory can give us a greater understanding of time as social, as collective, but also *how* we carry it within us as individuals.

We learnt through Covid how precious time with family and friends really was. We re-evaluated our lives and what mattered. Many people revised their sense of trust and care within a community and determined *to live* differently as social and economic worlds were transformed. But as the vaccines were discovered, by the beginnings of 2023, many wanted *to forget* what they had lived through and were finding it hard to engage with *how* their lives were disrupted, the people they were still grieving, and institutions unsettled with their futures threatened.

Philosophy and Social Theory: Global Ethics in Dangerous Times

The Covid-19 pandemic, along with the climate emergency, fundamentally challenged the globalised neoliberal world where it is only "me" that matters. We learnt to value "us". If it was a myth that "we are all in this together" because we faced different risks, we did learn that we *are* responsible for others. If it takes a village to bring up a child, it takes a more equal and just world to ensure that we can all be safe when the next pandemic arrives. But this was already a fundamental challenge within a world already threatened by climate emergency that was leading to climate refugees as parts of the world become uninhabitable.

We began to establish new routines and learnt to take contact on Zoom for granted. As author and journalist Sarfraz Manzoor wrote:

> …things that used to seem weird now feel completely normal. … My children understand the concept of a Zoom birthday party … (but) seeing my mother for the first time in more than six months, as I am doing this weekend, feels super weird… It was only when these ordinary things were taken away that I was reminded how much they meant.
>
> *(Evening Standard, Thursday 1 April 2021, p. 19)*

Sam Wells, vicar of St Martin-in-the-Fields in London noted:

> Keep in touch is such a strange expression… (referring to) things that don't involve touch at all... (but one) we've used this past year more than ever, because we all know how easy it is to catch the virus… and how fragile life is.

Writing on Good Friday, a day of repentance for Christians for a long history of excusing and participating in the spread of antisemitic rhetoric and behaviours, Rev. Wells draws a parallel with the scapegoating of East Asian people during the pandemic. He gives an example of his friend being "called names and blamed for starting the virus," and notes a wider trend for "(c)rowds on social media (pouncing) on those they could safely blame for all the grief of the pandemic" (*Evening Standard*, Thursday 1 April 2021, p. 18).

The Archbishop of Canterbury Justin Welby said Covid had taught us many things as ethical and vulnerable humans: showing us how we depend on each other, and acting as a reminder that "…no one is safe until we are all safe. Our lives are connected. We must not walk by on the other side, and love must prevail over fear when it comes to our global neighbours."

As a family, we were stretched across the UK, Brazil, the US and Canada, so we heard daily through social media, about the different *rhythms* of the virus, how different countries faced the threats. Often it was easier to deny fears that were taking shape. As ethical humans we were having to face vulnerabilities we had hidden from ourselves, and our moral and philosophical traditions had *not* prepared us for. These were unprecedented times, as we were to hear so often in the days to come. Our lives and commitments to others were being fundamentally challenged and we each carry our personal and family stories from these times that are stretched across time and space.

Guardian columnist Jonathan Freedland described the UK as feeling like a country "stripped to its essentials," with citizens having to quickly assess "what is indispensable and what is not." The essentials included: "nurses, doctors, care workers, delivery drivers, the stackers of supermarket shelves ... good neighbours." The dispensable: "celebrities" and "star athletes." Freedland perceives a new order of value, and the realisation that the most needed members of society are poorly compensated. He notes that at this time, "Leave or remain feels like an ancient divide," and that for that moment, "the only distinction that matters, is alive and dead" (*The Guardian*, 8 April 2020).

Elise Gould, at the Economic Policy Institute in Washington told *The Guardian*'s Chris McGreal about the effects of the pandemic: "It's not just about jobs or wages. It's about health and working conditions and access to health insurance. All of these things highlight that there's two different societies in this country." A year after the pandemic began, the BBC televised *Pandemic 2020* with part two entitled *The Great Divide*. It opened saying: "It takes one international flight to carry the Coronavirus around the world."

Demonstrations in the United States about the economic costs of lockdown were supported by Trump. In the UK, Boris Johnson hoped the AstraZeneca vaccine would redeem his government after the UK reported deaths were among the highest in the world. The daily figures on the news put the numbers of new virus reports and the dead against the numbers of those who had received the jab, as if the growing numbers of those getting vaccinated somehow erased the losses of so many families.

In spring 2021, activists called for changes in intellectual property laws to give people in poorer nations access to the vaccine. While some richer countries could deliver vaccines to all adults who wanted them, many of the world's poorest countries had not vaccinated a single person.

Winnie Byanlyima, executive director of UNAids and a UN undersecretary general said:

> Nine months ago, world leaders were queueing up to declare any Covid-19 vaccine a global public good. Today we are witness to a vaccine apartheid that is only serving the interests of pharmaceutical corporations while costing us the quickest and least harmful route out of this crisis.

Abhijit Banerjee and Esther Duflo authors of *Good Economics for Hard Times* and winners of the Nobel prize for economics for 2019, pointed out that the International Monetary Fund had calculated it would cost just $50 to ensure that 60 per cent of the world's population was vaccinated by the first half of 2022 (*The Guardian*, 5 June 2021, p.1).

They said in June 2021:

> As it stands today, vaccine access is deeply unequal. The US is starting to vaccinate children, even as health workers and elderly people are waiting for shots in most of the world. At the end of April, less than two per cent of the population

of Africa had been vaccinated while, 40 per cent of the population of the US and 20 per cent of Europe had received at least one dose. India, one of the largest vaccine manufacturers in the world, has fully vaccinated only three per cent of its population, and is still in the middle of a nightmarish second wave that has forced the country to stop exports of all vaccines.

(The Guardian, 5 June 2021, p.1)

A doctor in Khartoum told Reuters: "On a normal day in Sudan you can't find a ventilator. Those who have immunity will survive, and those who don't will have to pray."

When everyday routines of work and leisure were severely disrupted, many felt desperately isolated and concerned at the loss of employment. Parents were obliged to do their best to educate their children at home, but often without the necessary technological resources. The strain this put upon intimate relationships, when women were left to cope within an unequal gender division of labour, damaged physical and mental health. There were increases in sexual violence across the globe. People were under pressure. It was estimated that 100 million more people were living in extreme poverty compared to the start of the pandemic.

Vulnerable Humans and Fearful Futures

There were moments when scientists talked about the need to learn how to live with the virus, acknowledging that it could not be defeated. We were to learn *how* to live with a multitude of different viruses, rather than in a constant struggle *against* an animal nature as European Enlightenment modernities had so often framed it within the secularised terms of a dominant Christianity. As *ethical humans* we were also emotional and spiritual selves rather than simply rational selves who had transcended their animal natures.

There were some people, like the poet and children's author Michael Rosen, who recovered from Covid-19 after long weeks unconscious in an incubator. They spoke about having returned from the land of the dead. Many people are still suffering today from the effects of Long Covid, a condition which brings exhaustion and brain fog.

Covid-19 taught us *how* bodies can affect each other at a distance. It left us yearning for bodily connections we previously took for granted. It brought us closer to how Brazilian Indians conceive the person as a compound of other people who are their relatives, so tacitly questioning disembodied notions of liberal individualism that so often guide philosophical legacies in the global North that have served to legitimate colonising histories of violence of white supremacy.

Tribal leaders in Brazil said medical teams working to immunise indigenous villages met fierce resistance from some communities where evangelical missionaries were stoking fears of the vaccine.

"Religious fundamentalists and evangelical missionaries are preaching against the vaccine," shared Dinamam Tuxa, a leader of The Articulation of Indigenous

Peoples, or the APIB, Brazil's largest indigenous organisation. This was hardly surprising given the populist President of Brazil, Jose Bolsonaro, who identified strongly with Trump and appealed to the evangelical vote. He ridiculed Pfizer and fanned false rumours across social media saying sarcastically: "If you take the vaccine and turn into an alligator, it's your problem. If you turn into Superman or women growing beards, I have nothing to do with that" (*The Guardian*, 11 February 2021).

The virus killed people across Brazil's indigenous communities raising fears that alongside the toll of human lives, the pandemic would inflict irreparable damage on indigenous knowledge of history, culture and natural medicines. A *Guardian* report shared that among the Munduruku people, they lost ten *sabios*, or wise ones, losses reflected on by tribal leader Alessandra Munduruku: "We always say they are living libraries… It's been very painful" (*The Guardian*, 21 June 2020).

Indigenous leaders such as Tuxa, said the government was *failing* to protect the country's 900,000 indigenous people – many of whom live in small communities, where dozens often share the same house. APIB logged at least 332 Covid-19 deaths, and 7,208 Coronavirus cases across 110 communities. "We are facing extermination," said Dinamam Tuxa. He said Brazil's Funai indigenous agency had taken too long to send emergency food kits to people isolating in their villages, forcing them to risk infection by travelling to nearby towns for emergency government payments. They *carry* memories of how the tribes had been previously decimated by epidemics of measles and flu and many now feared the virus was being spread by 20,000 wildcat miners – or *garimpeiros* – encouraged by Bolsonaro who were overrunning Brazil's biggest reserve – the Yanomami.

Across the region, communities were advised to go into lockdown and evacuate outsiders. "Right now, the big issue is stopping this virus from reaching the villages. If this virus gets into the villages, it will cause a huge amount of death," said Sofia Mendonca, a public health official who worked in the Xingu. "We are talking about true genocide," she warned. She said taking flight at a time of epidemic was a longstanding practice for South American indigenous communities, a survival technique passed down from generation to generation," or acquired from personal suffering (*The Guardian*, 30 March 2020).

"This is part of their ancestral memory," she said, adding:

> People are panicking. They are worried – and they want to go back. But it is very important for there to be a quarantine process so you can (safely) return to your village, to your home. And this will require different strategies in each place.

As Diaz Mirabel, a member of the indigenous Kurripako people of Venezuela said, "Due to our community-based way of life, the transmission would be very fast and the mortality would be extremely high."

The Brazilian photojournalist Sebastiao Salgado called for wildcat gold miners and illegal loggers to be expelled immediately from indigenous lands. "We are on the eve of a genocide," he said. "Indigenous communities have been so under attack…The government has no respect at all for the indigenous territories." Critics accused Bolsonaro, who came to power in 2019, of stimulating the invasion of indigenous reserves in search for minerals and dismantling the government agencies supposed to protect them. The pandemic made an already bleak outlook even worse by paralysing what protective efforts remained (*The Guardian*, 3 May 2020).

As Salgado recognised: "When you endorse or encourage an act that you know will eliminate a population or part of a population, this is the definition of genocide… permission is being given for the death of these indigenous people."

Writing Sociology as an Art of Living

I was used to writing autoethnography and investigating connections between the personal and structural relations of power within a practice of sociology as *an art of living*. I had written on the impact of events like Diana's death, and the terrors of 9/11 in New York, the London Bombings of 7/7 where sociology was challenged in its languages of secular rationalist modernity, to illuminate the events and shape concepts that could engage the moral realities, we were living through.

Sometimes we need to withdraw to write as a way of *making sense* and working through what's happening in life. Writing can help make experiences *real*. Sometimes it is through finding words to communicate with others, that we can *take in* what we are living through ourselves and put things in focus. In this book, I share certain diary entries in real time, sharing the *process* of shaping concepts that can help to illuminate the uncertain realities we were living through. This has meant, at moments, drawing on journal entries to focus upon particular concerns, *as* they were taking shape.

What resources does sociology as a way of living gift to us? How does it learn from those who recognise sociology *as* an ethical practice in conversation with those who acknowledge philosophy as an art of living? How can we listen and learn from the painful experiences people have lived through about *values of care* that should inform an ethical and just society? What have we learnt to value? What is there that we feel we need to transform, both locally and globally in economy, politics, and society, now class, racial and gender inequalities and everyday violences have been exposed and rendered visible? They can *no longer* remain hidden and forgotten within a neoliberal "common-sense" that did so much in Britain to legitimate years of austerity and left the NHS so unprepared for a global pandemic many authorities had warned of.

Writing has been a way of making real my own shock. I was aware I was in a privileged position being able to work from home and living in a house with a garden. Everything changed when my younger brother Tony got Covid-19. As it turned out, he only had a few days to live.

The writing was put aside for a while. Tony died in Barnet hospital on 6 April 2020, 12 days after his diagnosis, in the midst of the Covid crisis. I was searching for words to express the suffering we were living through, aware that so many people in the UK and across the world were going through similar fearful experiences which were hard to voice. Suddenly Covid-19 was no longer a topic to be researched but an experience of grief that was being lived both individually and as a family. How was this to transform my writing and research as I lived through a grief shared by so many across the world? How does this help philosophy and sociology come into a revitalised conversation with everyday ethics and structural relations of power and domination?

Shared Grief, Multiple Deaths and Democratic Accountability

I was distressed at how the media counted deaths as numbers, with politicians saying "each death was a tragedy" before quickly moving on. It is difficult to comprehend and process *what* the enormous levels of pain, grief, and mourning means for us all. How are we to understand what we have lived through and the grief that so many are still suffering? How should we remember the dead? Acknowledging ourselves as vulnerable humans, how should we be caring for people still suffering? How can caring for others be made central to our responsibilities as democratic citizens and as ethical and vulnerable humans?

These issues are vital in recognising *how* experiences shared by Covid-19 Bereaved families for Justice in the Covid Inquiry are not simply personal narratives that remind us of the terrible losses suffered but should be recognised as evidence that have direct institutional and policy implications. On the opening day of the Inquiry chaired by Heather Hallett, a retired court of appeal judge, Hugo Keith, counsel to the inquiry, noted how Brexit planning has caused pandemic preparedness to stall and they had assumed they would be dealing with a flu epidemic. She emphasises the inequalities would be "at the forefront" of the investigations. "Those who have suffered the most want to know if anything could have been done to prevent or reduce their suffering." (*The Guardian*, 27 July 2022) But there are also questions about whether a "listening exercise" can do justice to the evidence that the bereaved offer.

We all carry our personal stories of survival, even if as time passes, we have often blocked them as we do our best to forget how fearful and unprepared, we felt. So many people around the world want Covid-19 to be put behind us. Perhaps they hope that *if* they no longer talk about it, it will be over. At some level they can take reassurance from the vaccine that life *can* return to normal.

We may *not* want to be reminded of the losses we suffered, the deaths of family and friends or the opportunities we lost in education and work that cannot be easily recovered. Children and students can *still suffer* from mental conditions and feelings of vulnerability that can be traced back to months of lockdown. It can feel easier to block out what we lived through and to place it firmly in the past, even though it constantly *makes* itself felt in the present disrupting our lives and shaping different futures, especially in a time of climate emergency with refugees seeking safe havens and liveable lives.

We are facing fundamental questions that inevitably challenge the philosophy and social theory that we so often take for granted. This is helping to create polarised societies and authoritarian governments that are building walls rather than creating bridges between communities. This is why it is so important to reflect and learn from the disruptions of the global Covid pandemic, both personally and politically, while we face the ongoing climate emergency.

Acknowledgements and Gratitude

Writing can be a practice of making sense, but it can *also* be part of a process of grief and mourning. It is a process in time and autoethnography as method often takes time as connections can slowly emerge and we can be questioned by our research in unexpected ways. Writing about Covid inescapably draws on the personal as we lived through these times in very different material conditions of risk. We could *not* know what might happen or when we might have our own personal stories of loss and griefs to live with and live through. We discover the different levels at which we are connected to other bodies and souls.

I lived through the loss of my younger brother Tony supported by the love and wisdom of my partner Anna. As I have been rewriting, Anna was suddenly to die just two years later, on Friday 11 March 2022, just as a family we were coming to terms with the loss of Tony. This has been a time of grief for Anna and it has been uncanny but not disturbing to read her presence in some of the stories I share.

It has made the writing more personal, but also hopefully more truthful to what so many have lived through with grief. Sociology *as* an art of living is a personal journey across different levels and layers of experience. It travels across times and spaces, as we often make unexpected connections between the personal and the political, the individual and structural relations of institutional power. We are also, always engaging the traumatic memories from the past as well as anxieties and uncertainties in the present.

I would like to thank family who have shared a difficult year of grief and mourning when we would so have wanted to have been able to be together able to hug and cry with each other. I want to thank Anna, Daniel, Lily, Lara and Rich who have always been there and lived through this time together. After Anna's sudden death we supported each other and after the birth of my granddaughter Iris – as a Brazilian grandpa – Vovo – we shared in the love and joy she brought with her into the family. Through these difficult and grief filled years are all so grateful for the loving support of family and friends who have gathered around and supported us in such a loving and generous ways.

I'm also thankful for all the conversations I have had with friends and colleagues in different communities as we have lived through these impossible times. I'm also thankful for conversations with students in different settings, including the Sociology Department at Goldsmiths, University of London, the Nylon postgraduate groups across London, Berlin and New York and the staff and rabbinic students at Leo Baeck College.

I would also like to thank the Moral Psychology Group in Boston, including Lawrence Blum, Anat Biletzki, Sally Haslanger, Adam Hosein, Lisa Rivera, Margaret Rhodes and Naomi Scheman and Christopher Zurn, for welcoming me online and all the conversations about what was happening in the United States through different phases of the Covid-19 pandemic. There was the philosophy reading group with Lawrence Blum and Megan Laverty and more recently the group with Lawrence Blum Clare MacCumhall, Mark Hopwood and Rachael Wiseman.

We were constantly in touch with family in Brazil as they lived through terrible scenes of multiple deaths, unfolding along with Bolsonaro's government inaction. I want to thank Marilyn and Sami Caro for their constant love, understanding and support, we also learnt from family in the US and Canada. Different groups have also provided invaluable support and insights as we came together online, including my long-standing men's group and my meditation group.

The workshop we organised with Johan Siebers on *Martin Buber and Communications* that drew so many people across the world was also an invaluable virtual space, as were the dialogues we had together as friends and convenors throughout that perilous year.

I would also like thank those who read chapters, shared ideas and experiences and gave invaluable advice, including Anna Ickowitz, Lawrence Blum, Megan Laverty, Lily Ickowitz-Seidler, Lara Hollander, Daniel Ickowitz-Seidler, Richard Budden, Hans Fink, Terry Cooper, Rick Morrison, Tony Dowmunt, Jane Foot, Martin Hargreaves, Patrick Nash, Mike Wibberley, Rob Senior, Claire Highton, Liene Ozolina, Katherine Robinson, Ruth Sheldon, Joanna Ryan, Polo Anteaga, Ros Schwartz, Andy Cowen, Zara Philips, Sara Da'Silva, Ulla Fink, Yoval Amit, Clive and Kerstin Lindley-Jones, Anita and Rasmus Sucksdorff, Jacob Krause-Jensen, Angelika Strixner, Tim Davis, Isobel Cosgrove, Lucy Goodison, Jonathan Truscott, Les Back, Ros Gill, Nirmal Puwar, Fran Tonkiss, Manali Desai, Michael Bull, Shani Orgad, Ben Gidley, Michael Keith, Paul and Barbara Morrison, Carol and Hilmar Schonauer, Teresa Ordorika, Benno De Keijzer, Adelina Sanchez, Tony Skillen, Lee Wax, John Launer, Rivka Gottleib, Shalom Bitan, Anthony Mobereola and Amir Moradi.

At Routledge I want to thank Grace Harrison for her initial support and inspiration and Rosie Anderson and Matthew Shobbrook for their continuing editorial guidance I owe a special thanks to my cousin Angela Singer who offered a detailed and careful reading of all the chapters at a crucial stage. She has helped to make the book more accessible to a wider audience. I also appreciate the insight, care and understanding Jessica Oliver of Lex Academic brought to the project at a vital moment, as well as the copy-editing skills and understanding of Rebecca Wise.

It took me almost nine months to make the move from the kitchen, after Anna's death, to the dining room where I could return to revising chapters on my laptop. It might sound like no distance at all, but it took all that time, inspired by Anna's love, compassion and wisdom, to move step by step through this time of grief. As a family we moved through this process of loss together. It made real to me the time to mourn that so many people across the world were living through and the need for a revisioning sociology in its relationship with philosophy to engage more deeply with our existence as vulnerable humans.

I had lost some of my skills on the computer and I had to learn to take first steps, like so many who had been harmed through the pandemic. As I interviewed people about their experiences of Covid-time, so many were reluctant to speak because they did not want to be reminded of their existence as vulnerable humans, unsure of whether they could make up for years they felt they had lived partly in hiding. Students felt they had lost vital years and possibly could not make up for the intellectual and emotional losses and compete.

But many were determined to make changes in their lives to actively respond to the climate emergency and biodiversity crisis. They wanted *to live* in a different relationship with themselves and with the natural world. They wanted to *create* alternative worlds, also inspired by the Black Lives Matter movement in the wake of the tragic murder of George Floyd on May 25, 2020 that in the middle of the Covid Crisis saw people taking to the streets to demand racial justice and a moral reckoning with colonial histories. Fundamental questions were being raised about how different generations could live in their present, as they shaped more just and equal futures. They also wanted to learn from the painful years they had lived through with the Covid-19 pandemic.

They felt angry at politicians who had failed them, but also determined with others, to learn the vital lessons about transforming, economic, political, and social lives and institutions, to play their active part across generations to create just and sustainable worlds. Aware of the interrelation between the Covid-19 crisis and the structural inequalities of race, class and gender it had revealed, and the climate emergency, they were prepared to take to the streets to help shape alternative futures as vulnerable humans committed to a politics of care, kindness and compassion and greater equality and justice between the Global North and Global South.

1

PLAGUES, FEARFUL MEMORIES, COUNTING THE DEAD AND GLOBAL HEALTH RISKS

Urban Histories, Cultural Memories and Fearful Hauntings

Samuel Pepys fastidiously kept a diary from 1660 to 1669, a period that included a severe outbreak of the bubonic plague in London. Epidemics have often haunted historical and cultural memories. These memories often returned *as* people searched for precedents to the coronavirus virus. In the midst of a global pandemic that they were struggling to come to terms with, they often felt imprisoned in their own homes, fearful of the threats in the world outside while identifying with those workers who were obliged to work on the front lines in hospitals and care homes and those who had no homes as places of refuge.

People had been forced to change their patterns of everyday life and were obliged to live differently with schools closed and children at home. Those who could work from home endeavoured to do so. Patterns of thinking, feeling and acting were interrupted and while this could lead to increases in domestic violence, it could *also* challenge people to re-imagine the lives they had been living: the relationships at work and at home they had learnt to take for granted as somehow beyond question.

For Pepys and the inhabitants of London, as Ute Cotz-Heumann, a medieval historian from the University of Arizona, reminds us: "There was no way of knowing whether an outbreak of the plague that occurred in the parish of St Giles, a poor area outside London's city walls, in late 1664 and early 1665 would become an epidemic" (*The Conversation*, 24 April 2020).

Pepys wrote his first entry about the creeping threat of plague in the city on 30 April 1665, but Cotz-Heumann notes that "…it was not until the beginning of June when he saw with his own eyes the houses 'shut up'… (and) 'marked with a red cross upon the doors, and 'Lord have mercy upon us' writ there.'" That was when he became increasingly troubled by the outbreak.[1]

DOI: 10.4324/9781003296874-1

The fear was communicated to him through observing corpses being taken to their burial through the streets and it *became personal* when a number of his acquaintances died, including his own physician. In late August, having drawn up his own will, he wrote of deserted streets and how pedestrians he encountered moved as if they "…had taken leave of the world." This echoes with changes in the way we have learnt to walk with fears of Covid-19, seeing others on the streets as zombies and potential carriers of the virus, even if they do not know it themselves as they could be asymptomatic. People we have to avoid as all costs, especially if we have more years and so are defined as at risk in the present plague.

In Pepys' London, the Company of Parish Clerks printed "bills of mortality," the weekly tally of burials that undoubtedly undercounted the dead, just as the daily figures of deaths in NHS hospitals *undercounted* the deaths in care homes and in the community, where testing was largely reserved to those admitted with symptoms of Covid-19 to hospital. Pepys documented the growing number of plague victims in his diary. At the end of August, he recorded 6,102 victims but feared a higher number of fatalities, closer to 10,000, mostly because the victims among the urban poor weren't counted. Those whose life is given enough value to have their deaths counted remains an issue. A week later he noted the official figure of 6,978 in one week, "a most dreadful number."

Pepys was alarmed that people were attending funerals and gathering in some public places as attempts to control the plague were failing. Quarantines were *not* being enforced and people were ignoring official orders. Although plague victims were supposed to be buried at night, this system broke down and Pepys complained that burials were taking place "in broad daylight."

In the 17th century, despite the scientific revolution that Pepys lived through, nobody knew that the *Yersinia pestis* bacterium carried by fleas *caused* the plague. Medical science rather theorized that the plague was spread through miasma, or "bad air" created by rotting organic matter and identifiable by a foul smell. Remedies available had to do with purifying the air by smoking tobacco or holding herbs and spices in front of your nose that you could breathe in.

Pepys records using tobacco for this purpose, but was clearly sceptical over the effectiveness of the various remedies discussed at the time. He was very concerned with his state of mind, constantly mentioning that he was trying to be in good spirits, so maintaining a good balance of the humours in the body, according to medical thinking of the time. Melancholy, which was through to result from an excess of black bile, was deemed to be dangerous to one's health so Pepys sought to suppress negative emotions, as we might say. On 14 September he wrote that hearing about dead friends and acquaintances "doth put me into great apprehension of melancholy… But I put off the thoughts of sadness as much as I can."

In 1722, Daniel Defoe published his book on the Great Plague of 1665 – *A Journal of the Plague Year* – claiming it was "written by a citizen who continued all the while in London." It took 60 years for people to realise that he had written it from testimonies of the time, yet it remains, according to David Roberts, Professor of History at the University of Georgia: "The most harrowing account of an epidemic ever published…We read about the containment orders published by the government and how people got round them. We share the distress of families denied proper funerals for their loved ones" (*The Conversation*, 6 April 2020).

Defoe's narrator, identified only as HF, is fascinated by what happened when the lord mayor ordered victims to be locked in their homes to protect the lives of others. Watchmen were posted outside the front doors who could be sent on errands to fetch food or medicine and took the keys with them, so people contrived to get other keys cut. Some watchmen were bribed, assaulted or murdered and Defoe describes one as "blown up" with gunpowder.

HF also became obsessed with the weekly mortality figures, though he was aware that people were reluctant *to admit* there was an infection in the family. After all, they might be locked in their homes to catch the disease and die. With Covid-19, people could also be reluctant to acknowledge that someone is ill, if they feel it threatens their chances to work and bring wages home.

But Pepys was also concerned, as a devout Christian, that some people were so wicked they deliberately infected others. He cannot square this with his kindlier view of human nature yet he hears many stories about victims breathing into the faces of passers-by, or infected men randomly hugging and kissing women in the streets. He was also troubled by the fact that the plague seemed to be *affecting the poor disproportionately* who lived in cramped conditions.

Not only, as Defoe recognised, were they more likely to suffer from ill health in the first place, but they had no means to escape to safer areas outside the city. Near the start of the outbreak in 1665, the court, and those with money or homes in the country, fled London in large numbers. By the time the idea occurred to others with means, you couldn't find a horse for love nor money.

Throughout the journal, HF says he hopes his experience and advice might be useful to others. He insists that the most dangerous time was when people thought it was safe to go out. A warning that speaks to the present Covid-19 – that this was when the plague flared up all over again. The appeal of such literature for the reader, as Roberts notes is a "feeling that you might sneak with him to the very edge of the plague pit and live to tell the tale." HF hands us a doggerel poem that sums up his feelings and possibly ours too at a certain time as we remember the fearful early times with Covid:

A dreadful plague in London was
  In the year sixty five
  Which swept an hundred thousand souls
  Away: Yet I live!

Communications, Fears and Lockdowns

Italy's experience of the spread of Covid-19 communicates lessons about the steps to isolate the virus and limit people's movements. These needed to be put in place early, with absolute clarity, then strictly enforced. But these lessons were *not* heeded in either the UK or the US because of the governments in power and their reluctance to recognise early enough the gravity of the situation facing them.

Italy had surpassed China as the country with the highest death toll, becoming the epicentre, at least for a while before the US took over, of a shifting pandemic. The government had sent in the army to enforce the lockdown in Lombardy, the northern region at the centre of the outbreak, where bodies had piled up in churches.

As Jason Horowitz, Emma Bubola and Elisabetta Povoledo reported in *The New York Times* communicating their warnings:

> The tragedy in Italy now stands as a warning to its European neighbours and the United States, where the virus is coming with equal velocity…Despite now having some of the toughest measures in the world, Italian authorities fumbled many of these steps early in the contagion – when it most mattered as they sought to preserve basic civil liberties as well as the economy. Italy's piecemeal attempts to cut if off – isolating towns first, then regions, then shutting down the country in an intentionally porous lockdown – always lagged behind the virus's lethal trajectory.

As they argue: "In the critical early days of the outbreak, the Italian prime minister, Giuseppe Conti and other top officials sought to play down the threat, creating confusion and a false sense of security that allowed the virus to spread."

They also recognised that:

> Even once the Italian Government considered a universal lockdown necessary to defeat the virus, it failed to communicate the threat powerfully enough to persuade Italians to abide by the rules, which seemed riddled with loopholes." And they note: "The difficulties of navigating Italy's divisions of power between Rome and the regions resulted in a fragmented chain of command and inconsistent messages…Politicians across the spectrum worried about the economy and feeding the country and found it difficult to accept their impotence in the face of this virus.

Something similar was to take place within neoliberal societies that had fostered notions of individual autonomy and ideas that people *are* in control of their lives and capable of planning their own futures. The speed with which any sense of future possibilities was to give way in face of the virus, helped to produce intense anxieties and fears of what the future might look like.

As Jason Horowitz, the Rome Bureau chief of *The New York Times*, also reported from Italy soon after the virus was to take such a firm grip:

> The mayor of one town complained that doctors were forced to decide not to treat the very old, leaving then to die. In another town, patients with coronavirus-caused pneumonia were being sent home. Elsewhere, a nurse collapsed with her mask on, her photograph becoming a symbol of overwhelmed medical staff.

He reports on the speed of the traumatic movement of the virus:

> In less than three weeks, the coronavirus has overloaded the health care system all over northern Italy. It has turned the hard-hit Lombardy region into a grim glimpse of what awaits countries. They cannot slow the spread of the virus and 'flatten the curve' of new cases – allowing the sick to be treated without swamping the capacity of hospitals.
>
> *(The New York Times, 12 March 2020)*

Already in early March in Castiglione d'Adda, a town of 4,600 in Lombardy, 18 people had died within the past two weeks and as of Thursday 5 March, 121 inhabitants were infected. The town's mayor Costantino Pesatori was waiting for the end of his 14-day quarantine period. He described the virus to journalist Angela Giuffrida, as "surreal" and "like living in a film." He noted that people even at that point had begun to break the lockdown rules out of frustration. Stefano Lovisetto, a 58-year-old from Vo Euganeo, was discharged from hospital after overcoming coronavirus. "I had no symptoms, not even a cough… people are saying that this is the plague, but it isn't" (*The Guardian*, 6 March 2020, p. 9).

Moreno Colombi, 59, also recovered from the virus, but said she was being treated by fellow residents in Truccazzano, a town of 6,000 near Milan, as if she had the plague. She was the only confirmed case in a town that was not yet under lockdown. "They are speaking badly about me – it's as if I did a robbery or something… all it is a virus that just so happened to affect me." She explained that her symptoms were minimal, and comparing herself with other who were very unwell with the virus, expressed the view that "most of those (suffering) have other pathologies" (*The Guardian*, 6 March 2020, p. 9).

Health Emergencies and Ethical Challenges

Things were to get a lot worse very quickly. "This is a war" said Massimo Puoti, the head of infectious medicine at Milan's Niguarda hospitals. He said the goal was to limit infections, stave off the epidemic and learn more about the nature of the enemy. "We need time." Jason Horowitz reported on the lessons learned:

> Italy's experience has now underscored the need to act decisively – quickly and early – well before case numbers even appear to reach crisis levels. By that point, it may already be too late to prevent a spike in cases that stretch systems beyond their limits. With Italy having appeared to pass that threshold, its doctors are finding themselves in an extraordinary position largely unseen by developed European nations with public health care systems since the Second World War.
>
> *(The New York Times, 12 March 2020)*

This was a lesson that neither the UK, a European neighbour, nor the US were to learn. It partly explains the high levels of deaths in the UK, even though the government persists in saying that they acted at the right time, when they evidently did not and it was only through the rapid construction of the new Nightingale hospitals that the health system wasn't completely overwhelmed.

The metaphor of *war* took hold, at least in Italy as the doctor, Daniele Macchini wrote: "The war has literally exploded and battles are uninterrupted day and night," calling the situation an "epidemiological disaster" that has "overwhelmed" the doctors. Fabiono Di Marco, a doctor in Bergamo, had taken to sleeping in his office. He said that doctors literally "draw a line on the ground to divide the clean part of the hospital from the dirty one," where anything they touched was considered contagious.

Dealing with the virus across Europe and the world, people had become acutely aware of what they *touched* and the dangers carried in that sense. It was hard to know what you could touch safely, especially when you left the house or entered a space like a hospital that had Covid-19 patients. Many patients with other critical conditions had declined to turn up to A&E departments or for treatment, leading doctors to anticipate that after the first wave of coronavirus passed, they would be inundated with cases of cancer and other critical conditions that would be reported much later and so probably, harder to treat.

Giorgo Gori, the Mayor of Bergamo, admitted that in parts of Lombardy the *gap* between resources and the enormous influx of Covid-19 patients "forced the doctors to decide not to intubate some very old patients," essentially leaving them to die. "Were there more intensive care units…it would have been possible to save more lives." Dr Di Marco disagreed with this mayor's opinion on this but did add that: "…it could happen that we have a comparative evaluation between patients."

There were guidelines on what to do in a period that bordered on wartime "catastrophic medicine". In the context of a grave shortage of health resources, the guidelines said intensive care should be given to "patients with the best chance of success" and those with the "best hope of life" should be prioritised. This faced doctors with impossible ethical choices, especially if they were treating people they knew.

The guidelines *were* framed in utilitarian terms saying that "in the interests of maximising benefits for the largest number," scarce intensive care resources should be given to those who had, first, "greater likelihood of survival and secondly who have more potential years of life." Dr Petrini said: "No one is getting kicked out, but we're offering criteria of priority. These choices are made in normal times, but what's not normal is when you have to assist 600 people all at once."

There was a lot riding on the notion of "criteria of priority" and though it was claimed that a similar crisis was avoided in the UK, in fact, with the overrunning of the health service, there were issues about elderly people in care homes who could *not* be tested for the virus and so were excluded from the figures. They were not offered the possibility of transfer to hospital because of their poor chances of survival with underlying health conditions. It was only towards the end of April 2020 that the health authorities were under widespread public and media pressure *to include* care homes in the daily tally of deaths. But given that there was a crisis in testing, many of the people dying in care homes were never seen by doctors who couldn't visit because of the threats of the virus and many were not registered as Covid-19 deaths on their death certificates. Later many were certified as dying *of* Covid when in fact they had died *with* Covid.

Italian lawyer Carlo Palermo, who represents public hospital doctors, said it helped that it was a public system, even though, as in the UK, it had suffered from years of budget cuts. Had it been an insurance-based system, there would have been a "fragmented" response, he said. He did acknowledge that if the virus spread south, as it did with poorer health conditions: "The system won't hold, and we don't be able to assure care."

The Italian Government was to regret allowing flights from the infected regions in the north to the south. Tullio Prestileo, a doctor of infectious diseases at Palermo's Benfratelli Hospital, noted that the government should have "track(ed) and register(ed) people who came to the south from the red zones of northern Italy in order to avoid spreading to the southern cities of the country" (*The Guardian*, 7 March 2020, p. 11).[2]

Communications, Risks and Democratic Authority

"The Italian disease is becoming a European disease and Trump, with his decision (to close flights to foreigners coming from Europe), is trying to avoid this becoming an American disease," said Romano Prodi, a former Italian prime minister and president of the EU commission. "In any case I think that coronavirus is already also an American problem," he said, adding that, because of the differences in the health care system, "it may be more serious than the European one" (*The New York Times,* 12 March 2020 – updated 17 March 2020).

On Sunday 5 April, initially at least, as journalist Lloyd Green reported:

> There was no White House briefing on the president's public schedule. But the bad news kept coming. Coronavirus deaths continued to climb and reports of the heartland being unprepared for what may be on its horizon continued to ricochet around the media.

Green also reported being informed by an insider to the administration that it was: "...simply collapsing. He's killing his own supporters." The journalist described Trump as "(appearing) incapable of emoting anything that comes close to heartfelt concern. Or just providing straight answers" (*The Guardian*, 5 April 2020).

As Robert Reich, a former US secretary of Labour under Clinton recognised:

> The utter chaos in America's response to the coronavirus pandemic – shortages of equipment to protect hospital workers, dwindling supplies of ventilators and critical medications, jaw-dropping confusion over how the $2.2 trillion of aid in

> the recent coronavirus law will be distributed- was perhaps predictable in a nation that prides itself on competitive individualism and hates centralised power.

President Donald Trump was clear in denying responsibility for the slow rate of Covid testing in the US. As David Smith, Washington Bureau chief for *The Guardian*, reported: "When the celebrity businessman has his back to the wall, he calls for the cavalry of corporate America." At his press conference on Friday 13 March, it was described that he:

> … rolled in business titans to save the day, treating them to plenty of handshakes and little social distancing. 'You're going to be hearing from some of the largest companies and greatest retailers and medical companies in the world,' presumably hoping to reassure the stock market.

Trump announced the "drive-thru" testing centres that would be set up in parking lots at CVS pharmacies, Target, Walmart and Walgreens stores.

When asked on Friday 3 April if he could assure New Yorkers that there would be enough ventilators next week when virus sufferers were expected to overwhelm city hospitals, he replied: "No. They should have had more ventilators." In a federal system, Trump had consistently chosen *to blame* state governors for the crisis that was unfolding on so many different levels. At the same time, he was urging them to consider an early opening up of the economy. Trump told governors to find life-saving equipment on their own. He refused to create a central bargaining agent, arguing in neoliberal market terms that the federal government was "not a shipping clerk". This left states and cities bidding against each other, driving up the prices of ventilators, gloves, masks, infusion pumps and portable X-ray machines.

According to Reich, citing Trump's tendencies to dismiss events as "hoaxes," including alleged Russian influence in his election and his own impeachment: "The real hoax is Trump's commitment to America." His conclusion is that the pandemic proved another opportunity for the former President to cling onto power at any cost.

Nick Cohen, writing for *The Observer* (22 March 2020, p. 54) noted that the crisis "has revealed the emptiness of leaders who manufacture nationalist fears to maintain their power…Trump looks as out of a luck as a cornered conman." At the same time, he recognised: "To see how a pandemic can be used to ensure that supplies of politically useful rage keep flowing, look at how US Republicans are constructing a cover story. They have plenty to cover up."

On 22 January Trump made the claim: "We have it under control. It's going to be just fine." As Cohen notes, the US population were offered little more than "bluff and bombast to make the virus seem a minor nuisance and then, as reality dawned on the president's narrow mind, to ensure that blame went to anyone else but himself."

Fox News had long worked as the media outlet that acted as a front for Trump's administration. At the beginning of March, criticisms of Trump's inability to see a national emergency when it was staring him in the face were met by Fox presenters pushing impeachment conspiracies and minimising the health risks presented by the virus.

In the same article, Cohen highlights the swift change in the perception of the virus in the Trump administration, when it became clear how dangerous and contagious the virus was. He suggests that this could have been an opportunity for the administration to honourably admit to their earlier failures, but that ultimately within the wider context of the culture wars waged by the Trump camp, that honesty would have jeopardised their re-election prospects. Further evidence that the administration was leaning into their divisive impulses came in the form of the rampant use of the term "Chinese virus," infuriating Trump's liberal opponents and inviting his base to retaliate.

Trump's supporters will insist that everyone knows the outbreak started in China because of China's appalling treatment of animals and the Chinese Communist party having done its best to hide the outbreak's existence and put pressure on the World Health Organization (WHO) to go along with it. In shaping a populist common-sense he will have persuaded many of his core voters to blame the multiple deaths *on* the Chinese so taking attention away from his own failures to prepare for the virus heading in their direction.

Cohen notes that the repercussions don't end there. Should the blame be placed on China for the virus, any domestic critics of the administration are labelled as traitors supporting Chinese communists. By 19 March, Trump publicly accused journalists asking tough questions of "siding with China." This, as Cohen observed, became an opening for "nationalist tricksters to wrap themselves in their tattered flags."[3]

Mass Media, Politics and Failing Control

"The US response will be studied for generations as a textbook example of a disastrous, failed effort," Ron Klain, the American attorney who fronted the fight against Ebola in 2014 and who later served as White House chief of staff under President Biden, told a Georgetown University panel. "What's happened in Washington has been a fiasco of incredible proportions."

Jeremy Konyndyk, who worked at USAid (The United States Agency for International Development) from 2013 to 2017 said the White House had all the information it needed by the end of January to act decisively, but that Trump repeatedly played down the severity of the threat, later blaming China for what he called the "Chinese virus." That CDC – the US Centre of Disease Control and Prevention – botched the rollout of testing was the first indication that the Trump administration was faltering as the health emergency gathered pace (*The Guardian*, 28 March 2020).

Valerie Griffeth was a founder member of one the new online start-ups that were trying to fill the Trump void. Set up by emergency department doctors across the country, GetUsPPE.org sought to counter the top-down chaos that was putting front line health workers like herself in danger through a lack of protective gear. She was an emergency and critical care doctor in Portland, Oregon. Early on in the crisis, Griffeth said it dawned on her and many of her peers that the federal government to which they would normally look to keep them safe was nowhere to be seen. They resigned themselves to a terrible new reality in what was supposedly a leading global power.

But she had also witnessed the emergence of something new, an explosion of American citizens, like their counterparts in the UK, facing similar shortages of PPE doing it for themselves and working at home sometimes to make the missing items, like protective masks. "People are stepping up all around us… I'm amazed by what has happened in such a short time. It gives me hope."

Konyndyk said the stark outcomes between different countries in terms of illness and death had been determined not by Covid-19 itself, but by *how seriously* each government took the risk and how early they acted. "On that score we failed badly… You can have the best system in the world, but if you give the virus an eight-week head start it will eat you alive." This was starkly revealed for the UK on BBC Radio 4's *Any Questions?* on Saturday 2 May. Anthony Costello, professor of Global Health at University College London, made it clear that the UK now accounted for one in ten of the world's Covid-19 deaths and a death rate five times that of Germany. That was his response to a question from John Hopkin in Birmingham: Did the panel agree with the prime minister saying that people will be looking at "our apparent success."

Costello reported the *Financial Times* saying that the rate was actually eight times worse than Germany because if you added in the deaths in social care, it would be 48,000 deaths in the UK. Looking back, he said, the British Government set up a group of scientific experts but half of them were actually government employees, so it was hardly independent. As the Covid Inquiry was to hear in June 2023 planning for a no-deal Brexit had prevented government efforts to plan for a pandemic. They didn't have a single public health specialist or anyone internationally from the Far East that *could* have given them strong advice on the basis of their own experience, for example in South Korea that had kept deaths figures relatively low.

Apparently when SAGE (the Scientific Advisory Group for Emergencies) met for the first time at the end of January they were thinking on the lines that this was like pandemic influenza where you *don't* test, and they said we didn't have the scale to test and trace so the modellers didn't look at that as an option. This was the first mistake.

Secondly, when we came to 12 March when the prime minister, Boris Johnson and the chief medical officer, Chris Whitty and chief scientific advisor, Patrick Vallance announced a policy of stopping all community testing and tracing with no lockdown, they said they wanted us to get this infection. They said that it was good for us all to be infected because we would get "herd immunity".

That was at exactly the same time that Korea had launched a successful testing and tracing policy that enabled them to suppress their epidemic in three weeks with 250 deaths so far and Greece did a complete lockdown before they had a single death. On 10 March we had fewer than ten deaths and about 500 cases and we let it run for another two weeks. They might have thought we wouldn't comply with a lockdown and there possibly wouldn't be a vaccine, but they were wrong, so we've ended up with 48,000 deaths in a terrifyingly short period of time.[4]

Costello was still not clear whether the government was going for real suppression of the virus or whether they were split, with some ministers wanting to open the economy sooner so they going to attempt to manage this as they flattened the curve, acknowledging that we would still have the virus over the next two years. As Costello argued, we had more time to prepare and had the example of Italy to follow but we failed to listen and to learn. Now he argued we "should go for it" and acknowledging we got it wrong in the beginning, go for a policy of aggressive suppression.

Naomi Oreskes, a history of science professor at Harvard, saw the unfolding crisis in the US as the fulfilment of her worst fears:

> When we first heard about coronavirus, I and several of my colleagues worried that Trump would not attend to scientific advice. This is a man who has exhibited a reckless disregard for scientific evidence over climate change. If he could do that, there was always the question of whether he would take seriously any science.

As she noted: "What we've seen is that for people in power in this country, ideology beats even an imminent threat." As Ed Pilkington of *The Guardian* reported: "He would dig into the tried and tested Republican playbook of showing hostility to science and expertise, reining in government intervention and prioritising the money markets" (*The Guardian*, 4 April 2020).

"This will be regarded as the worst public health disaster in America in a century," said Eric Topol, at Scripps Research in San Diego. "The root cause of the disaster was the lack of readiness to understand where, how and when the disease was spreading. We now know there will be well over 100,000 deaths." Topol said: "A vast majority of those people will have been unnecessarily lost because of the lack of preparedness of the United States. As a leader, Trump had to accept responsibility, which of course he won't." It was hardly surprising that Nancy Pelosi, the top Democrat in Congress, accused Trump directly of "costing American lives" on CNN and said: "As the president fiddles, people are dying."

Communications, Uncertainties and Post-Truth Politics

In an article for *The Atlantic* entitled "Why the Coronavirus Is so Confusing" (*The Atlantic*, 29 April 2020), Ed Yong acknowledges that so many things about the pandemic are still maddeningly unclear. "Why do some people get really sick while others do not? Are the models too optimistic or too pessimistic? Exactly how transmissible and deadly is the virus?" Clearly these vital questions remained unanswered partly because of how rapidly and widely the pandemic spread.

Yong considers the statistics at the time of writing that 3.1 million across the globe were infected with Covid in a quarter of a year, wreaking havoc on the global economy and stalling millions of lives. People who wanted to feel in control of their lives were suddenly confronted with fear and uncertain futures, owing to the "...variability of Covid-19... perplexing doctors." This, he states, resulted in a particular challenge to assemble statistics on coronavirus: "...of its case-fatality rate (CFR) – the proportion of diagnosed people who die – have ranged from 0.1.50 to 1.5 per cent." Doctors are trained to work with firm numbers so that often, in a crisis situation like Covid-19, they are relying on their iPads as a source of security, fearful of really engaging with the patients themselves.

It is the numbers that have an objectivity, even if they are abstractions, and this is what medical students often rely upon to give them a sense of what they are dealing with rather than observing symptoms themselves. "Folks are talking about CFR as this unchangeable quantity, and that is now how it works," said Maia Majumder, an epidemiologist at Harvard Medical School. In any case, the total cases depend on how thoroughly a country tests its population, which has been a real issue in the US and UK.

"We've never faced a pandemic like this before, so we don't know what is likely to happen or what would have happened," said Zoe McLaren, a health-policy professor at the University of Maryland. "That makes it ever more difficult in terms of the uncertainty." She also acknowledged: "Clinicians are under tremendous stress, which affects our ability to process information. Is this actually working, or does it seem to be working because I want it to work and I feel powerless?" These were uncertainties that doctors were not trained to handle, especially with their patients.

Many of the disease experts seemed to misjudge the odds that the epidemic would become a full-blown pandemic. Even Anthony Fauci a presidential advisor and critical voice that warned Americans of the real dangers when it hit, said on 26 January that the virus posed a "very, very low risk to the United States" and was a concern for public-health officials, but not the public. He quickly changed his tune, even if it brought him into conflict with Trump.

As Ed Yong notes: "We hunger for information but lack the knowhow to evaluate it or the sources that provide it." Zeynep Tufekci, a sociologist at the University of North Carolina described coronavirus as "the epistemological crisis of the moment. There's a lot of expertise around, but fewer tools than ever to distinguish it from everything else. Pure credentialism doesn't always work." As he insisted: "I hope the lesson people take from this is not 'Experts were wrong'. If you followed the right people, they were overwhelmingly right. We just didn't put them in the right place so we could hear them."

Yong also pointed out that the narrative that experts underplayed the risks wasn't fully correct either. On 26 January Thomas Inglesby of John Hopkins Bloomberg

School of Public Health tweeted: “We should be planning for the possibility that (the coronavirus) cannot be contained.” He followed with a list of recommendations.

It might have been initially true that the risks were low, but Inglesby said: “Officials should have noted that the true extent of the disease was unknown, because tests weren’t in place; that the virus has already spread globally; and that control measures such as airport screening and travel bans have historically been unsuccessful.” He said the fuller statement took longer to explain, but that’s how it was in outbreaks. Inglesby said: “There’s a lot of uncertainty, and we shouldn’t try to tidy it up.”

He acknowledged that the impulse to *be* reassuring was understandable. This was especially so with Trump’s post-truth politics which had long denigrated science, particularly in relation to the climate emergency. “The most important thing is to be as accurate as possible,” Inglesby said. “We should give people information so they can do what they think is right. We should tell people what we don’t know and when we’ll know more.”

Ed Yong affirms:

> If officials – and journalists – are clear about uncertainties from the start, the public can hang new information onto an existing framework and understand when shifting evidence leads to new policy. Otherwise, updates feel confusing so when the CDC (Centers for Disease Control) suddenly reverses its position on wearing masks, without having previously clarified why the issue was so divisive, it seems like an arbitrary flipflop.

As Kate Starbird at the University of Washington who studies information flows during a crisis told Yong: “That’s a dangerous way to communicate. It communicates diminishing trust in organisations. And when people don’t have a place they can go for trusted information, it makes them vulnerable to disinformation.”

She recognised that when a disaster happens people tend to share information that is useful to their communities. “When an earthquake happens, you talk to your neighbours and in a few days, you’ve figured out what’s going on. For Covid-19, the uncertainty is persistent.” As Yong also noted: “The pandemic’s length traps people in a liminal space,” and this can be particularly stressful to people brought up within a neoliberal common-sense that stresses the control that people *should have* over their lives and encourages people to constantly plan for their futures.

But when people are locked-down and forced to self-isolate as households at home, uncertain about the future but also about how to secure the safety of their families – is it safe to go outside and when? – this creates deep fears and anxieties as the routines that have ordered their everyday lives and helped to give them a sense of control over their futures, have suddenly disappeared. They’ve vanished into a thin air that carries its own threats of illness and possibly death. People are suddenly living in new moral worlds that they find hard to navigate. They can feel lost and unknowing about what they can communicate. Though China imposed quarantine measures, placing 45million people under lockdown, the immediate response as Mark Honigsbaum, a medical historian, noted "was that it could never happen here. Even though quarantines had been employed in Europe since the14th century, few of us thought that citizens of mature western democracies could be persuaded to accept similar restrictions." He thinks this "imaginative failure arguably lay at the heart of Britain's decision of pursue a herd immunity strategy" (theguardian.com, Sunday 11 July 2021).

While historically people might have struggled to get helpful information in a 24/7 media culture, as Yong notes:

> Now people struggle because they're finding too much. It does not help that online information channels are heavily personalised and politicised, governed by algorithms that reward certain extreme claims over correct but nuanced ones. On Twitter, false information spread further than true information, and at six times the speed.

The repercussions of online chatter to how people thought about the pandemic were considerable. Di Riesta from Stanford University who studies *how* narrative spreads online, said: "For a lot of people, what is true is what the people I've chosen to trust in my community say is true." Those dynamics meant that, at least initially, liberal and conservative Americans had very different understandings of the pandemic.

As Yong noted: "The daily briefings from the White House have only exacerbated confusion. Trump has repeatedly tried to downplay the pandemic and rewrite his role in mishandling it." As he also recognised about Trump: "His playbook is his usual one: Deny responsibility, find a scapegoat, incite a culture war, and bend reality to his baldly stated version of it (even when that version contradicts itself)."

Jay Rosen, a journalism professor at New York University, also argued that the media's default position of constant piecemeal updates was ill-suited to covering a pandemic.

> Journalists still think of their job as producing new content, but if your goal is the public understanding of Covid-19, one piece of new content after another doesn't get you there… It requires a lot of background knowledge to understand the updates, and the news system is terrible at (providing that knowledge).

Starbird recommends slowing down and taking a moment to vet new information before sharing it. She herself is spending *less time* taking in every scrap of pandemic news and more time with local sources. It's the equivalent, she says, of "hand-washing for the infodemic." And it might dispel the illusion that the pandemic can be tracked in real time.

This rapid and constant flow of new data in those crucial first months of the crisis made it almost impossible to monitor the situation and provide accurate reporting. Yong reflected on the inaccuracy of daily infection rates, and the major factors impacting this: "…the number of tests being done (which is still insufficient), the lag in reporting results from those tests (which can be long), and the proportion of tests that are incorrectly negative (which seems high)." Reportage on fatalities furthermore was unable to give "a real-time glimpse at the virus's toll. Because of delays in reporting, they tend to be lower at weekend… (the) numbers I see say as much about the tools researchers are using as the quantities they are measuring."

But somehow, we have learnt to be *reassured* by the numbers, as if they carry an objectivity that can take us away from our fears and anxieties of our everyday lives. Even if they don't have a reality that politicians and researchers often rely upon because of their training, they allow for a sense of control over a world that can feel so fearful and out of control.

Yong explains the particularly insidious nature of the aftermath of the virus, making the point that some natural hazards, in his example hurricanes and earthquakes, have "evident" dangers and "visible" immediate consequences, which makes it easier to navigate paths to relative safety. In the case of viruses and pandemics, they "lie below the threshold of the senses." Citizens have to rely on information rather than what they see to feel comfortable and safe enough to emerge from the wreckage.

Counting the Dead

As Jacqueline Rose also acknowledges in *Pointing the Finger* on Albert Camus's *The Plague* (*London Review of Books* Vol 42, No 9, 7 May 2020):

> When trying to track the spread of a virus, tallies…are always approximate and imperfect, but knowing this seems to make no difference to their quasi-sacred status. It is as if intoning numbers according to the same recognisable formula, however scary, allows us somehow how to feel on top a situation which everyone knows – and not just because of government incompetence – is out of control.

One of the things *The Plague* conveys, she notes:

> Is that, at the very moment we appear to be taking the grimmest reality on board, we might also be deluding ourselves. Counting is at once a scientific endeavour and a form of magical thinking. It can be a way of bracing ourselves for and confronting an onslaught, and at the same time a doomed attempt at omnipotence, a system of classifying the horror and bundling it away."

I stopped listening to the daily numbers of the dead in hospital when my younger brother Tony was taken into London's Barnet Hospital with breathing difficulties. Within 12 days, during which I was able to speak to him, he died, on Monday 6 April at 10.45 in a crowded hospital with none of the nurses – very understandably, because they were rushed off their feet – having any time to sit with him and no possibility of his close friends and family visiting. At roughly the same time, Boris Johnson was in an intensive care unit receiving oxygen with two nurses sitting with him throughout the night to enable them to adjust his oxygen levels. There was no such care and attention for Tony.

Somehow it took me time to realise *how* our personal family grief was tied up with so many other deaths in the country. The daily news briefings would talk about regretting each single death, whether they be in a hospital or the much- neglected care sector where so many of the elderly and frail were left – abandoned to die often without really being identified *as* Covid-19 deaths.

With a community of the dead *absorbed* into the daily numbers, it was as if Tony had disappeared into nowhere. There was a silence with the government failing to develop a shared narrative around the losses that so many of us were suffering. The speed with which people were dying created its own shock across personal lives and the wider community. There was little public acknowledgement of what people were going through in their loss and grief.[5]

It was the family that was left to grieve and mourn on our own, even though Tony was a person who had absorbed the early government messages, repeated by Johnson and Trump, that there was little to worry about and that it was like the flu and no bad thing if you got it if you were relatively fit, as Tony was, as it would give you immunity and allow you to return to work. This was a message I heard from him when he told me had got the virus.

Tragically he was to learn a different truth. But absorbed into the daily death numbers, *who* was to take responsibility for these early messages? They were never to be fully acknowledged once the pandemic took hold and they never formed part of a shared narrative. Rather it was more convenient for the government to forget and deny and to delay any public accountability.

At the time, the government strategy – whatever efforts they have subsequently made to deny it – was for people in the country to get the virus and so gain 'herd immunity' – an impersonalised term that treated the population as a 'herd'. In this way, the government remains responsible since they were going against scientific advice coming from the WHO and so they must be held to account for the many deaths that need not have happened if they had followed "the best scientific advice" at the time, as they falsely insisted they were doing. As the Covid Inquiry was to hear, Boris Johnson told senior advisers that the Covid virus was "just nature's way of dealing with old people" and he was "no longer buying" the fact that the NHS was overwhelmed. The chief scientific advisor, Sir Patrick Vallance, noted in his diaries that Johnson seemed "obsessed with older people accepting their fate" and letting young people keep the economy going (theguardian.com, Tuesday 31 October 2023).

Rose also notes the disparity – one of many:

> Between the medical care of the prime minister, assigned an intensive care bed at a time of acute shortage, while still fit enough – or so we were initially told – to govern, and the negligence suffered by Thomas Harvey, a nurse from East London who had worked in the NHS for 20 years. His family was advised that he didn't need to go to hospital (they called four times) before he died gasping for air in his bathroom.

As Rose recognised, it is the moment in *The Plague* when the disease is nearing its end in the Algerian city of Oran, when the numbers no longer add up or make sense. With inconsistent shifts in daily numbers and districts reporting very different numerical fates, Camus' narrator remarks that the plague *was losing* "its self-command, the ruthless almost mathematical efficiency that had been its trump card hitherto."

Rose notes: "Mathematics flattens. It is a killing art. Counting humans, alive or dead, means you have entered a world of abstraction, the first sign that things have taken a desperate turn." But she is also aware that:

> Of course counting can mean the exact opposite. If someone counts, they matter, with the further implication that they can be held answerable for their own deeds. Not to count, on the other hand, is to be overlooked or invisible, like the Arabs of Oran, whose virtual absence from Camus' portrayal is its most significant failing.

Notes

1 Some helpful historical reflections into ways that epidemics have often been marginalised in historical accounts that often focus upon wars and revolutions see Sheldon Watts *Epidemics and History: Disease, Power and Imperialism* (New Haven: Yale University Press 1999); J.N. Hayes *Epidemics and Pandemics: Their Impacts on Human Histories* (ABC-CLIO 2005) and Mark Honigsbaum *The Pandemic Century: One Hundred Years of Panic, Hysteria and Hubris* (London: C. Hurst and Co 2019).

2 An investigation of how the Coronavirus challenged Italian society as the first country in Europe to be attacked by it and to acknowledge our human frailties in face of it is given in Max Police *Italy and Europe at the Beginning of the Coronavirus* (Italy: Independently published 2021) As a history and philosophy teacher he sees the pandemic also as an opportunity to seek out new ethical and value imaginations.

3 An account of the early years of the Coronavirus in the USA that also investigates Trump's responses is Lawrence Wright, *The Plague Year: America in the Time of Covid* (New York: Penguin 2021). See also *The Pandemic Divide: How COVID Increased Inequality in America* ed Gwendolyn L. Wright and Lucas Hubbard (Duke University Press, 2022) challenging the initial idea that "We're all in this together" they show how Black and Latinx populations suffered illnesses and deaths at much higher rates. Those working in low-paid jobs and living in confined housing were particularly vulnerable. They highlight steps that could have been taken to mitigate the full force of the pandemic but weren't.

4 A helpful discussion about the failures to plan and respond to a pandemic that had been anticipated is provided with a certain insider view by Jeremy Farrar and Anjana Ahuja *Spike: The Virus vs. The People* (London: Profile Books 2022).

5 Attempts to engage with the suddenness of so many deaths and the difficulties of grief when you could not be with people through their death process were offered by Jennifer Haupt (ed) *Alone Together: Love, Grief, and Comfort in the Time of Covid-19* (Central Avenue Publishing 2020) These essays, poetry and interviews were messages of hope in community in a time of isolation and despair. The pandemic has brought losses, death, and changes to everyday life on a global scale. See also *Narratives of Covid: Loss, Dying, Death and Grief during Covid-19* (Milton Keynes: The Open University 2021).

2

MASCULINITIES, WARS, MIGRATIONS AND IN/VISIBILITIES

Metaphors of War, Illness and Death

It is when we write, as much as where we write, that makes a difference to *how* we write. This is the historical and cultural moment in which we try to make sense of the world and anticipate different futures. Writing on the 75th anniversary of VE day – the declaration of Victory in Europe on Friday 8 May 1945 – carries a particular significance for me, not least because I was called Victor as were many men born then.

For my parents, Jewish refugees seeking sanctuary in London, my name was also a claim to belong, as well as an act of appreciation. At the same time, they were having to come to terms with hearing about deaths in their families as a result of Nazi violence and the terrible, unspeakable deaths of the Holocaust – the Shoah. This was barely utterable *as* a war against the Jews of Europe in any way separate from the Second World War into which it was somehow folded.[1]

On 5 April, giving an address to a world in the grip of a global pandemic, Queen Elizabeth II quoted a line evocative of wartime resilience and hope: "We will meet again." Recalling the refrain from the song popularised by the 'Forces Sweetheart', singer Dame Vera Lynn, the use of the phrase connected with a grieving population, reeling from being separated from loved ones. In advance of the 75th anniversary of VE day, the author Kate McLoughlin reflected on the history and enduring power of Dame Vera's signature song: noting that she "turned a song about absence in any situation into a classic expression of wartime optimism."

As the singer wrote in her 1975 memoir, *Vocal Refrain:* "Ordinary English people don't, on the whole, find it easy to expose their feelings even to those closest to them." *We'll Meet Again*, would go "at least a little way towards doing it for them." The phrase "ordinary English people" has its own resonance as to who was included in the early post-war years and who was excluded. I doubt that refugee

DOI: 10.4324/9781003296874-2

families felt embraced by that phrase, but they hoped that in time and if they made appropriate efforts and compromises, they could feel somehow feel included.

McLoughlin highlights how "We'll Meet Again," with its "swooping and strangely haunting melody," has so thoroughly affected popular culture, noting its "ironic" usage in Stanley Kubrick's *Dr Strangelove*, and the "alienating" sampling of it on Pink Floyd's song *Vera* on *The Wall.* In an interview, Vera Lynn shared how she felt like a "personal family representative" when she visited British servicemen in hospital in what was then Burma… and how important it was to look attractive to wounded soldiers who hadn't seen their womenfolk for months, even years.

McLoughlin felt: "The Queen understood that what keeps us going in times of war and pandemic is the thought that we will be reunited with our loved ones, when the blue skies drive the dark clouds far away" (*The Conversation*, 7 May 2020).[2] While the government remained uneasily silent, Queen Elizabeth was reaching out with words people needed to hear.

This is very much a *generational* vision, and it passes over in silence the many families whose relatives and friends had died in the Second World War, as they have died in the Covid-19 pandemic. The generation abandoned to die in care homes were those who carried memories of the war. VE day was being celebrated for the sacrifices they made. The way government figures talked about the curve of infections and deaths flattening, and the notion that we had possibly reached the peak and it had started to descend, was itself a form of *denial*. It worked as an abstraction to conceal the pain of multiple deaths. It hid the anger that people felt at the government's early messages, that the virus was no worse than the flu and that if you got it, it would be no bad thing because you would gain immunity. This proved a terrible policy and governments are still to be held accountable.

These were messages responsible for the deaths of many. They had taken the early messages to heart and learned the hard way about the dangers they faced. It did *not* make it easier when Boris Johnson suggested the country *was* fighting a second Battle of Britain and Trump pretentiously called himself a "wartime president".

By the time Trump finally took note of rising death rates in the Unites States, governments around the world were assuming emergency powers and human rights were being limited. Memories of wartime were being invoked with governments still *actively* forgetting colonial histories and the contributions of colonial forces from the Caribbean and the Indian sub-continent. This was till the global demonstrations in response to the brutal murder of George Floyd, in Minneapolis in the midst of the Covid-19 pandemic, firmly placed issues of racial inequalities and police brutality into the wider context of class and racial histories of colonialism and empire.

Masculinities, Enemies and Risk Taking

Guardian writer Simon Tisdall contemplated the perils of using the language of war when confronted with crisis, as institutions were responding to the pandemic with "wartime metaphors, images and language."

He recognised how French President, Emmanuel Macron's continuous references to "We are at war" not only appealed to a particular vision of heroic masculinity that could produce its own insensitivities to the risks and dangers people faced with Covid-19 but *also* ignored that "any talk of war is inherently scary." Tisdall also recognised *how* war rhetoric "divides communities at the very moment you need to pull societies together around a sense of common purpose" (*The Guardian*, 21 May 2020).

Tisdall warns of politicians who resort to invoking the "invisible enemy" as a tool to fuel fear, and who embrace "collateral damage" as "unfortunate but inevitable." He adds that this has a political dimension where virus victims are people who are especially vulnerable to the decisions of the government: that some are "more innocent than others." He is rightly wary of newspaper headlines "summoning up the Blitz spirit, recycling 1940s propaganda."

He also recalls Camus' warning: "Plagues and wars always find people equally unprepared… people say: 'It won't last long, it's too stupid'. And war is certainly too stupid, but that doesn't prevent it from lasting. Stupidity always carries doggedly on." This can make it more difficult, especially for young men firmly raised within neo-liberal masculinities, to really take in threats they face.

The *Slate* journalist Aymann Ismail profiled David Vega, a young medical student, who contracted Covid while partying in Florida in early March 2020. Vega described his lack of care and precautions, despite seeing masked people around him, and his own education path. He explains that he thought his youth and healthy lifestyle would protect him, and cites a not-unusual attitude to pandemics as being a remote prospect "…in school, you hear about these pandemics, the Spanish flu… it's hard to really conceptualise that it's real until either you… a loved one or someone who you know experiences it. And for me, unfortunately, it had to be me going through it, to have a take-home message from all that."[3]

At the very beginning he thought it was a little crazy to take all these extra precautions, reflecting that as an African who had spent two months in hospitals in Africa where resources are scarce, he should have known better. He shared that a "shocking" turning point for him was the cancellation of the NBA (National Basketball Association), when he started to realise the seriousness of the situation.

Asked by Ismail: "What do you think you needed to hear or to experience to believe you could get the coronavirus too?" David responded:

> I think if I just would've seen the repercussions that we are now seeing and living day by day, I would not have done what I did. I would have taken all these steps way more seriously. We can't be frivolous about our lives and the lives of others. This is where we really gotta support each other.

Simone Weil in her *Notebooks* reflects on values of self-worth and how they are contextualised through relations of power. She notes how a young man who feels that he has counted for something in school, can be deeply *shocked* by his first day working on an assembly-line, where he is made to feel that he counts for nothing. Across the world people were shocked by the quickness of deaths that came with the Covid-19 pandemic. Nothing had prepared them within a scientific medical culture that too often assumed it could solve any problem they were confronted with. This resonates with how people have often shared experiences of hope as they signed up to go to war, thinking it would be over soon, only to be shocked by the everyday realities they are suddenly thrown into.[4]

Empire, War, Migrants and In/Visibilities

As author Wendy Webster discovered in her research, the migrants and minorities involved in keeping essential industries going as war workers, and serving in the armed forces, as well as nursing the sick, were celebrated in the British wartime media. But as she notes, when the war was over, they were rendered invisible and they were written out of the histories taught, when the "national story" was produced, and the picture narrowed, omitting the stories and contributions of global citizens who served wartime Britain (*The Conversation*, 7 May 2020).

Webster raises the point that at the start of the war, people of non-European descent were rejected for service by both the British Armed Forces and those in the Commonwealth, including Canada and Australasia.

Webster notes that almost a century on, at another crisis point, coverage of the pandemic made the diversity of the NHS clear. Of the weekly "clapping ceremony" shared by thousands across the country, she pointed out that some were participating in the celebration of the work of people who had, for perhaps the first time, been "made visible," having been "devalued in an economy where human worth has been measured by the wage you can demand."

Under a heading "Thank you and goodbye" Webster predicted that these celebrations would be short lived, considering the appalling post-war treatment of troops and workers from the Empire who were swiftly demobbed by the British government to avoid settlement in Britain. This created a deliberately hostile environment for people who had uprooted and risked their lives for a country that quickly forgot about them. Renee Webb, who served as a pilot – first in Jamaica and then in Britain – remembered: "I was terribly concerned at that time that people should have forgotten so easily…I mean of the many questions that were asked of me, one of the main ones was: 'When are you going back?'" [5]

Under the "hostile environment" policy shaped by Home Secretary Theresa May, many young men and women from the Caribbean were told by the UK government to go back. Some were sacked from jobs in the NHS.[6] Others, who were detained and threatened with deportation, had arrived in Britain as children to join mothers who were working as NHS nurses.

Webster cites studies showing that BAME (Black, Asian and minority ethnic) doctors were disproportionality affected by the shortages and insufficiency of PPE: 64%, compared with 33% of their white colleagues, felt pressured to carry on with their work despite having reservations about the effectiveness of their own equipment. The appalling statistic that emerged indicating that BAME healthcare workers were significantly more likely to die during the crisis than their white colleagues was a damning indictment of a system in which workers were afraid to voice their concerns about safety protocols, for fear of losing their job security.[7]

Part of this group of doctors who were working around the clock to save lives are defined as highly skilled migrants but have no access to public funds should anything go wrong. As Amina Chitembo from De Montfort University reminds us: "Their condition for being in the UK is that they fend for themselves and do not seek any help from the public purse" (*The Conversation*, 2 April 2020).

They were *not* included in the measures announced to help those affected by the Covid-19 pandemic and who died in the line of duty. The shortage of critical workers would have been much worse if they had not been dedicated to their work, which partly explains Home Secretary Priti Patel's announcement during the crisis of automatic visa extensions for 2,800 NHS personnel and other critical care staff.

Many had spouses and children depending on then and were also subject to lockdown conditions. As Chitempo reports: "What these migrants don't know until they arrive in the country, is that strict rules mean that should they fall ill and are unable to work, they will have no access to financial support." The hostile environment was still very much a feature of their everyday lives, even if they were being celebrated with applause on the doorsteps weekly on a Thursday at 8pm.

Awareness grew that people had been treated unjustly in being obliged to work on the front line with Covid-19 patients *without* the state having provided them with the necessary protective equipment to keep them safe.[8] This threatened a narrative that the government was working hard to defend – that it had done everything with the best advice of scientists and that it had acted effectively and at the right time.

As Sean Lang, a historian at Anglia Ruskin University noted:

> The image of victory in a just war is important because inevitably the current pandemic, like every other crisis Britain has gone through since 1945, has been compared to the war... It is inevitable that people still facing a deadly enemy should seek solace in the heroic memory of VE day.
>
> *(The Conversation, 6 May 2020)*

But the myths around VE day also need questioning because many people were too tired and exhausted to celebrate in May 1945. They knew that the war was continuing in the east against Japan. So many young people had died and so many families were in grief. Henry Irving, historian of the Second World War, noted during the celebrations of the 70th anniversary in 2015 that in 1945: "The events came after a week of frustrating rumour and were an anachronism to many who had lived through the war" (*The Conversation*, 7 May 2015).

It seems that it was people who hadn't fought directly and those who had not been exhausted by losses who celebrated the most. Interviews for the research organisation Mass Observation found that: "The majority of the people interviewed felt that this has been badly handled." According to reports at the time: "Every anti-climax added a little to people's slowly increasing apathy and frustration." This points to the dangers of identifying the efforts mobilised against the coronavirus with the war.[9]

Irving speculates that VE Day failed to live up to the expectations of it owing to the very nature of the war, as it did not "mark a sudden, glorious victory." A contemporary *Daily Mirror* article reported "a glorious night" while reflecting on the continuing conflict in Japan.

We need to be careful about invoking the metaphor of war when it comes to the struggle against the Covid-19 pandemic. We are uncertain, given that this is a new virus, what the future will bring and how long it might cast its shadow over everyday life which cannot "return to normal." We might find it hard to imagine what a "new normal" might look like. But what has also been exposed, as happens during war, is that the risks and burdens do *not* fall equally.

The *structural inequalities* that have so long remained invisible within a national rhetoric of the country "united" and "pulling together" against a common enemy till victory is achieved, can too easily lead us *to forget* the contributions different communities made. It can also make it easy to ignore and displace the grief and mourning that so many families are affected by. There are deaths in war as there are in a pandemic but, as Camus appreciated, it is wrong to put them aside as we take refuge in moral and political abstractions as we talk *too easily* about victory and the sacrifices that were necessary to achieve it.

Global Inequalities, Ethics and Facing Death

Writing at the time of the Ebola crisis and the fear of its spread in 2015, *Guardian* journalist Ed Vulliamy was moved to respond to the Albert Camus novel *La Peste* (*The Plague*): a text among a body of work marked by a rare closeness to the subject of death, vividly and epically depicting humans confronting and cohabiting with death.

Vulliamy reads the novel at a moment of surging Ebola cases, nothing that it: "works on the literal as well as metaphorical level… Like every good metaphorical or allegorical work, it can represent beyond its intentions; including pestilences both moral and metaphorical that have happened after Camus' own lifetime" (*The Guardian*, 5 January 2015).

Vulliamy understands: "Nowadays, *La Peste* can tell the story of a different kind of plague: that of destructive, hyper-materialist, turbo-capitalism." Camus explores our relationship with the absurdity of modern existence. It can describe very well the plague of modern society. Millions come aboard tomb ships or move across murderous deserts, in search of empty promises. They help to destroy nature, the constant against which Camus measured human mortality. Essential to Camus' existential isolation was the discrepancy he noted between the power and beauty of nature, and the desolation of the human condition.

For Vulliamy in *La Peste:* "Absurdity is a source of value, values and even action. The group of men gathered around the narrative represent all human responses to calamity." He notes that much of the novel's power lies in a central act of resistance: the characters can do little to halt the spread and severity of the plague, but they are empowered by their own witnessing and testimony. In an early essay, *Le Desert,* Camus talked about "repugnant materialism." Vulliamy alludes to Meursault, anti-hero of *L'Étranger* (*The Stranger*) who recognises what he has done in killing an Arab on the beach. He says: "I understand that I had destroyed the harmony of the day." He notes everything humanity does in a turbo-capitalist age, with his ravaging of nature, destroys the harmony of the day.

For Camus, we seem already, without knowing it, involved in a struggle for some dimly fathomed *moral justice*, even though we have ceased to be able to define it. At the end of the novel, his wife having died of illness elsewhere unconnected with the plague, Dr Rieux watches families and lovers reunite when the gates of the Algerian city of Oran are finally opened. He reflects upon the possibilities of inner peace for those "who knew now that if there is one thing one can always yearn for, and sometimes attain, it is human love." But he has already recognised that for those others "who aspired beyond and above the human individual towards something they could not even imagine, there has been no answer."

Yet as Vulliamy recognises, there is: "No answer. No description, even of what that something else might be. And yet it nags, it makes demands on us, and those who identify with Rieux know what it is, though we have abandoned a definition." In *The Rebel* written four years later in 1951, Camus writes in the opening chapter: "In every act of rebellion (*révolte*) the man concerned experiences… a feeling of revulsion at the infringement of his rights."

Jacqueline Rose analyses the following passage from *The Plague,* which depicts the aftermath of the plague death of a child, discussed by Rieux and a priest, Father Paneloux:

> "There are times when the only feeling I have is one of mad revolt."
>
> "I understand," Paneloux said in a low voice. "That kind of thing is revolting because it passes human understanding. But perhaps we should love what we cannot understand."
>
> "No, Father. I've a very different idea of love. And until my dying day I shall refuse to love a scheme of things in which children are put to torture."

In this passage, Paneloux powerfully rejects Christian notions of love that would pass over, render invisible and somehow even excuse the deaths of so many of the poor, as a matter of fate, when many of them were avoidable in a more equal and just world. Rose indicates that the plague "sparks a revolution in the blood." She describes the novel as a "protest" or a "warning," addressing the same concerns thrown into sharp relief by the Covid-19 pandemic: noting that these crises illuminate the "truth of social deprivation." Rose cites author Arundhati Roy's own similar observations on the revelatory power of crisis to uncover the truth of inequalities. In a 2021 article for *The Guardian*, Roy criticised the governmental response to the pandemic in India, which saw city workers in their millions flee to the provinces, furthering the spread of the virus. Roy strongly condemned the catastrophic mishandling, stating: "We are witnessing a crime against humanity."[10]

"Something is being registered which many people had turned a blind eye to before," Rose wrote. Camus documents the horror of the cruelties and atrocities humans inflict on others, in full awareness, a horror that should not be lost on us at this moment. We are living through a time when refugees are allowed to drown in the Mediterranean while governments refuse to allow ships to rescue them, even holding captains responsible if they break the law and insist on saving lives.

During the course of Camus's novel, people starve as the profiteers move in to take advantage of the shortages and the gulf between rich and poor widens; which resonates with how the Covid-19 lockdowns around the world unfolded. Camus' own damning words illustrate this: "Thus whereas plague through its impartial ministrations should have promoted equality among our city's folk, it now had the opposite effect and, thanks to the normal play of different forms of selfishness, it sharpened the sense of injustice in the hearts of mankind." When the poor of Oran take to the streets under the banner "Bread or air" their demonstrations are met with instant and brutal suppression. Rose summarises the message of the novel: "It is a delusion to suggest that death is the great equaliser."

She notes that in the rhetoric of crisis, "we," or the notion of unity is losing credibility in the face of glaring inequalities: in her example, "families with gardens and those housed in airless, cladded tower blocks," but is also complicated by new distinctions. She gives the example of how quickly the police went from publicly paying tribute to the NHS for their services to attacking and detaining peaceful protestors who included numerous healthcare workers objecting to the lack of PPE. This *is* exactly the kind of contradiction Camus encourages us to reflect upon.

Illnesses, Deaths and Impossible Choices

An Uber driver died from Covid-19 after trying to conceal his illness for fear he would be thrown out by his landlord. Even if this eviction threat was not strictly legal, it was widely reported, and illness left many people homeless who had no wages coming in to pay their rent. Rajesh Jayaseelan, a married father of two who had come to London from India about a decade earlier, died alone in Northwick Park in Harrow on 11 April. His friend Sunil Kumar, an NHS IT worker, told Robert Booth, social affairs correspondent of *The Guardian* what happened (*The Guardian,* 18 April 2020, p. 7).

Kumar said Rajesh's fear was based on an earlier experience of eviction when his previous landlord ordered him to leave because as a minicab driver, he worried he would spread the disease to him and his family. Rajesh, aged 44, had "starved" for several days in his rented lodgings, telling his wife by phone that he did not want to leave his room because other residents might realise he had Covid-19 and he would be told to get out if the landlord got to know.

Booth reported that Jayaseelan had slept in his car on consecutive nights while ill, and after he drove himself to hospital, he was immediately placed on a ventilator, in a critical condition. He tragically passed away after Kumar arranged a video call so that Jayaseelan's mother and wife, who were both in Bangalore, could say goodbye to him. In those initial months of the pandemic, multiple Uber drivers died of Covid-19.

The lack of clear guidance and protection for mini-cab drivers left them highly vulnerable. They had to leave home in order to work and support their families and there were fears they could bring the virus home with them. Yaseem Aslam, general secretary of the App Drivers and Couriers Union, said: "It is very distressing. The migrant workers in particular are vulnerable because they feel forced to work because they are not entitled to government benefits."

Uber said it would compensate drivers up to £100 a week for up to 14 days if they were diagnosed with Covid-19, placed in quarantine or asked to self-isolate. But many drivers had accepted the early government message that it was not worse than a bad flu and some were afraid to set up plastic barriers in their cars in case this might breach their licence, so it took time to really take in the dangers they faced every day at work.

Many felt they had no alternative, but they were worried and fearful. Kumar said Jayaseelan came from poverty and had hoped to move his family to London but could not yet afford to. He travelled to Bangalore to see his mother, wife and children, aged four and six, for two months each year. He had been worried about catching Covid-19 and called Kumar asking him how to stay safe.

Around 20 March, Jayaseelan was admitted to Northwick Park with dehydration but was discharged after receiving intravenous fluids, Kumar said. It appears that he went back to work, and his last fare was at Heathrow airport on 25 March, after which he fell ill again. "He was finding it difficult to breathe," Kumar said. "He told his wife he wished he had someone that could look after him even for a week and give him some food and take care of him. In the last week he really starved." When his condition worsened, he refused to call an ambulance because he might alert others to his sickness and cause him to be thrown out again, Kumar said. He felt obliged to conceal what was happening to him and did his best to render himself *invisible* because of his fears.

Virgilio Castro, 63, who told the Grenfell inquiry that he tried to fight the blaze at the outset and suffered from breathing problems thereafter, also died from Covid-19 on 9 April. He was one of at least 29 coronavirus victims up to that point, from the UK's Filipino community, many of whom worked in the NHS as nurses and porters. Of those who had lost their lives by then, 18 worked in the health sector. Castro, who worked as a maintenance supervisor, told the Grenfell Inquiry that he lost many people he knew in the fire. "The Grenfell Tower fire; it shouldn't have been allowed to happen and I want the public inquiry to ensure that it can never happen again," he said.

The fire had *made visible* the stark inequalities in living conditions in London's richest borough of Kensington and Chelsea where the negligence of the authorities has been exposed. It has since been made clear that there was more concern in the refurbishment over the look of the building to other people in the borough, than with the safety of the residents whose protests were ignored.

Castro lived on the 17th floor of the 24-storey building for 26 years. He moved there with his wife in April 1991 just after their daughter was born. His wife died a decade ago. He told the inquiry: "I have watched my daughter grow up in that flat and have many fond memories living there as a family." He said that he had cried at a CCTV image, provided by the police, of him leaving the tower that night. "I still find it difficult to look at that photograph" (*The Guardian*, 18 April 2020, p. 13).

As Ben Quinn reported for *The Guardian*: "Echoing concerns elsewhere, there is anger that Filipino workers are among those bearing the brunt of a shortage of personal protective equipment." John Alagos, a nursing assistant aged 23, fell ill at Watford General hospital after a 12-hour shift. He was caring for coronavirus patients and is possibly the youngest British medic to have died from the virus. Melujean Ballesteros, 60, who was a nurse at St Mary's hospital, Paddington died on 12 April after being admitted to hospital with a fever. For a long time, it was difficult for anyone to get tested, even if they worked in the NHS, unless they had symptoms of the virus and were in hospital.

When police knocked on Emylene Suelto Robertson's door in Dunbar, on Scotland's east coast, they confirmed the news she had dreaded. Her uncle Donald 'Dondee' Suelto, an NHS nurse, had died alone in his London flat of suspected coronavirus. He was 51. The grief was difficult to enough to take on, but she didn't realise how difficult it would be to locate her uncle's remains.

As Aina Khan reported for *The Guardian*, for coronavirus victims without an "official next of kin," "laying them to rest (was) fraught with bureaucracy." Emylene Suelto described the painful uncertainty her family (based in the Philippines) was faced with. When they contacted her daily for updates, she was unable to respond to them.

He had worked as an NHS nurse for 18 years after migrating here and worked in the chemotherapy department of Hammersmith hospital. His niece described him as a "fun, joyful, dedicated and caring" man. Three days after treating a patient who tested positive for Covid-19, Suelto was sent home to self-isolate. His niece was in regular contact with him on Facetime and text and he began to report mild symptoms three days later. "My uncle said to me: 'I will catch the virus, because my patient coughed in front of me, and I had no mask."

When she hadn't heard from him for five days, she informed the police on 7 April. They broke down the door of his flat that evening and found him dead. She criticised the NHS in the aftermath of her uncle's death, in their negligence in providing the appropriate PPE, and added: "my family struggled to find the body. Why was nobody responsible for him?" His body was finally located in Poplar Coroner's Court, which at the time of *The Guardian* article was yet to rule on the cause of the death (*The Guardian*, 18 April 2020, p. 17).

What is so disheartening and makes you angry is the predictable response of the spokesperson for the Imperial College Healthcare NHS trust that refused to accept any responsibility and took refuge in the abstractions Camus rebelled so firmly against. The statement issued by the trust in response to Mr Suelto's death was formulaic, and attempted to suggest familiarity with the use of his first name. The Trust used the opportunity to state they were following guidelines on the use of PPE, and to deny that Mr Suelto was working in a space where patients with the virus were being cared for: *end of story*. So much for the democratic idea that people have equal worth and dignity in their lives as they do in their deaths.

Covid Ethics, Exposing Inequalities and Life Risks

As columnist Kenan Malik recognised: "In a crisis, a society often reveals both its best aspects and its worst." He illuminates the lessons around systematic "hypocrisy" that can be learned from the Covid-19 pandemic. The pandemic revealed the selfishness of hoarding on one hand, and on the other the selflessness of mutual aid groups. In a crisis too, issues that policymakers have long ignored suddenly become visible and urgent. The pandemic laid bare the insecurity of work and the cruelty of welfare policy. He analysed the line "we're all in it together," frequently heard at the height of the crisis, bookended by periods of harsh and callous policy that disregarded the plight of society's most vulnerable (*The Observer*, 22 March 2020, p. 45).

On social distancing policy, Malik observes that its "economic burden" has primarily fallen to the worst-off in our society. The poor feel obliged to carry on working just to provide food for the family, and at the same time are fearful about bringing the virus home with them and infecting their families. They feel placed in an impossible and fearful situation where each day they feel stressed and anxious but feel obliged to carry on working. Low paid work, as Malik recognises "has allowed supermarkets and shops to stay open, or on zero-hours contracts delivering food and other items to those safely self-isolating at home."

With the coming of the pandemic, policymakers have suddenly discovered that those normally consigned to the margins of the labour force as "unskilled workers" are crucially important to the functioning of the economy. Cleaners, shopkeepers, delivery drivers – those are the people, often migrants or women, on whose invisible labour society depends upon and whose efforts are usually treated with contempt, that are, at least for the time the crisis lasts, recognised as essential workers. As he acknowledged: "The government list of 'key workers' is a list largely of jobs in which workers get paid derisory sums for doing vital work. Low skilled has become as much a measure of moral worth as a job description" (*The Observer*, 22 March 2020, p. 45).

The impact of the pandemic also made visible to many that statutory sick pay was just £94.25 a week. The health secretary, Matt Hancock, admitted on BBC Television's *Question Time* that he could not live on that. "But you expect others to live on it," Fiona Bruce, the chair observed. But even that meagre sum was *not* available to two million lower-paid workers, those on zero-hours contracts or the self-employed.

The issue of whether workers feel able to take sick leave, Malik notes, may be acute in a pandemic situation, but has "long confronted thousands of self-employed and gig-economy workers." But as Torsten Bell of The Resolution Foundation also pointed out, unemployment benefits are worth less in real terms now that they were in the early 1990s, amounting to what Malik terms "state-sanctioned poverty within our benefits system."

Successive governments since at least the 1980s have stigmatised claimants and made the welfare system harsh and mean-minded. Ian Duncan Smith who, as Secretary of State for Work and Pensions from 2010 to 2016, is responsible for the disasters of the universal credit scheme, has continuously argued against *any* form of universal basic income, as a "disincentive to work". This argument is often used *to reduce* benefits to the bare bones. What could have been a reasonable reorganisation of the benefits system, in Duncan Smith's hands was turned into a punitive one, something made all too visible in Ken Loach's film *I Daniel Blake* which made painfully clear the everyday hardships, cruelties and moral damage inflicted by the benefits system.

Even though the government announced a three-month delay before landlords could order evictions for those who have lost wages or their jobs, this merely delayed rather than eliminated the problem. The fear of eviction and homelessness is an issue for many on low wages. This is part of a wider, systematically implemented policy of building precarity into social life, Malik acknowledges this and states that far from creating it, the crisis has "made visible and exacerbated a pre-existing problem."

During the resolution of the 2008 global financial crisis, significant amounts of public funds were utilised, but the burden of that generosity fell upon the working class and public sector employees, through a decade of austerity measures. Malik expressed hope that once the pandemic was contained, the public should be incentivised to address issues such as low wages, precarious employment and insufficient social benefits. The strikes across the public services, including the NHS, in the winter of 2022/3 showed how little was learnt, whatever was promised.

Minicab driver Zubair Chaudry used to pick up 12 or 13 passengers a day from Luton Airport. After the pandemic struck, he and the other 90 Addison Lee drivers were lucky if they got two fares a day from the few flights that now landed. He discussed his feelings of helplessness, saying "If we don't work, we can't live." They each had to pay £210 a week to rent their vehicles and they had to cover their own fuel costs. Chaudry lamented the rapid loss of income, saying: "We don't know how we are going to put food on the table for our families."

They were among the millions of low-paid workers with precarious livings who stood to gain little from the government's package of emergency measures. Jason Moyer-Lee of the Independent Workers Union of Great Britain said the government *had* excluded workers in the gig economy. "They are saying they will do 'whatever it takes', but precarious workers have been completely left out." His statement noted that little assistance had been offered to those in "bogus self-employment," and those on zero-hour contracts (*The Observer*, 22 March 2020, p. 10).

Emanuele Barbaro, 37, had worked in the Newcastle branch of Carluccio's Restaurant for six years but now he had been laid off without pay. "We have got a mortgage and we've got a little one. We have got another child coming in July… Even if they freeze the mortgage payments, there will be only one person to pay all the bills." In some London restaurants, contract hours had been slashed to just four a week. A waiter who earned around £12 an hour with tips told the journalist Tom Wall that higher earning directors and shareholders should take the hit, rather than low-paid staff. "I will not be able to afford my rent and my bills and food shopping on four hours a week… I'm scared" (*The Observer*, 22 March 2020, p. 10).

Neoliberal Capitalism, Crises and Everyday Philosophy

Considering key differences between the economic crisis prompted by the pandemic, and the Great Crash of 2008, journalist Andrew Rawnsley summarised how the latter narrowly avoided a repetition of the Great Depression with "Near-zero interest rates, quantitative easing and bank bailouts." He notes that in the latter, people learned the lessons of the "negative social consequences" and "deep public alienation" that came from witnessing the "spectacle of shameless financiers" walking away wealthier from the chaos they had caused all too slowly. He did *not* think with the depth of structural inequalities and injustices that were clear to see with the pandemic that politics could go back to business as usual (*The Observer*, 22 March 2020).

While he thought it was too early to make any confident predictions about the long-term ways in which this crisis would *reshape* society, he said it had *already* upended many of the assumptions that "have governed politics here and elsewhere for decades." Thc coronavirus does not respect national borders, political ideologies or even conventional thinking.

As governments scramble to try to contain the pandemic and mitigate the fallout on economies and societies, "the previously unthinkable is suddenly transformed into the essential," as Rawnsley frames it. It has been especially challenging, he thinks, for politicians on the right who have been animated for decades by the creed that the only good government is a small one and the notion there is no problem to which the market cannot supply the answer (*The Observer*, 22 March 2020, p. 47).

As Rawnsley argued:

> A philosophy rooted in the conviction that individualism and competition are the wellsprings of healthy and productive societies is found wanting when confronted by a crisis that can only be endured and resolved by rediscovering the virtues of collectivism and solidarity.

There were profound challenges to a neoliberal common-sense as the risks being taken every day by key workers raised questions about why they were so poorly paid when they were shown to be "essential". It has been hard for an instinctive libertarian like Boris Johnson to accept the case for the active and well-resourced state, which was why the UK was slow to lockdown with such dreadful consequences of well over 30,000 deaths.[11] A note by Patrick Valance in his diaries presented to the Inquiry, after a meeting in December 2020, hinted at the power wielded by the right of the Conservative party during the pandemic: "PM told he has been acting earlier and the public are with him (but his party is not)… He says his party 'thinks the whole thing is pathetic and Covid is just nature's way of dealing with old people – and I'm not entirely disagreeing with them. A lot of moderate people think it is a bit too much." (theguardian.com, 31 October 2023).

Johnson had to learn the bitter lesson that only government "can provide a safety net for workers deprived of the ability to earn their living because they are trying to do the right thing by isolating themselves or because their employer is in trouble." As he noted: "The alternative was to see a massive and rapid surge in unemployment that would have overwhelmed the welfare system and threatened serious civil disorder."

In the wake of Rishi Sunak's first budget as then-Chancellor in 2020, columnist William Keegan commented that the government appeared "hell-bent on not seeking an extension of the period for Brexit negotiations," despite contending with "a calamitous virus – for which the austerity-struck NHS was hopelessly ill-prepared." Furthermore, he noted the wonderful irony that: "Objections to freedom of movement were a vital factor in the Brexit vote, yet, while EU countries have temporarily suspended freedom of movement, the British government did not clamp down and, in effect, invited more of the virus in" (*The Observer*, 22 March 2020, p. 58).[12]

Notes

1 As people were taking in the enormity and dangers of the time they were suddenly living through and the dangers they were facing people looked back to earlier times in the hope that country could pull together and learn from traumatic histories and memories. I share some of my family history in Victor Jeleniewski Seidler *Shadows of the Shoah: Jewish Identity and Belonging* (Oxford: Berg 2000).
2 Kate McLoughlin in theconversation.com, 7 May 2020.
3 Aymann Ismail in Slate.com, 12 April 2020.
4 Simone Weil *The Notebooks of Simone Weil* (London: Routledge, 2003). She was described by Albert Camus as "the only great spirit of our time".

5 Some reflections on post-war migration are offered in John Salt and Hugh Clout (eds) *Migration in Post-War Europe: Geographical Essays* (Oxford: Oxford University Press 1976); David Olusoga *Black and British: A Forgotten History* (London: Pan 2017); Ian Sanjay Patel *We're Here Because You Were There: Immigration and the Land of Empire* (London: Verso Books 2021); Paul Gilroy *There Ain't No Black in the Union Jack* (London: Routledge 2013) and Stuart Hall *Familiar Stranger: A Life between Two Islands* (London: Penguin 2017). See also Stuart Hall *Essential Essays, Vol2 Identity and Diaspora* (Durham NC: Duke University Press, 2018) and Tony Kushner *The Persistence of Prejudice: Anti-Semitism in British Society during the Second World War* (Manchester: Manchester University Press 1989) and *Remembering Refugees: Then and Now* (Manchester: Manchester University Press 2014).

6 Hannah Jones, Yasmin Gunaratnam et al. *Go Home? The Politics of Immigration* (Manchester: Manchester University Press 2017).

7 Addressing Impact of Covid-19 on BAME staff in the NHS (england.nhs.uk).

8 How Covid-19 impacts BAME workers in the NHS (ukri.org); Royal College of Nursing report "BAME Nursing staff experiencing greater PPE shortages despite COVID19 risk warnings".

9 For a study of the original mass observation project that includes the first detailed historical study of the formation of ordinary people's 'racial' attitudes in Britain see Tony Kushner *We Europeans?: Mass-Observation, Race and British Identity in the Twentieth Century* (London: Routledge 2004).

10 Arundhati Roy 'We are witnessing a crime against humanity' (*The Guardian*, The Long Read 28 April 2021).

11 This figure is suggested in Yury E Khudyakov ed. "Estimating the effects of lockdown on Covid-19 Cases and deaths in England: A counterfactual modelling study", *PLoS One*, 2022; 17(4): e0263432.4.

12 Through the pandemic it was being made clear how the promises made for Brexit were being exposed and how different sectors of the economy, including the NHS and care sector, were finding it hard to recruit workers and that prices of imported goods were rising. Rather than being short term issues that would sort themselves out, as those who supported Brexit were arguing, people were seeing how responses to the pandemic were undermined. For reflections on the aftermath of the Brexit referendum see Victor J. Seidler *Making Sense of Brexit: Democracy, Europe and Uncertain Futures* (Policy Press: Bristol 2019).

3

GLOBAL INEQUALITIES, MIGRATIONS, DEPRIVATIONS AND DESPAIR

Thinking Austerity, Institutions and Health Inequalities

How should we think about inequalities of health within a liberal democratic society that promises equality of health provision? Does this become an issue of social justice? In BBC Radio 4's "The World this Weekend" there was an illuminating interview with Professor Michael Marmot, Professor of Epidemiology at UCL and chair of the report Fair Society, Healthy Lives. That interview followed reflections on how the North-East of England had become the new centre for the outbreak of Covid-19. Presenter Johnny Diamond opened with the stark announcement that: "The poor are dying of Covid-19 at twice the rate of the rich." Then he asked: "Is a decade of cuts showing its face in the North-East?"

The latest regional analysis reveals a brutal truth: "the rich are likely to get better and the poor more likely to die. Deprivation and death from Covid-19 walk hand in hand." The latest Office of National Statistics breakdown *shows* that deprived urban areas of England have suffered far higher death rates than prosperous or rural locations.[1]

We know that underlying health conditions are a significant contribution to coronavirus death rates, but these are also interrelated with processes of deindustrialisation in the North-East. John Tomaney, Professor of Urban and Regional planning at UCL, argues that the traditional industries like coal mining and ship building produced well paid jobs, particularly for men but they were often jobs that produced diseases and ill-health, so they have their own health legacies. Once these industries have gone it can be difficult to find new jobs of equivalent status and pay that *can* sustain masculine identifications with being breadwinners for their families.

Tomaney traces how we can see these experiences of *despair* that helps create new kinds of diseases, including drug dependency, suicide and alcoholic liver

DOI: 10.4324/9781003296874-3

disease as people take refuge in drugs, including alcohol, as they are haunted by feelings of inadequacy and failure as they can no longer provide for their families, so losing a sense of self-respect and self-worth. Rather than reaching out to others for help and revealing your vulnerability, it can seem easier especially for men giving prevailing masculinities, to take their own lives.

These "diseases of despair" as he names them, help to shape patterns of ill health. Because of the nature of the work you did, for example in mining and then the despair you can feel at the closing of the pits, but also the defeats of the miner's strike, people's bodies can seem much older than their chronological age and so much more susceptible when they get pneumonia or a virus like Covid-19. But also, people living in poverty are likely to have a poorer diet and can have a tendency towards obesity so that we have to be careful when doctors are trained to talk of obesity as a "risk factor" and *not* to treat it independently from the industrialisation and high sugar-content in foods that it is easy to be addicted to at some level.

Rather than thinking of obesity as a 'life-style choice' we have to *question* medical training and the ways health professions learn to think of independent variables in abstracted terms that are *not* grounded in the everyday realities of structural inequalities that have been intensified and exacerbate through years of austerity since the global financial crisis of 2008, that was to see areas like the North-East as badly hit when those responsible for the crisis were rarely held accountable within the criminal justice system.

When doctors talk about the prevalence of obesity in the North-East, they often treat it abstractly as a 'risk factor' that operates independently, even when they acknowledge that exposure to childhood adversity makes you more likely to be obese as an older child, as a teenager and as an adult. The fact that your parents might have been in prison or had mental health issues 'can really have a long-term impact on your health.' But as Johnny Diamond then tries to frame it, saying that "the medical odds are already stacked against people in places like Middlesbrough" and "then there is the pattern of employment in the region," as if they are *not interrelated* as part of a social and economic context.

As Tomaney notes:

> These are communities that are disproportionately dependent for their employment on 'essential services and key workers' so they have to go out to work everyday day. They cannot work from home. The area lacks higher-skilled white-collar jobs. To say, they have "a particular challenge in this respect" – the language of 'challenge' carries its philosophical assumptions that too often individualises and takes us away from exploring the everyday realities of structural inequalities which show themselves in patterns of consumption including drug and alcohol abuse.[2]

One revelation that has come out of this crisis, as he explains it "is how much we have neglected the funding of essential services and the protection of key workers."

These issues, he argues "are going to become vital across the whole country but they are particularly significant for areas that have been badly hit by the pandemic which already had underlying social and economic challenges."

This was also affected by years of austerity and cuts. Local government funding was slashed by central government during Prime Minister David Cameron's Tory coalition years. The responsibility for failing services appeared to lie with local authorities, thus protecting the government from people's anger at the injustices and systematic structural neglect they were suffering. In a report submitted to the Covid Inquiry, Paul Nowak, the general secretary of the TUC, said: "In the NHS and social care, funding cuts put staff levels in the danger zone. Cuts in social security pushed many more people below the poverty line, leaving them more vulnerable to infection…Austerity cost the nation dearly" (theguardian.com, Sunday 4 June 2023).

At the same time, public health came into the local authorities' remit in 2013, transferred from the health service. It was in the right place but had come ten years *too late* when austerity was biting hard and deep cuts had been imposed. It was also at a time when there were severe cuts in the health service itself which meant it was unprepared for any pandemic to come.

For people obliged to work in essential services social distancing was hard to sustain. Likewise for multigenerational households, with shared kitchens and with no access to outside spaces. The poorer you are, the harder it has proved to be to socially distance and the *more vulnerable* you are to the virus which has been the case in many migrant and ethnic communities, not only in the North-East but across the country. People often *felt abandoned* by a national rhetoric that showed *no* awareness of the *everyday realities* of their lives. The notion that 'we are all in this together' was so evidently flawed that it could intensify peoples' feelings of isolation within their own communities.

As structural inequalities and levels of poverty and deprivation have been rendered visible, so people are faced with fundamental moral and political questions about the kind of society they might want to create in the future. They saw the high death rates in poor working-class migrant and ethnic communities.

As Michael Marmot, director of the UCL's Institute of Health Equity and chair of the report *Fair Society, Healthy Lives* and its recent review that showed a very clear social gradient in mortality (BBC Radio 4 World at One interview with Johnny Diamond). The more deprived the area the higher the mortality and that has *got worse* over the last ten years of austerity. He notes that for women in the most deprived areas life expectancy was declining and things had got consistently worse in terms of health inequalities.

Marmot says:

> …you could be misled by the Prince of Wales being infected, the prime minister being infected, into thinking this was the great leveller, but this was not true at all. Once the pandemic took hold, we saw an exposure of the underlying health inequalities and an amplification of them.

Johnny Diamond who is also the BBC Royal Correspondent came back saying, "At least the lockdown has to affect everyone equally – everyone has to be locked down?" This was said before the scandal of the multiple parties in Downing Street that showed over months how there was one law applying to those who make the law and seemingly a different law for everyone else.

But Marmot insists, "It is the opposite of people being affected equally." People in hospitality reported before the lockdown that only 10% could work from home, while in communication and media 53% said they could work from home. When lockdown came many people in food and hospitality lost their jobs. The money that would have gone to people working in restaurants and hotels was now being transferred up the income scale to those able to work at home who were now spending less. As Marmot notes, "If you are locked down in a one-bedroom flat that you share with a partner and two or three children it's real hardship."

He drew attention to issues in social care pointing out that the reduction in adult social care spending over the last decade was 7% in real terms but in the most deprived 20% areas the reduction was 16% and in the least deprived 20% the reduction was 3%. We might be concerned about the deaths of the elderly and workers in social care, but we just haven't been spending, so as he says:

> …there is a clear line between our lack of preparedness in the health care system, in social care system and in community resources more generally, the decline of support for the voluntary sector – a clear line between austerity and our lack of preparedness to cope with this pandemic.

In the Foreword to the "10 Year Review of Health Equity in England" written just before the pandemic Michael Marmot paints a picture of a "faltering" United Kingdom, where life expectancy has "slowed dramatically, almost grinding to a halt" since 2011.[3] He sees a correlation between this and years of austerity, which has left a nation underfunded and undereducated, turning to increasingly precarious working and living arrangements, and resulted in an alarming increase in homelessness and food bank use which has left "ignored communities with poor conditions and little reason for hope." Crucially, he identifies these consequences as ultimately likely to affect generations, and particularly dire for "minority ethnic population groups and people with disabilities" (p. 5).[4]

Marmot endorses what he wrote ten years earlier in the Marmot Review, that "health inequalities are not inevitable and can be significantly reduced", and attending to them is a "matter of social justice… (this) inaction that cannot be afforded, for the human and economic costs are too high." His report submitted to the Covid Inquiry notes, "the UK entered the pandemic with its public services depleted, health improvements stalled, health inequalities increased and health among the poorest people in a state of decline." Kate Brackwell, council to the inquiry, read from the report, which said Government austerity policies after 2010 had an adverse effect on health inequalities (edp24.co.uk, 6 June 2023).

Marmot sees issues of inequality as inseparable from the challenge presented by climate change, for the creation of a "just and sustainable" future, and cites New Zealand as a concrete example of pursing a political path that places "wellbeing, not growth, at the heart of its economic policy: enabling people to have the capabilities they need to lead lives of purpose, balance and meaning" (p. 7).

Race, Migration, Ethnicities and Risks

Asking the question, "If Coronavirus doesn't discriminate, how come Black people are bearing the brunt?" writer Afua Hirsch acknowledged her desire to believe the constant refrain of the pandemic, that "we are all in this together…. bearing the strain equally." Possibly this would have made it easier to accept the lockdown and the restrictions on everyday freedom that were being imposed, knowing that in a democratic society in which citizens are guaranteed equal legal and political rights, we would all equally be playing our part in a national emergency.

Hirsch goes on to unpack how this myth of togetherness came to fall apart, particularly on matters of class. The glaring chasm between mild inconvenience for some, and others in states of sheer desperation, "living hand to mouth" became increasingly apparent. For some, self-isolation was not a realistic prospect. Like Marmot, she recognises the lethal effects of poverty, despairing over the statistics that living in deprivation quadruples the chance of a person dying from "avoidable causes": a figure likely to increase if policy fails to change (*The Guardian*, 8 April 2020).

Turning the discussion to race, which she notes should have been had nationally 'from the outset', she reflects on the "alarming rate" that Black, Asian and ethnic minority people became critically ill with the virus. Of a study sampling 2,000 covid patients in a critical condition, 35% were ethnic minority people: double the figure that a general population sample would give.

She reflects on the significance of the fact that the first four UK doctors who succumbed to Covid-19 contracted on the frontline of patient care were all Muslim men of African or Asian heritage: Dr Amged El-Hawrani and Dr Adil El Tayar of Sudanese heritage, Dr Habib Zaida of Pakistani heritage, and Nigeria-born Dr Alfa Sa'adu. Hirsch considers this reflective of how the NHS has "always been heavily dependent on ethnic minority staff … (who comprise) 40% of its medical workforce – more than double their proportion in the UK population."

She notes how coverage in many newspapers has been designed to show NHS workers as almost entirely white and how significant this is. This profoundly dishonest whitewash matters because how we remember these moments, "also build narratives about our society, about who serves, about who deserves recognition."

The virus is having a disproportionate impact on Britain's minorities in terms of reduced access to health treatment compared to white people, lower incomes and relying on precarious work and zero-hours contracts as well as having insecure housing so living with threats of eviction. In all these ways migrants and ethnic minorities are placed at greater risk also in relation to Covid-19. As Hirsch says more generally, claiming to be "race neutral" in policy has the dangerous consequence of failing those who would not otherwise get the support needed, and that "treating everyone the same can embed inequalities."

Hirsch also describes the "colonial mindset" of the response to the virus: drawing attention to the initial reluctance of policymakers to adopt precautions when advised by East Asian countries on how to deal with the threat. Writing in April 2020, Omar Khan, director of the Runnymede Trust reflected on the "life and death" matter of racism, long preceding the coronavirus pandemic, with BAME communities experiencing enduring key social disparities.

He described the pandemic as highlighting the "harsh realities" of these injustices, particularly through the appalling statistics showing disproportionate rates of critical illness and fatalities in BAME covid patients, and "making it clear why race should be viewed as a social determinant of health." He points out the statistics of those early months that 35% of the covid patients in critical care over the age of 85 were BAME, significantly disproportionate to the general BAME population in that age bracket: 2–3% (*The Guardian*, 20 April 2020).

He also reports the striking statistic, that it was actually the first ten doctors who died of Covid-19 and two-thirds of the first 100 health and social care workers came from ethnic minorities. As Khan notes, although ethnic minorities are more likely to work in these sectors, the mortality figures far exceed their representation in health and social care. One likely reason, as he explains, is that ethnic minority staff face a higher likelihood of being on the frontline, exposing them to greater risks of virus exposure, performing undesirable and comparatively risky tasks, and thus professional discrimination appears to be a significant factor contributing to their increased susceptibility to serious illness from Covid-19.

Though Kahn is right to say that these long-standing inequalities have profoundly influenced the severity of the virus among BAME patients, the positivist methodology that he shares with Marmot can also make it harder to understand *relational* aspects of health and it can fail to challenge ways doctors are trained into particular ways of thinking about "risk factors" and "variables" in ways that mean they can read up a person's health status from the numbers on their iPads without really having to listen to their emotional and social histories. They don't really have to engage in a process of listening because they supposedly already know from their numbers what they are going to learn.

Kahn draws attention to the "limited understanding" in the UK of structural and institutional racism. At the same time, we need to think carefully about the interrelation at different levels of different forms of explanation so questioning the positivist terms in which causal explanations are too easily assumed when we talk of the "social determinants" of health. Khan draws too categorical a distinction when says, "Instead of suggesting individual or 'cultural' explanations for these outcomes, the evidence shows that the social and economic inequalities faced by ethnic minorities lead to poor outcomes in health."

We might need to take account of a whole range of different factors, operating at different levels, but often their relative significance can only be made clear when doctors learn how to listen to the different levels of experience that their parents are sharing with them. Often this is rendered almost impossible within the short time consultations allowed when doctors no longer look at their patients, or their bodily responses, as they speak because they are trapped behind their computers that have captured their attention.

Khan eloquently expresses the concern widely held at the time that the government's response to Covid-19 would be lacking, especially the political history of neglecting racial inequalities in policy. He expressed the fear that inequalities would deepen with increased state powers and reduced individual rights. He recognises that whenever the coercive power of the state is extended, those in power are most likely to be applied to ethnic minorities, including younger Black men in particular. And if citizens feel empowered to report on each other, he notes "that too is likely to lead to unequal reporting of who is a threat, given existing public attitudes about race and criminality."[5]

Inequalities, Discriminations and Vulnerabilities

Rebecca Solnit reported from the US in April 2020 with uncertainty of how nationwide vulnerabilities would be amplified in the pandemic: in healthcare, of course, but also in "economic, social, political and racial" spheres.

So little was known and people across the world were suddenly living with fearful of uncertainties and unsure how to protect themselves and where exactly the dangers were that could threaten their lives. As she traces the pandemic she recalls, "Age was the first factor most of us in the west heard about in the unequal impact of the virus." The virus was for the most part mild in children and younger adults, and was more serious in older people, which gave rise to misinformation in the early stages that it posed little danger to the young. As cases rose, the media produced "cautionary tales" of seriously ill young people that soon provided a counterpoint to this narrative.

Solnit expressed the hope that an increasing awareness of intersectionality would lead to more nuanced understandings of how individuals would be differently affected by the virus. She gives the example of the varying economic impacts of lockdown on different communities. Some people suddenly lost jobs while key workers were under enormous pressure to work in potentially hazardous circumstances.

Even though people were instructed to "stay at home" some people lived in overcrowded conditions with shared bathrooms and other people had no homes to stay in. Those in prison found it hard with their lack of freedom to sustain social distance. Solnit focuses on the dilemma faced in San Francisco: a city where homelessness is endemic, where officials tried to place unhoused people, but created a situation resulting in "70 residents on one impromptu shelter testing positive for the virus" (*The Guardian*, 17 April 2020).

She also recognises the digital divide's impact on school and university students, where students needed equipment and internet connections at home to even participate. At university where students couldn't gather in a shared and equalising context, it became clear, as Les Back in the department of Sociology at Goldsmiths, University of London reported, teaching on zoom brought home the very different living conditions that students had at home. The overcrowded spaces that could make it hard to focus upon your studies, especially when there were so many fears and anxieties about sickness and family members. Students had very different caring responsibilities for children and elderly parents in families where parents were obliged to work because their work was defined as essential and that they could not leave to self-isolate at home.

Solnit notes the swiftness with which universities acted to remove the students from campuses: assuming that those students had somewhere to go "home" to, a prospect terrifying to those with challenging home lives, or without family.

She also records how those who live alone have been reporting devastating *loneliness*. People who live with others have reported everything from exasperation to fear, including the anxiety of others not doing enough to minimise the spread of the virus, or behaving in ways that would guarantee this spread. There were also *gender issues* about responsibilities within a changed household where children had to be educated and food has to be prepared and where it is hard for anyone to escape for more than a limited exercise period outside. Among Black men, she notes, there could be an anxiety around mask-wearing feeding into negative racist stereotypes around criminality.

In her reflections of health disparities due to racism, and how they increased the chance of becoming severely ill or dying, Solnit shows a political sensitivity to the interrelation of different factors when she writes of the risks experienced disproportionally by black people across the US:

> Higher levels of diabetes and hypertension… linked to the stress of racism; asthma and respiratory problems… to polluted air of many urban and industrial areas; and lack of long-term access to good medical care and food sources (due to poverty and discrimination).

As Solnit looks to the future, she recognises the global nature of the pandemic, speculating that it will touch "Nearly everyone on Earth," but will affect all to varying degrees of severity depending on a wide range of social factors. In a time of gathering awareness about a global climate emergency, the pandemic was potentially intensifying a sense of interdependency at a global level.

She recognises some will face racism outside the home or violence within it. The pandemic is a spotlight that illuminated underlying problems – economic inequality, racism, patriarchy. As she notes, compassion "begins with understanding the differences," and inequalities are "chronic illnesses that weaken us as a society, morally, imaginatively, and otherwise."

Risks, Racial Inequalities and Racial Justice

The Office of National Statistics in the UK, as reported by journalists Robert Booth and Caelainn Barr, has found that, taking into account age, measures of self-reported health and disability and other social-demographic characteristics, "black people were still almost twice as likely as white people to die a Covid-19 related death," with Bangladeshi and Pakistani males being 1.8 times more likely to die from Covid-19 than white males.

As Zubaida Haque of the Runnymede Trust describes, the results as alarming: showing the severity of the impact of racial discrimination, but pointing out that this was "not taken into account in most statistical modelling of Covid-19 risk factors." These groups have been shown to face higher levels of unemployment and child poverty than white groups. They are also more likely to experience overcrowding in housing and so would find it harder to maintain social distancing and would feel more compelled to continue going to work even if this is unsafe for them.

Helen Barnard of the Joseph Rowntree Foundation, said these "stark" findings, alongside projections for "the deepest recession on record" should prompt societal soul-searching on issues of "justice and compassion" (*The Guardian*, 7 May 2020).

Booth and Barr note fears of "pre-existing health inequalities" risk factors among ethnic minorities, including diabetes, cardiovascular disease and hypertension affecting survival outcomes for patients in need of ventilators.

But research by Ben Goldacre at the University of Oxford also shows that the increased risk among BME people cannot be explained by people having a higher risk of cardiovascular disease or diabetes. As he reports, "That is not the explanation," finding that people from deprived social backgrounds were also at a higher risk and again this finding could not be explained by other risk factors.

In an analysis of Covid-19 fatalities by the ONS in relation to occupation it has been shown that men in low-skilled jobs are almost four times more likely to die from coronavirus than professionals. Security guards, care workers, construction workers, plant operatives, cleaners, taxi drivers, bus drivers, chefs and retail workers are all at a greater risk of dying. One *Guardian* report by journalists Caelainn Barr and Phillip Inman outlined statistics that suggests a higher number of fatalities among workers on lower salaries: tending to be more practical and public-facing that higher-paid roles. In turn, it reports that these roles are disproportionately occupied by ethnic minority workers. It is evidently so much safer to be able to work from home and it is those who are obliged to stay at work that have been put at most risk.[6]

As John Phillips of the GMB trade union said, the figures were "horrifying" and "stark," and suggested that "Ministers must pause any return to work until proper guidelines, advice and enforcement are in place to keep people safe".

Neil Pearce, a professor of epidemiology at London School of Hygiene and Tropical Medicine, described Covid-19 as an "occupational disease," criticising the pressure on people to return to workplaces that were potentially unsafe, or unable to minimise the risks of exposed, people-facing professions (*The Guardian*, 11 May 2020).

Risks, Deprivations and Despair

Dr Micheal Head, a researcher in global health at the University of Southampton assesses the research, giving a summarising example that of two people of a similar age, a "male diabetic Asian bus driver" faces a greater risk compared to a "female healthy Caucasian company director."

Working class deprivation is multi-ethnic and is reflected in health inequalities in different parts of the UK. Public Health Scotland has shown that the highest proportion of confirmed cases of Covid-19 was among the most deprived 20% of the population (*The Guardian*, 11 May 2020). Inverclyde local authority, on Scotland's west coast has the highest Covid-19 death rate in the country, at 12.7 deaths per 10,000. This is more than double the national rate at 5.1.

Stephen McCabe, a Labour councillor has asked the Scottish government to address regional disparities. He says, "We have high-density housing, high levels of people with co-morbidities, a high proportion of older people living here, so we knew we were going to be hit, but what surprised us was that we were out in front" (*The Guardian*, 11 May 2020).

Chris McEleny, an SNP councillor describes local anger over Inverclyde topping the "wrong league tables." The impact on the community has been tangible, says Reverend Fraser Donaldson, of Hope Community Church in Greenock, who describes a visible decline in morale within the community in the face of news coverage describing the area as the "capital" of both "deprivation" and "corona" (*The Guardian*, 6 May 2020).

One Greenock resident, Martin Callander, sees evidence of the coronavirus death toll all around, describing the constant local news coverage and word of mouth: "My friend's wife is a funeral director: today she has seven funerals, one every hour." Beyond the official tallies, he described the wider effects on people's wellbeing: tragically sharing news of the suicides of two of his friends. But then there are also ways that the community has come together in acts of kindness and support (*The Guardian*, 6 May 2020).

At the Crawfurdsburn community centre volunteers come together to help distribute food. Laura Reilly who runs the packing efforts shared her lack of surprise at how tough the community were finding the lockdown: especially those unused to asking for support, giving an example of a Port Glasgow resident who "was down to his last banana." They have delivered 2,00 food boxes, 3,000 hot meals and 500 prescriptions, as well as setting up a daily keep-in-contact phone service, bicycle repairs and fundraising for laptops for children struck at home without any technology.

The organiser, Stephen Henry says: "If you look on social media, you can see the impact that this is having on the community and the loss people are feeling." So often the focus on numbers of dead in the daily national briefings doesn't really engage the grief and mourning that is so hard to bear when people feel separated and isolated from family and friends in hospital. Henry has plans to set up temporary memorials – wooden love hearts where people can write the name of someone who has died – in parks and on the esplanade, which residents can visit on their daily walks.

"There's a lot of negativity around Inverclyde," says Henry, "but if you scratch the surface there's some amazing stuff going on. People are engaging with each other at a human level." The pandemic was helping to renew a sense of community in some areas as it was intensifying anger as social inequalities were being made visible.[7]

A Global Pandemic and Health Injustices

While the data was still emerging in the United States, it has become clear that Covid-19 deaths are falling disproportionately on the Black community. African Americans are more likely to live in urban areas that have been hit the hardest by the pandemic and many live in southern states whose governments have been slow to respond to the current crisis. But as in the UK, and more so because of a lack of nationally funded health service that is free at the point of need, the pandemic is revealing long present racial disparities in health.

As Devan Hawkins, an instructor in public health, reports, structural racism in areas such as accommodation, healthcare and social support causes a drop in living standards more likely to result in Black Americans developing co-morbidities that severely affects the outcome of recovery from Covid-19.

Hawkins notes, also resonating with research in the UK that has a very different racial history of Empire, that "occupational segregation" has further increased the risk of the virus to Black Americans. He cites research showing that Black workers are over-represented in essential services, with a 37.7% employment rate in these industries, while only 26.9% of white workers work in similar sectors. In the healthcare industries this figure rises to around 50% in health and social care, and 40% in hospital settings, compared with white workers. They are employed in jobs across the country with a higher likelihood of having to work through any lockdown and so of being exposed to a dangerous virus.

Black workers comprise a disproportionate share of bus drivers and postal workers, two essential occupations that require close contact with the public combined with a high risk of infections. They are also less likely to be employed in jobs that provide paid sick leave, so they have less access to benefits and are less likely to be covered by government schemes to help those unemployed through the pandemic.

As Devan Hawkins notes, "Black workers are not only vulnerable to the direct health impacts of Covid-19, but also more likely to be vulnerable to the economic fallout of this pandemic." He recognises "In a country where so much insurance coverage is insurance-based, large job losses will likely only exacerbate racial and ethnic disparities in access to insurance" (*The Guardian*, 16 April 2020).

Writer Alana Lentin has noted, "as BAME people die and suffer disproportionately from the virus, it is clear 'race' is about power", which she notes goes against a dominant "discourse in the west that for decades has claimed that 'making it about race' unnecessarily sensationalises an issue. Some treat the connection between race and the virus with derision"[8]

David Green, chief executive of Civitas argues in a Comment piece in the *Daily Telegraph* (4 May) entitled Campaigners are twisting BAME Covid-19 data to further their "victimhood" agenda." He argues:

> The Coronavirus crisis initially led to a great surge of national solidarity symbolised by Thursday evening clapping. But this sense that we are all in this together appears to have been intolerable to the inequalities industry, whose unrelenting strategy is to identify statistical disparities that can be portrayed as manifestations of victimhood.

Lentin recognises the weakness of

> a conversation around race that is defined by "free speech rationalists" pitted against "irrational antiracists." These antiracists see race everywhere, supposedly demonising and silencing everyone with "concerns" about migrants, Muslims or Black people – the same people who are now dying disproportionately of Covid-19.

She recognises "race is not a category that antiracists impose on the world, or a debating point about individual morality: it is a factor that shapes the lives of the people who are racialised" (*The Guardian*, 12 May 2020).

Deepening Inequalities and Impossible Choices

Journalists Max Fisher and Emma Bubola reported in *The New York Times* on the pandemic's deepening effect on inequality, felt globally. The reporters express alarm at the "a self-reinforcing cycle" increasing the virus's lethality, and putting in place dangerous conditions to reinforce "right-wing populism, racial animosity and deaths of despair – those resulting from alcoholism, suicide or drug overdoses." Expert in public health Nicole Errett of the University of Washington noted the "interconnected" nature of these phenomena, explaining a trend that following disaster that sees "Pre-existing social vulnerabilities" sharply rise in intensity.[9]

Because each low-income families, including racialised African Americans and Latinos are often, because of the nature of their work, forced to accept a higher risk of exposure that can infect others.[10] By contrast, those with the privilege of working from home in professional middle-class jobs can also reinforce their barriers with the outside world that can start at their front door. They learn to regulate any food or parcel that crosses the threshold, making sure that they clean it well so that it cannot carry any virus into the safety of home. They self-isolate and make sure that delivery workers place any parcels at a safe distance.

The people who are forced to work outside their homes – which includes a higher proportion of BAME people – are obliged to take risks to bring bread home.

At the same time, they are worried and anxious that they might catch the virus but also that they might bring it home and infect their children, particularly if they are known to have a weakened immune system. They are left in impossible situations where there is no "reasonable choice" open to them but to hope that somehow, possibly because of their age or because they don't have an underlying health condition that somehow things will be fine. But it is a matter of luck and when you know other people who work with you have come down with the virus, it can leave you deeply concerned but unable to do anything about it.

Fisher and Bubola quote Domenico Marra, a factory worker in Milan who spoke on behalf of his colleague who were desperate to carry on, but feared putting their families at risk. Lorenco Tacco who works in the same factory said they went on strike because of their employer's failure to provide sufficient health protection as the epidemic spread, and noted that it was the most financially insecure who shouldered the burden of having to take the greatest risks, with the wealthy able to "run away" (*The New York Times*, 16 March 2020).

Lara Fulciniti, a waiter residing in a Milan suburb, was already struggling to make ends meet, before the epidemic struck, and when it did, it was disastrous. "I am not ashamed to say I did not pay my bills this month," she confided: a dilemma shared by many. She expressed worry that her son's school would reopen before was able to earn enough to cover travel and his school lunch.

Like people around the world, in very different material circumstances and exacerbated by the everyday racism that so many people of colour confront, many people feel that the governments have been more concerned to support businesses than really provide for the many who are forced to live hand to mouth or survive within the informal economy.

Unequal access to health care in any country makes getting sick especially expensive for the poor. In the US, as Fisher and Bubola report, the number of people entitled to paid sick leave in the top quartile of earners is at 90%, compared to 47% in the bottom quartile. They note that health experts fear that health costs will accelerate outbreaks of Covid-19 particularly as stories circulate about the *cost* for coronavirus testing or treatment. People will *not* want to know that they have symptoms because they know that they cannot afford to get sick so they will keep on regardless, at the risk of passing on the virus to those they come into contact. People will carry on going to work while minimising the threats of the virus for fear of losing their jobs.

Because communities tend *to cluster* by economic status, with concentrations of working-class poor ethnic communities, Dr Errett[11] said the people who are both at the greatest risk of infection and likely to suffer most from the virus are all in proximity, multiplying the risk. Even small pockets of mutually reinforcing poverty and ill health make everyone more susceptible. Because diseases do not respect the barriers that separate rich from poor, even if the rich do their best to stay apart and isolate themselves, health inequality is a risk for everyone. In Delhi, a city of acute inequality, the slums provide the perfect environment to expediate outbreaks of disease. Dr Errett encourages people to think more widely about public health, not only at an individual but at a societal and public level. "If there's one person can't get treatment, that person is posing a risk to everyone."[12]

Spreading Death and Denial

Imported by the Brazilian elite vacationing in Europe, the coronavirus is now ravaging the country's poor, ripping through tightly packed neighbourhoods where the disease is harder to control. Public health data show a shift in recent weeks from the wealthy boroughs of Sao Paulo and Rio de Janeiro to the urban favelas that exist around the cities.[13] Brazil was set to become a *deadly* hot spot of the virus as the poorest areas often lack running water, septic systems and healthcare facilities, find it impossible to cope with what has hit them so hard and at such an accelerated speed.

With President Bolsonaro playing down the seriousness of the disease for so long, people got the message that it was no real threat and carried on crowding the streets. "For those who haven't been through it, it's like the disease doesn't exist," said Paulo do Santos, 43, who lost his father to the virus in Brasilandia, a poor district at the north end of Sao Paulo (Reuters, 1 May 2020).

William de Oliveira, a community leader in Rio's poor hillside favela, Rocinha, can rattle off the names of several friends killed by the virus. Yet it was clear that life was continuing very much as normal, with shops and bars bustling, which he lamented. Oliveira said, "We can reverse economic problems… but we can't reverse deaths."

Writing when President Jair Bolsonaro was still in power, and in a state of dangerous denial on the severity of the crisis, journalist Tom Phillips reported on the staggering covid death tolls in Brazil, contradicting Bolsonaro's complacent briefing citizens that "the worst of the crisis was over." Under-reporting and a lack of testing also means that the true numbers are almost certainly much higher than those officially reported. The Amazon state of Pará responded to 4,472 cases and 369 deaths, with lockdowns in ten cities, including its capital, Belem. Helena Brígido, of the state's infectious diseases society, painted a hellish picture of hospitals, and queues of citizens outside official buildings attempting to receive emergency payments, saying "People need to be scared of this virus… People need to wake up" (*The Guardian*, 6 May 2020).

Bolsonaro had told reporters when Brazil's Covid death toll rose to 77, revealing his own form of class racism and white supremacy, that he didn't think Brazilians would get the virus. He explained his theory, without providing evidence or detail, that Brazilian's were miraculously immune to illness, after seeing "some bloke jumping into the sewage, he gets out, had a dive, right? And nothing happens to him." Without offering any scientific evidence, Bolsonaro continued to speculate that the virus may have already infected large swathes of the Brazilian population, providing them with the "antibodies that help it not to proliferate," again, providing no evidence or justification for such a statement (*The Guardian*, 6 May 2020).

His flippant response to the crisis, initially following in the footsteps of Trump whom he admires and aspires to identify with – which he had dismissed as a fantasy and media trick – has been widely condemned, but this did not mean that many of his supporters did not take his dangerous message to heart and lived in firm denial of the threats around them. Kim Kataguiri, a right-wing congressperson who supported Bolsonaro before his 2018 election, has since become a critic, saying the president's "erratic, irresponsible and populist" antics were putting Brazil at risk. "It's pretty clear he is primarily interested in his re-election and very little about actually fighting coronavirus," Kataguiri said (*The Guardian*, 8 May 2020).

Notes

1 Michael Marmot is a health researcher whose writings show there is nothing inevitable about health inequalities include *The Health Gap: The Challenge of an Unequal World* (London: Bloomsbury Paperbacks 2016); *Status Syndrome: How Your Place on the Social Gradient Directly Affects Your Health* (London: Bloomsbury 2015); Leo S. Olschki *Fair Society, Healthy Lives* (ci.nii.ac.jp, 2013) and with Sridhar Venkatapuram *Health Justice: An Argument from the Capabilities Approach* (Cambridge: Polity 2011). See also Solomon Benatar ed. *Global Health: Ethical Issues* (Cambridge: Cambridge University Press 2021) which addresses global health in the context of the accelerated destruction of the planet and draws upon cross-cultural dialogues to make practical recommendations to promote global health.

2 BBC Radio 4 "The World this Weekend" interview. See also John Tomaney and Andy Pike "Brexit, devolution and economic development in 'left-behind' regions", *Welsh Economic Review*, 03/12/18, https://doi.org/10.18573/wer.231.

3 Marmot, M, Allen, J., Boyce, T., Goldblatt P. and Morrison, J. Health Equity in England: The Marmot Review 10 Years On (Institute of Health Equity, 2020).

4 For an understanding of different times of austerity in Britain and how they continue to echo see, David Kynaston *Austerity Britain 1945–1951: Tales of a New Jerusalem* (London: Bloomsbury 2008); Mary O'Hara *Austerity Bites: A Journey to the Sharp End of Cuts in the UK* (Bristol: Polity Press 2019). She investigates the effects on everyday lives of a raft of austerity measures that had profoundly damaging effects on much of the population. She dispels the notion that "we are all in this together". Kerry-Anne Mendoza argues in *Austerity: The Demolition of the Welfare State and the Rise of the Zombie Economy* (Oxford: New Internationalist 2015) how the pain of a financial crisis caused by bankers and speculators was being borne by ordinary people – and by the poor and disabled most of all. It provided an opportunity for a neoliberal government to pursue its project to shrink government and privatise resources.

5 For a study which explores the influence of race and gender on the health status of a diverse group of non-white women in the United States see Marcia Bayne-Smith (ed) *Race, Gender and Health* (Los Angeles: Sage Publications 1996). The work brings together different disciplinary perspectives to encourage the development of new paradigms of care.

6 Caelainn Barr and Philip Inman "Low-paid workers more likely to die from Covid-19 than higher earners" (theguardian.com, Monday 11 May 2020).

7 Discussions that help expose growing inequalities in the UK and globally are offered by Polly Toynbee and David Walker *Unjust Rewards: Exposing Greed and Inequality in Britain Today* (London: Granta Books 2008). They show how the widening gap is tearing apart the fabric of society, made evident in the strikes across the public sector in 2022/3. See also Danny Dorling *Inequality and the 1%* (London: Verso Books 2019) who argues that since the 2008 global recession the 1% has only grown richer while the

rest find life increasingly hard. He lays bare the extent and true cost of the division in our society. Inequality is more than just economics. He shows that it is the 1% that threatens us with the most harm and why the balance urgently needs to be addressed. See also Clare Bambra, Julia Lynch and Katherine Smith *The Unequal Pandemic: Covid-19 and Health Inequalities* (Bristol: Policy Press 2021).

8 Quoted in Alana Lentin "Coronavirus is the ultimate demonstration of the real-world impact of racism" (theguardian.com, Tuesday May 2020).

9 Explorations of how racism takes a toll on individuals and the health of the nation in the US are offered by Linda Villarosa *Under the Skin: Racism, Inequality, and the Health of a Nation* (New York: Anchor 2023). She shows how Black people in the US have poorer health outcomes than white people at every stage of their lives. She shows how coping with the daily scourge of racism ages Black people prematurely in a process of "weathering." She explores the truths of racialised trauma showing how structural violence has physical and mental ramifications. See also Stephen Bezruchka *Inequality Kills Us All: Covid-19 Health Lessons for the World* (New York and London: Routledge 2022). If capitalism generates and deepens inequality, inequality shortens lives across the world even among those who celebrate capitalism. He documents how Covid-19 is a sped-up version of global health inequalities and how living in a society with entrenched hierarchies increases the negative effects of illnesses for everyone.

10 Max Fisher and Emma Bubola "As Coronavirus Deepens Inequality, Inequality worsens its spread" (nytimes.com, 16 March 2020).

11 Dr Nicole A. Errett is a public health expert on extreme event resilience at the University of Washington.

12 For an investigation of the Covid-19 pandemic and its devastating effects in India see Abantika Ghosh *Billions Under Lockdown: The Inside Story of India's Fight against Covid-19* (New Delhi: Bloomsbury 2021). When WHO first declared Covid-19 a global pandemic in March 2020, there was apprehension about how India, the country with the highest TB cases and diabetes, with an inadequate health infrastructure and a population of 1.3 billion, would fare. See Rajib Bhattacharyya, Ananya Ghosh Dastidar and Soumyen Sidkar (eds) *The Covid-19 Pandemic, India and the World* (New Delhi: Routledge India, 2021) which shows how the pandemic contributed to considerable suffering and affected socio-cultural relationships including Hindu-Muslim conflict, domestic violence and issues of identity, gender and vulnerability. See also Chandra Kumar Sharma and Resmi Banerjee (eds) *Coronasphere: Narratives on COVID 19 from India and its Neighbours* (New Delhi: Routledge India 2022). As they report Covid-19 has been "the most critical health calamity of the century since the Second World War, which has destroyed both lives and livelihoods. It is a human, economic, and social crisis…its lethal impact has been disproportionately felt by the poorer and the marginalised sections of every country and region in the world." Migrant workers were often stranded in the cities without food and shelter, and many were forced to return to their villages involving a fearful trek. The pandemic had a devastating effect on migrant labour and the informal sector.

13 This was an early strain of the virus; Reuters 1 May and *The Guardian*, 6 May 2020.

4

SHOCKS, ISOLATIONS, LOCKDOWNS AND FEARFUL FUTURES

Shocks, Fears and Insecurities

Tuesday, 14 March 2020. A day after the Prime Minister Boris Johnson shifted gear in his response to the coronavirus and the atmosphere in the streets had changed, I could feel my own bodily anxieties. I had seen the BBC News at 10 where they announced the new measures and I stayed up to watch Newsnight on BBC 2, something I had tried to avoid doing since the exhaustion of the Brexit crisis. It left me feeling uneasy as I listened to a health minister finding it impossible to respond to questions about how unprepared the National Health Service was after years of austerity and how slow they had been to respond to the first signs of a global pandemic in China.

The crisis was upon us, but the NHS did not have anywhere near the number of ventilators that they needed, and they had asked manufacturing companies whether they could change production to cope with the need. This was not the only sign of a wartime economy to come.

I felt my own sense of unease as I was thinking about what risks I might be taking in getting a haircut in Golders Green in North London. Why was I feeling so nervous and uneasy? Were we not still in the early stages of the pandemic in the UK? But could I really think this after the serious announcements to limit social contact and the advice to people to avoid pubs, clubs and going to theatres. I had already seen the empty shelves in the supermarket and the panic buying that so many people were engaging in – saying to themselves that if other people are doing it, then we have to do it ourselves.

The empty shelves of toilet paper were last week's reality but since then there had been empty shelves across different aisles in the supermarket and queues outside before opening times. It was as if people could deal with their feelings

DOI: 10.4324/9781003296874-4

of insecurity and anxiety by making sure that they at least had stocks of essential goods at home, just in case.

When I came home from my haircut, I noticed an advertisement on the side of a red double-decker bus saying: "Something you cannot see can still harm you." It seemed to be a message about the corona virus and possibly it was something that I would not have noticed on another day. It was as if my anxiety drew the line to me. Opening my iPad, getting prepared to write, I received a tweet from Rob Edwards@robthemhnurse-1d saying: "Lad at Asda, aged 13–14. Put the final two bags of pasta in his basket then realised an older lady who was also trying to buy some would go without. He promptly put them in her trolley with a 'You need 'em more than me, love'. Then told his mum they've sold out."

There was another tweet that came out that showed how people were anticipating the comforts they might need in an uncertain and fearful time. Beth@bltwistxo said: "We are in the middle of a pandemic and Netflix have decided to take off all the Shrek films? That big green ogre is an essential key to the happiness in many people's lives. This is a despicable decision. And I for one am not happy. NOT HAPPY AT ALL." This got 12.8K retweets and 86.2K likes.

One turning point for many that March was the winding down of sports fixtures, leaving fans "shocked, concussed, even a touch bereft," as sportswriter Jonathan Liew recognised (*The Observer*, 15 March 2020). That month brought the virus home to the UK in myriad ways: from the "grisly" initial reports and footage of the virus's devastating effects in China to the unprecedented lockdown in Italy and nationwide school closures in Ireland, Britain braced itself. Liew movingly notes that for the British people who build their lives around sport, embracing it not only as a way of "passing the time", but as "offer(ing) a liturgy, a structure on measure the passing days and seasons," the cancelling (in his example) of "Fulham v Brentford" was a rupture in the "veneer of normality."

Dwelling further on the relationship between sport and the passage of time, Liew details the moments that added up to a dramatic pause to the entire industry, reporting that at this point in the span of a couple of weeks, it seemed that "every hour (brings) more jolts to a system that on some level we all took for granted," an accelerated news cycle gearing up to a period of total silence and enforced inertia.

With some insight and empathy for other sport support, Jonathan Liew suggests:

> Perhaps during these long weeks ahead, we could all use a little patience. Perhaps even a little humility, especially in the face of unfolding human tragedy… Little by little, the galaxy of sport will blink back into life, and it will feel like a benediction and an irrelevance all at once, a reminder that of all the things that don't matter, sport matters most of all.
>
> *(The Observer, 15 March 2020, p. 3)*

Another watershed moment in March, as reported by journalists Sean Ingle and Justin McCurry (in *The Observer*) was the uncertainty surrounding the Temple of Hera-set ceremony, lighting the flame of the Olympic torch ahead of the doomed

Tokyo 2020 Olympics. The ceremony, with ancient roots, unfolded with a sense of pomp and drama that "could have been directed by Cecil B DeMille," but the occasion was haunted by uncertainty that the games would take place: and even "whether the flame (would) reach its final destination, Tokyo's National Stadium on the 24th of July" (*The Observer*, 15 March 2020 p. 6).

Paul Macinnes in *The Guardian* also recognised this sense of urgency through the lens of sport, exploring the plight of British football facing up to the realities of a "prolonged spell of financial and legal uncertainty."

Within the Premier League, the effects of the virus were immediately felt, with a number of high-profile faces publicly withdrawing after contracting the virus. Among them was the Arsenal manager Mikel Arteta, whose statement in response to media and public interest in his own condition thanked supporters, and dwelled on the "huge and unprecedented challenge," underscoring the importance of health and wellbeing, and advised people to "Protect each other by following the guidelines and we'll come through this together." He praised the Premier League "for making the right decisions." (*The Guardian*, 14 March 2020, p. 2).

Social Distance, Isolations and Everyday Ethics

Families, villages, communities, towns and even countries were dealing with the everyday realities of separating out from each other and so being in a situation of quarantine, sometimes for an indefinite period. The term quarantine is derived from the Italian *quaranta giorni*, in reference to the practice during the 14th century of requiring plague-infected ships from Venice to sit at anchor for 40 days before landing. I wonder whether it was connected to the idea of certain groups being forced to separate themselves and live apart, as was the situation for the Jews of Venice who were obliged to live in the ghetto in Venice. Each night they were ordered to return to the space of the ghetto and so live in a form of quarantine. The Venetian government created a sequestered habitat, a city within a city, putting the Jews under surveillance.[1]

Tracing historical lessons imparted by how people have dealt with the containment of plague, journalist Peter Beaumont noted with irony that "it was a quarantine in China (a 1910 plague outbreak in Harbin) that would inform most modern approaches, not least in China, where it became embedded in myth." This particular outbreak was notable because of its horrifying outcome: 95% of those who contracted the plague at this key fur trade location succumbed to the disease (*The Observer*, 15 March 2020, p. 13). He notes:

> The quarantine was managed by a celebrated doctor named Wu Lien-teh. He implemented not just a strict lockdown, including the suspension of transport links with Russia and Japan, but introduced measures still used, including dedicated quarantine centres and hygienic burials. Lien-teh's methods were preserved for others to learn from with his "meticulously" kept recordings and notes.
>
> *(The Observer, 15 March 2020)*

With the current coronavirus – it was to take time before we were to learn to identify it as Covid-19 – many people around the globe were now being asked to self-isolate and so take responsibility for the conditions of their own quarantine. But this was proving difficult in the UK because people could not easily be tested unless their symptoms were severe, and they were admitted to hospital. Drawing on experience teaching at Leo Baeck College in London, on Wednesday, 18 March 2020, in a small group of five people, two were unsure of whether the symptoms, which could include a cough and high temperature, meant that they had the virus. Since a teacher at the college had come down with coronavirus, this only added to the anxiety. They already had suspicions that the symptoms they had could be interpreted as signs of the virus, so what to do?

This is the insecurity that shaped the unanticipated everyday ethics that we were all living with as we had entered the corona-verse, and where everyone reported that they have been talking about nothing else. Suddenly life was taking on a new fearful and unexpected form. People everywhere in their relationships and on the internet had been looking for an authority to give instructions. Soon many people realised that they were going to have to make their own decisions about whether to self-isolate because it was going to be difficult to get tested.

A doctor with long experience who suspected she might already have it was concerned that she must not spread it. Suddenly everything in her life seemed challenged as she faced moral decisions about who to stay in contact with. Across the planet we were gradually becoming aware that we were moving into a different moral universe, which would give shape to its own rules. We were suddenly made aware of the economic, social and cultural differences, between the global North and South and their health systems, which would shape our futures as vulnerable humans. We were learning that reality is always framed in moral terms, even if we remain largely unaware of the workings of structural inequalities within the common-sense of a liberal moral culture that insists on the neutrality, universality and impartiality of morality.

The doctor was the person who contacted me late at night to tell me that the class had moved on-line and that she no longer felt able to attend it in person, as she had been planning to do. She was feeling helpless and without the control that she had assumed herself to have over her life.

She reminded me of the man I met walking in the park the day before who wondered whether it would not be better for him to get the virus, because at least then he would know where he was and would gain a certain immunity. This would give him more control of his life and a feeling that he could then help others and so regain a sense of purpose now that he was no longer working. People were thrown as they felt attacked by an unfamiliar sense of uncertainty and a fear that they were living in a time without a familiar sense of futures. It felt dangerous and people felt insecure because they no longer knew what was expected of them and how to relate.

A student had joined the Zoom from Northern Italy where they had already been in lockdown for a few weeks, and she could let classmates in London know the terrors they might expect. She talked about how isolated people felt, even when they were in contact over social media. She was bringing news from a future that could soon be shared across the world and she was introducing us to the everyday ethics we could soon be living.

At some level, she shared, this could reinforce a sense of isolation, especially knowing that doctors you knew were having to deal with impossible decisions about life and death. This in a short time was to become agonisingly familiar. Who was to be given the chance of a ventilator and who was going to be denied access because of their age or an underlying medical condition, meaning they would have less chance of survival?

In Italy, she was looking after her mother, but she was also concerned that people could not visit their elderly parents or friends in old-age homes because of the fear of passing on the virus. There was a tense atmosphere within the populist politics that had taken hold in Italy over the past few years, a pressure to look for someone to blame. Someone had to be responsible for the spread of the virus. How else could they live with not having been able to visit their dying relatives in a hospital or care home, sometimes not having been able to be present at the funeral that was organised?

There was an abiding feeling of helplessness among people within a neoliberal culture who had for years been taught to be independent and self-sufficient and in control of their lives and relationships. Now they were being forced to isolate themselves. There was also an anger that somehow it had come to this. Who was to be blamed? Why did the state authorities not take drastic action earlier? We had whole cities, regions and countries in quarantine – in lockdown – so that you could not leave the isolation of home without a document from the state that gave you permission for being on the street. This was the situation in Italy, France and Spain who had all moved to forms of national quarantine as a way of gaining some control over the spread of the virus.

Research seems to show that the virus was spreading in Italy for a while and that people tended to minimise the dangers they faced, when across Europe some medical authorities were saying that if you got Covid it was no worse than bad flu and that each year thousands died from influenza. They were slow to really test for the virus and so to trace people who had been in contact with it. The virus can be contagious before symptoms show, which can make it difficult to trace its spread.

In the group, a student from the United States talked about how it was impossible to know what the future might bring so that our relationship with time had been disturbed. We were going to have to quickly learn how to live in time and space differently, as we learned to constantly engage with risks. He had been involved for a while in planning a wedding but now it seemed an impossibility. They could not know what was going to happen next week, let alone next month. There was an ethical anxiety spreading about the risks we were suddenly and unexpectedly confronted with in everyday life.

It had become impossible to anticipate what the future might bring and for him it felt so much worse being isolated from his family who were dealing with the virus in the United States. He was in regular contact with them on Skype and felt an acute sense of loss because this was exactly the day that his mother had died two years ago. He had been living through grief which was suddenly to become an experience shared by so many through these Covid-19 times. Sadly, so many people across the world were also unable to sit with their relatives while they died, and many people couldn't attend funerals.

He shared the news of his mother's death after noting that it was exactly a year since the group had all met, so establishing a sense of emotional connection with everyone in the supportive group. He was not there with his father and the rest of his family to mark his mother's death and so to live through another stage in the long path of grief and mourning. Somehow, he felt more acutely the limits of Skype and the screen contact he had with them. He could hear about what was happening, but he could not really contribute through doing things for others that could support them in their lives.

Talking about generations, another student shared how it wasn't always a younger generation that was ignoring the dangers of the virus and getting on with their lives as usual, possibly because as a younger age group, they did not feel endangered and threatened by the virus in the same way. In her experience, younger people were taking note and she had read the report by Professor Neil Ferguson from Imperial College that had warned that there could be 200,000 deaths in the UK if they did not change the course they had set.

He had stressed the importance of really engaging with what was happening in Italy that was shifting the variables in the models they had shaped through what had happened in China, where far more people were getting seriously ill and needing to be treated on ventilators for two weeks in hospital. She said reading the report was scary and immediate dangers felt very real. In her experience, it was now often the older generation who were saying that they had lived through the Second World War and 9/11 so they felt they would get through this. To her it seemed as if they "just didn't get it" and she hoped they soon would, and if they did not, reading the report would make a difference and help them "get it".

Eugenia Tognotti, a historian of quarantine, who wrote an essay on the subject for the US Centres for Disease Control and Prevention, and who was then on lockdown herself in Italy, argued that successful quarantine required "social acceptance".[2] She said it also depended on other conditions that varied according to geography and political context. She pointed out in response to Peter Beaumont's article that they were rarely uncontroversial. "Let's not forget that quarantine measures raise many ethical issues," she said, referring to the Sars outbreak in 2002, an even more deadly, if less widespread, coronavirus.

There were reports that it was the deadly impact of the Sars virus in places like Hong Kong that had helped the population there readily accept the restrictions of quarantine that they were asked to accept. Their experience with Sars meant that many people immediately understood the dangers they were facing and the necessity to close schools, restaurants and clubs almost instantly. There was a general social acceptance of the measures that were necessary, despite the years of political challenge to the local social state administration in Hong Kong.

Eugenia Tognotti also noted: "In China, compared to other infected countries, there was stronger control of the social strata at risk. Village-level authorities were empowered to isolate travellers from Sars-infected areas and enforce quarantine on people suspected of having had contact with Sars patients." As she also acknowledged: "That raises many questions regarding the impact of isolation and quarantine measures, and possibly discrimination against certain social categories and minorities. The present emergency and rigid measures adopted pending the Covid-19 epidemic will give us more lessons."

This made her also wonder about the question raised for many leaders in liberal democracies: "Can the kind of quarantine applied in China – with the rigid measures – work in western democratic countries?" She answered her own question with a big "IF". One that became increasingly apparent across European countries that had, according to the World Health Organization, become the new centre for the spread of the virus now that some Asian countries seemed to have got it under a certain control. As she recognised, in a comment now of global significance, as the Covid-19 spread to South Africa and South America – "Only if countries were not caught unprepared and if they recognised the enormous importance of planning."

This involved communication across populations about the dangers that the virus brings so that it was not only vital to stress the importance of hand washing and not touching the face and mouth but it was also critical to maintain a "social distance" with others, particularly the elderly and those with underlying health conditions that put them in immediate danger if the virus was passed on to them.

Tognotti added:

> We can learn from the past. In time of plague and cholera, well-trained and experienced public health officials were quick to recognise the crisis and launch an emergency public health response to contain outbreaks. A well-organised educational campaign to inform and calm a panicking and frightened public, and combat misinformation and fake news, is extremely important. It's the effort that Italy is making right now with some success.

But it was also clear that in a time of social media and a populist politics that had developed its own means of communication, there had not only been racist and xenophobic targeting of Chinese populations, wanting to hold them responsible for the outbreak and for the fear and anxieties that so many people were understandably feeling, but also that there had been widespread misinformation and fake news. Many people had sought to profit from remedies that had very little scientific or complementary support. There had been rumours of people wanting to gain access to houses by offering testing for the virus.

Democracy, Fears and Distrust

On Thursday, 12 March 2020, things suddenly got serious in the UK and there was an orchestrated plan to inform the population and get them on side. Reporting on a briefing delivered by Boris Johnson, Professor Chris Whitty and Sir Patrick Vallance, journalists Toby Helm and Robert McKie noted that the then-Prime Minister and the expert advisors seemed to be performing "calm reassuring authority," while delivering the stark warning: "Many more families are going to lose loved ones before their time" (*The Observer*, 15 March 2020, p. 6).

While Johnson recognised that the spread of coronavirus was a generational catastrophe, he wanted to assure people that the UK government was following the best scientific advice available to them and that they were in control of the situation, with a "clear plan," involving a distinct number of phases that they would move on when the time was appropriate. One of these phases was to impose a week-long quarantine period for those with "persistent coughs or fevers." Those over 70 or with underlying health issues would soon be told not to venture out, and families were to be quarantined if one member had a cough.

The journalists noted that the internal logic of the message may have been flawed, and even that those pushing the message had their disagreements with it. The Covid Inquiry was to hear from Lee Cain, the former Downing Street director of Communications, that Boris Johnson had the wrong "skill set" to lead the country in the pandemic. His senior aids were left "exhausted" by him constantly changing his mind on crucial decisions. He said, Johnson was hard to work with "just because he will oscillate, he will take a decision from the last person in the room" (guardian.com, Tuesday 31 Oct 2023). Indecision seriously impacted on the pace of the government's reaction and many people were to lose their lives as a consequence.

On the subject of large gatherings, Vallance suggested that forbidding them was unlikely to have a "big effect" on infection rates, citing an increased likelihood of transmission at smaller scale, such as "watching football in a pub" above attending a stadium match, regardless of crowd size (p. 6).

Yet within a few hours, these calm assurances began to look shaky and obviously out of step with what was unfolding in Italy where much more radical action to restrict mass gatherings had been taken. Within a couple of days, the Premier League, Football League and Scottish Football Association announced that they were all suspending their seasons until early April.

There was tension in the atmosphere as people wanted to know more about the data upon which the government was making its decisions. Why did it seem to be out on its own, in comparison to policies being taken in France and Spain? This did not help to build the trust that the government needed to establish with the wider population and the "social acceptance" they would need if people were going to follow the suggestions that the government was making. It was easy for people to be sceptical saying: "These are only suggestions" and in any case "we have lived through much worse in the past" so why should they stop going out drinking with their mates in a pub and so break the habits of a lifetime?

The government seemed to be on the back foot, whatever image of careful and steadfast planning they sought to put out. They had little option but to follow the decisions already made by the football authorities and already, by the weekend, Whitehall was briefing that mass gatherings would, after all, be banned from the following week. This change of heart was also spurred by scientists wanting to know more about the methodology that was being followed.

There were questions from scientific and social researchers as to whether it was realistic for the government to talk about spreading immunity in the population by allowing possibly younger people to get the virus so building up what was called 'herd immunity' – a term usually applied to situations where there is a virus for a condition, for example measles where the proportion of the population inoculated falls below a certain level.

Politicians started asking questions about the strategy. Tory minister Rory Stewart called for the schools to be closed, even if meant that parents, including health workers, might have to stay at home to look after their children. He cited previous pandemic research on early school closures and preventing large groups of people meeting having a more positive outcome, "(stopping) the peaks of this kind of disease."

The Lancet editor-in-chief, Richard Horton, criticised the government for "playing roulette" signalling that if medical researchers and scientists obviously disagreed with the policies being taken, the government was possibly being less than honest. They were implying that there was a scientific consensus when there clearly was not, and were insisting that there was in order to gain trust because they were following the best scientific advice available.

It was Horton who was to argue in *The Lancet* that people should think of Covid-19 not as "a pandemic" but simply as an infectious disease where the focus needs to be on cutting lines of transmission. As he wrote:

> …we have learned so far tells us that the story of COVID-19 is not so simple. Two categories of disease are interacting with specific populations…clustering within social groups according to patterns of inequality deeply embedded in our societies…The syndemic nature of the threat we face means that a more nuanced approach is needed if we are to protect the health of our communities."
>
> *(The Lancet, 26 September 2020)*

Fears, Indecisions and Institutional Failures

Jeremy Hunt, a former health secretary and chair of the health committee in the House of Commons at the time, criticised the "concerning" decision not to ban mass gatherings. Politicians were choosing their words carefully not wanting to be seen as criticising the government at a moment of national health emergency that was also being gradually recognised as an economic emergency with possibly lasting consequences. These could be worse than the global financial crisis of 2008, even though this time it did not start with a crisis in the financial sector and the banks were potentially in a much stronger position to offer support to the "real" economy.

Critics insisted that the government learn the lessons of Wuhan, the centre of the coronavirus outbreak and where the Chinese authorities blocked all outdoor activities and halted the escalation. Professor of Genomics at the University of Birmingham Alan McNally ruminated on the success of social distancing in East Asia during the outbreak, but also called for "extensive testing" and an intensification of quarantine measures, even the use of "dedicated quarantine facilities" to fight the spread of transmission" (*The Observer*, 15 March 2020, p. 7).

Johnson, as a libertarian suspicious of extending state intervention, was doing his best to win support for carefully controlled interventions, possibly aware of the limits of what you can suggest to people, let alone legislate, or use the criminal justice system for in a liberal democracy. There was an obvious concern on the part of the government's advisors that if you acted too quickly towards a lockdown, you would not be able to sustain it over time and that people would in the end refuse to comply. They were mistaken in their anticipations, as most people were ready to comply when they realised the dangers they faced and that the numbers in hospitals were rising, along with deaths.

Possibly the government was also heeding the warnings of global health experts, such as Dr Michael Head of Southampton University who reminded us that, in contrast to China and other regimes with different cultural and political traditions and modes of rule, the British people have a high degree of autonomy in their day-to-day lives, and that long-term "high population compliance" could therefore not be guaranteed.

As scientists speculated about social life, they often did not refer to any sociological evidence but somehow drew upon their status as scientists without really qualifying what specific expertise they had. Head showed a certain scientific superiority within a democratic culture, disputing the British population's ability to follow rules that compromised their sense of control, suggesting that compliance was likely to decrease over time. He anticipated that "More stringent interventions (would) come, and potentially very soon."[3] He recognised that strategy would have to change to reflect the expectations of the UK population, that it was "not providing the evidence base" to provide enough justification for measures. Adam Kucharski from the London School of Hygiene agreed: "It's easy to say, 'Let's just do what Wuhan did'," but he cited that those measures proved "unimaginable in scale and impact." There are moral and political questions that interrelated with each other than can't be resolved by an appeal to a scientific consensus that obviously didn't exist.

He noted that measures in China included a lockdown imposed on nearly 60 million people in Hubei with strict quarantine and travel restrictions for hundreds of millions of people – both citizens and foreigners and was doubtful about their sustainability. He was also concerned that the vast majority of the population in Wuhan is likely to remain susceptible to Covid-19 as they have isolated themselves from contact.

He speculated on the new risks that could arise from the cessation of these actions, including another surge in new cases, especially in the light of territories that had effectively contained outbreaks, such as Singapore and Hong Kong, suddenly experiencing significant increases in infection rates. However, China was determined to maintain its policy of zero tolerance of Covid-19, including strict lockdowns and quarantining those who tested positive and their close contracts, even in major cities like Shanghai and Beijing, until it was forced to change tack, after widespread protests at the end of 2022.

Professor Mark Woolhouse of Edinburgh expressed worry early in 2020 that where "total lockdown" had been implemented, there was now a particular challenge to assemble "exit strateg(ies)" to reverse the measures. But at the same time Jonathan Ashworth, Labour's health spokesperson, was concerned that the public's confidence in the government's handling of the crisis was fragile and questions were increasingly being posed about key aspects of its strategy.

While agreeing that steps had to be taken to slow the speed of transmission to prevent overwhelm of the NHS, he noted: "People are increasingly questioning if the UK is following international best practice" and questioned the withdrawal from the "continued testing" model of patients with symptoms that had been endorsed by the WHO (*The Observer*, Sunday 15 March).

Ashworth argued for greater governmental transparency in keeping the public informed, highlighting the importance of "total clarity to maintain public confidence." Within days, after action by the football authorities against mass gatherings, the government, under criticism about its policies, was forced to move much more quickly into more restrictive measures than its key scientific advisors had recommended.

Global Health Crises, Authorities and Legitimations

As *Observer* columnist Simon Tisdall noted (Sunday 15 March, 2020), the adage "Politics isn't working" is frequently cited in our time, but gained particular currency as the pandemic unfolded, as political failings and weaknesses were unflinchingly brought to light. Tisdall reports on the exceptional backlash against Chinese president Xi Jinping's own detached response to the initial outbreak in Wuhan, detailing his fight to "contain the political and human fallout."[4]

The death of the young doctor Li Wenliang from Covid-19 – the person who had struggled so much with the authorities to take the dangers of the virus seriously and who had sounded the alarm in Wuhan in December only to be gagged by Communist party officials – sparked a widespread online revolt in the country. It took Xi till the middle of March before he felt able to visit the city to offer what almost sounded like an apology.

Over in America, Xi's counterpart gave a "predicably" Trumpian response: making the pandemic "all about him." For a time, Trump was also in denial about the seriousness of the pandemic and insisted it was a fake Democrat plot to harm his re-election chances. Ignoring the expert advice of scientists, as he had done so many times, he dismissed the threat and claimed his Mexican border would have somehow immunised Americans, and consistently referred to the "Chinese virus".

This was even when challenged at a press conference on 18 March, when the United States had long had time to shift gear and take on the crisis they faced, not only in health terms but also economically where memories of the Great Depression of the 1930s were being recalled. Trump refused the question of whether it was racist to keep calling it the 'Chinese virus' insisting – with an eye to the election in November – that this was where the virus had come from. It remained part of a "foreign invasion" against which the United States had to defend itself. Tisdall described Trump's political shortcomings as "embarrassingly obvious" in the face of crisis, but not unique in its "knee-jerk reaction in pulling up the drawbridge and blaming others." Tisdall compares his response to that of former Chancellor of Austria, Sebastian Kurz, who "hastily" shut down the borders to the country and imposed bans on the flow from specific countries, which Tisdall notes "recall Europe's chaotic response to the 2015 migrant crisis," which revealed a total lack of unity and concord in how it could be dealt with (*The Observer*, 15 March 2020, p. 10).

Tisdall notes how the pandemic was turning into a political nightmare for the European Union. The commission in Brussels was struggling to keep up, relaxing rules on deficit spending that had already been broken. Piecemeal, national-level policymaking is a gift to Eurosceptics, not least right-wing populists keen to exploit splits. He fears this "could have lasting consequences for European coherence. Public confidence may take a big hit."

There is no doubt that politicians faced genuine and impossible dilemmas. Italy's prime minister, Giuseppe Conte, was initially attacked for doing too much, by ordering widespread testing in Lombardy, and subsequently for doing too little. Italy also complained about being left out in the cold with very little help from the rest of Europe when it had to decide first to lock down the region around Lombardy and then the whole country.

As Tisdall recognised, when Italy was in total lockdown, "It is being studied like a laboratory guinea pig." German Chancellor, Angela Merkel's assessment that Covid-19 would infect two out of three Germans and there was not much that governments could do about it was less than reassuring. She did rightly call for "solidarity, common sense and open-heartedness" but her calls for Europe-wide cooperation could hardly ring true when Germany and France had limited exports of protective masks and equipment to safeguard domestic supply – hardly an act of solidarity with neighbours. Nor was Germany rushing to bail out floundering eurozone partners.

The statistics about the early evolution of cases can be confusing because some countries were slow to test or late to announce results. Italy's first case was at the end of January 2020, but the disease is thought to have been circulating there from the middle of the month. Likewise, the step rise of cases in Iran suggests it was spreading long before the first positive test. Many of the countries that had most success in containing the disease are the ones that had been affected by Sars in 2002–2003. In Hong-Kong, for example, there were strong social and cultural memories of Sars, and people had voluntarily stayed home when they could and used masks and hand sanitisers when they had to go out.[5]

In Singapore there was an early and exhaustive testing regime for anyone with flu-like or pneumonia symptoms where all possible contacts of those infected were tracked. Tests were free and there was a huge public education campaign that urged people even with mild symptoms to see a doctor. The government covered medical bills for suspected or confirmed cases, so there were no financial risks to getting tested. Taiwan brought in checks on travellers from Wuhan at the end of December 2019, after reports of a mystery, pneumonia-like illness. Restrictions on travel from mainland China even when the WHO said they were not necessary also helped. Extensive testing and contact-tracing also prevented the disease from spreading.

It was also that governments could draw upon a history that had been devastating just a few years back as well as cultural practices that made it easier for governments to feel that their suggestions would be respected and acted upon by a population who knew the dangers and had also suffered deaths in recent memories.

As Emma Graham-Harrison reported in *The Observer*, widespread testing in South Korea resulted in very low mortality rates, at the time of reporting, around 7,800 confirmed cases, with resultant deaths at below 1%. The country's most important tool in limiting the numbers of deaths had been its testing system. Testing was nearly ten-fold that in the UK. Many of those tested were members of the Shincheonji religious sect, whose members in Daegu city accounted for more than half of the cases. It showed the importance of spatial locations.

Even though the virus spreads so easily across space, like previous contagions, it can be concentrated in specific areas, which is possibly why in the UK with a concentration in London, other parts of the country could feel under less threat and so not take to heart the advice to socially distance. But they were also quick in South Korea to close schools and recognise that children can pass on the virus without really showing symptoms. As Graham-Harrison noted in the *Observer*: "Emergency childcare in classes of no more than 10 is offered to those who must work. Home working has been encouraged, with subsidies for companies that offer employees the flexibility to manage new care responsibilities" (*The Observer*, 15 March 2020, p. 11).

Notes

1 See the discussion of the Ghetto in Venice in Richard Sennett that tells the story of urban life through bodily experience in *Flesh and Stone: The Body and the City in Western Civilisation* (New York: W.W. Norton & Co. 1996). He shows how Christian ideals of community were challenged as non-Christians and non-Europeans were drawn into the

European orbit. These threatening differences were brutally articulated in the creation of the Jewish ghetto in Venice and the fear of touching that the ghetto exemplified.

2 Evgenia Tognotti is quoted in Peter Beaumont's article in *The Observer*, Sunday 15 March 2020.

3 Head is a global health expert (theguardian.com, Sunday 15 March 2020).

4 The coronavirus pandemic started in Wuhan, home of the leading lab studying the SARS virus and bats. Was that pure coincidence and how does it relate to China's history in bringing contagious diseases under control? Whoever achieves global leadership of the gene-editing industry will accrue great power and wealth. See Jasper Becker *Made in China: Wuhan, Covid and the Quest for Biotech Supremacy* (London: C. Hurst and Co. 2021).

5 For some investigations into the history of SARS in Hong Kong and Mainland China and its impacts, see S.H. Lee *SARS in China and Hong Kong* (Ontario: Nova Biomedical 2006); Jasper Becker *Made in China: Wuhan, Covid and the Quest for Biotech Supremacy* (London: C. Hurst and Co 2021). Becker asks if it was pure coincidence that the Coronavirus pandemic started in Wuhan, home of the leading lab studying the SARS virus. He points out that whoever achieves global leadership in the gene-editing industry stands to harvest great power and wealth while questioning the obsessive secrecy of a centralised political regime.

5

AUTHORITY, TRUST, BODIES, RISK AND CONTAGION

Questioning Authorities and Neo-Liberal Politics

George Monbiot, the eco-activist and writer, reflected that the systems of government in place across the world at the time of the pandemic were completely unsuited to the task of protecting the public from its effects. He drew attention to ruling administrations in the United States, Australia and the UK being guided by a politics of "dismissal and denial of risk," overseeing ecological destruction, the harm caused by an increasingly obese population and deprivation and then, the spread of Covid with the same slackness and lack of urgency (*The Guardian*, 18 March 2020, Journal p. 1).

Monbiot notes that it is unsurprising that these countries produced Covid responses that were "woefully unmatched to the scale of the crisis." He cites the UK government's early flirtation with pursuing "herd immunity" and then the lack of effectiveness of 'track and trace" and a disastrous roll-out of PPE equipment that was wholly inadequate as evidence of this carelessness, resulting in the entirely avoidable loss of so many lives.

Neo-liberal politics that had become the common-sense of many countries across the globe before some turned to more populist and authoritarian leaderships, as Monbiot explained, evolved into becoming an exercise in "public relations… politics is the means by which they are justified and promoted." Prime Minister Margaret Thatcher in the UK and President Ronald Reagan in the US, influenced the world to believe that a politics that led with social responsibility and care was an "interference," alternating between dismissive descriptors such as the "nanny state", "health police" and "elf'n' safety zealots." This led to a culture, in Monbiot's view, of demonising research and modelling as promoting "unfounded fears," "risk aversion" and ultimately resorting to "scaremongering."

DOI: 10.4324/9781003296874-5

As the political discourse shifted against so-called "red tape" and as neoliberal common sense was promoted across the mass media, it seemed that the very idea of government was "a mortal threat to freedom," and furthermore, a hinderance to providing solutions to problems in healthcare and the environment (*The Guardian*, 18 March 2020, p. 2). In so doing, Monbiot argues, this neoliberal agenda was making the case for "shrinking the state" and stemming the funding of public services by attacking and mocking the underlying ideology of the government working to actively protect its people, and in the process "crippling its ability to govern."[1]

This is what Monbiot calls "the pollution paradox": the more detrimental to public interests a company's activities are, the more spending is required to see that "it isn't regulated out of existence." While it is not in anyone's "commercial interest" for Covid to spread, the conditions that have been built to favour them, valuing perception over action, have enabled exactly this. An example Monbiot gives of this hypocrisy at governmental level was the high proportion of Johnson's front-bench ministers having worked at some point for the IEA (Institute of Economic Affairs): an organisation significantly financed by the tobacco industry.

Monbiot traces the recent history of Johnson's party's fortunes, increasingly divided between an older base with traditional and "conservative" values, and its polar opposite, the risk-taking radical right. He speculates that Brexit was an attempt to "bridge the great split" between these factions that had its root in the "rising power of dirty money."

Leaving the European Union permitted a reconciliation between these very different interests. But this has simultaneously meant threatening food standards and environmental controls, as well as price controls on medicines and other crucial regulations. Brexit has also raised barriers to immigration and integration with other nations, all the while using the language of "destiny and exceptionalism" while a real threat of trade impoverishment on the world's stage loomed.[2]

Monbiot acknowledged that though neoliberal common-sense could seem plausible and logically consistent, at times of crisis it creates the worst possible conditions from which to navigate back to stability. The architects of "hands off" government then must reckon with the discrepancy between the theories they place so much faith in, and the dire realities they lead to. He reminds us of Australian Prime Minister Scott Morrison's response to the Australian fires and Boris Johnson's belated engagement with the British floods: as governments that "flounder in the face of this pandemic." Damningly, he concludes that it is an impossible challenge "to govern (knowing only) that government is the enemy" (*The Guardian*, 18 March 2020, p. 2).

Fears, Brutalities and Cultural Memories

These fears are given historical credence by David Edgerton, author of *The Rise and Fall of the British Nation*[3] who reminded in a *Guardian* editorial of a storied history of British responses to crises with "cold calculation" that has led to a governmental belief that only the "cure" for virus could be "worse than the disaster itself."

Writing at the time, he perceives Johnson's team as unsure in their first assessments of how to deal with the virus, moving away from a "mitigation" to a "suppression" of the virus, according to new modelling evidence, which suggested that building up "herd immunity" would result in the overload of hospitals and the deaths of hundreds in a few weeks, as it had done in northern Italy.[4]

It is worrying that Johnson did not fathom the depth of the danger and even if he insisted that he was being led by science, the reality is that it was a political decision to transform everyday life and close down large sections of the economy. As an editorial in *The Guardian* noted, the then-Prime Minister was at odds with a public that "perceived a greater risk to their health than he seemed to assess" (*The Guardian*, 18 March 2020, p. 2).

The editorial noted presciently the landscape had quickly and dramatically changed: with a population facing an uncertain and lengthy lockdown with no end in sight, the government had to rely on the people's goodwill to "self-police" and maintain "discipline" without being made to feel an "infringe(ment) on (their) rights." But as the piece suggests: "individual fortitude, human kindness and local solidarity cannot replace the radical national effort required" to "equalise sacrifice across the population" (p. 2).

But the leader writer also recognised that the analogy with a "wartime situation" only worked so far. "Wartime maximises production. Lockdowns minimise production. The solution is not to dwell on GDP. That will inevitably fall in a shutdown, which requires us to transact less intensely. Instead, we need to focus on social wellbeing and health outcomes" (p. 2).

Edgerton reminded us of the "minimal preparation" made by Neville Chamberlain and Harold Macmillan's administrations when facing the threat of bombings during the Blitz and the Cold War, respectively, using the logic that adequate preparative would unsettle and scare the population (*The Guardian*, 18 March 2020, p. 3). During the Second World War, as Edgerton questions the balance between priorities, rather than pouring resources into bomb shelters, the government funnelled money to produce munitions, and build up the armed forces: a decision that influenced the lacklustre response two decades later when the British were faced with a new and wildly unpredictable threat: the hydrogen bomb.

The pandemic demanded another moment of decisiveness on the matter of whose lives were worth protecting and at what cost. For a time, it was obvious that Johnson was ready to disregard the deaths of the elderly in his search for herd immunity. His ethical values were exposed, and he was forced to change position. The Inquiry was to learn how Johnson was constantly changing his mind. As Matt Fowler co-founder of Covid-19 Bereaved Families for Justice notes:

> Back then we were often criticised for being unfair on the government when we raised our concerns. It's clear now we weren't being anywhere near critical enough. In March 20 when I was panicking over reports coming out of Italy and how best to protect my family if Covid-19 struck the UK, Boris Johnson was

said to be "laughing at the Italians" and joking "we were going to be great (at Covid-19)".

(openDemocracy.net, 3 November 2023)

Edgerton remarked that further into the Cold War, the British government of the 1980s came under fire for the publication of the booklet "Protect and Survive", which advised citizens at a time when nuclear warheads were being amassed by the superpowers, to "(paint) windows to reflect radiation, (stay) at home and (find) the safest place in the house to shelter." As with the Coronavirus, it was home that was to be a place of safety. People's relationships with their homes changed through lockdown. It became a place where adults had to work while children were educated. There were high demands for tradespeople who could help to redesign these spaces.

In the 1980s, the government's advice was ridiculed by the Campaign for Nuclear Disarmament (CND) as a ludicrously inadequate response to the threat of nuclear war. As Edgerton comments: "Yet these criticisms rather missed the point. The pamphlet wasn't a serious response to the nuclear threat, but a public relations exercise in light of the real policy. No shelters would be built" (*The Guardian*, 18 March 2020, p. 3). We might say that the focus on social distancing took attention away from the inadequate supply of ventilators in the NHS and the reality that after years of austerity and decades of underfunding, the NHS had been left unprepared for the crisis to come.

Tracing this history, Edgerton concludes, paints an uncomfortable picture of a state ready to "preside over catastrophic losses of life" rather than "overinvest in expensive (and potentially unnecessary) defences." These decisions were symptomatic of the government's long view: it was taking a gamble in the present, based on a belief about the future. Speculating on how this attitude could manifest in the pandemic response, Edgerton warned: "There is a huge difference between favouring a utilitarian calculus to minimise losses overall and heeding this principle when dead bodies start piling up" (*The Guardian*, 18 March 2020, p. 3).

Fearful Bodies and Traumatic Memories

Saturday 21 March 2020. The sun is shining, and it feels as if everything will be easier as long as the sun shines and we escape the endless greyness that shadowed a week that journalists insisted on calling "unprecedented". Hearing the events of each day rehearsed on BBC Radio 4's *World at One* this week it seemed that in no time at all, we had entered a different moral universe of fear and uncertainty. As I walked along Green Lane in North London towards Brent Park the streets were all but empty but even so, I noticed how I was keeping a "safe distance" from the few people I passed.

This was the Jewish sabbath – Shabbos – and the streets are often empty as groups of people walk to their local synagogues, but this was something else. I was struck as an elderly woman swerved and bent her body to make sure we were far enough apart.

I talked to a middle-class Jewish man who I had met the previous week and he told me their plans to spend a week with family in France had to be cancelled and Mother's Day would have to be on Skype. Somehow, we got talking about ancient history and the shared myths between different religious traditions. He said how the plagues, marked each year in the Passover meal, which was also supposedly Jesus's last supper, reflect different gods in Egypt.

He was disturbed to hear that Turkey's prime minister had resorted to anti-Semitism, blaming the Jews for the virus. Myths that stretch back to the Black Death are being re-worked within the present crisis as people, in their fear and insecurity, look to someone to blame. With the rise of authoritarian populism and nations become increasingly divided and polarised, there *is* a global rise of racism and anti-Semitism. With new technologies and social media, it becomes so much easier to create figures of hate to blame for difficulties in everyday lives.

We talked about the details of self-isolation and how his adult children left food for them on their doorstep. This was a concern that my niece had shared the previous night in a phone conversation – living on her own, who would be there for her if she was to get ill? She wasn't sure that even her sisters would come through for her, as they were self-isolating because of their own underlying health issues, or they had small children. I could feel my own emerging suspicions of others, fearful that they could pose a threat. I realised that I was shaping an ethnography of Covid that focussed on transformations in everyday ethics in a time of crisis and drawing upon auto-ethnography as an embodied methodology.[5]

As I was walking, it reminded me of family narratives, as fearful atmospheres in the present bring back memories of the 1930s and what my parents, as Jewish refugees, lived through. I had not previously felt able to feel the connection. After Hitler came to power in 1933, Germans were told to avoid all contact with their Jewish neighbours who were presented as a source of infection. They had to keep their distance, even if they would acknowledge their presence as they walked past them in the street, at least if others could *not* see them.

Growing up in post-war Britain it was hard for me *to identify* with the fears my parents from Austria had lived with. In my attempts to belong and so become like everyone else, it was easy to accept that these histories belonged to them alone. I might know about them intellectually, but I often found it hard to identify with them emotionally. The fears that were gathering around the isolations of everyday life during a time of Covid somehow brought me to reflect upon the very different *terrors* my family had lived with in the 1930s.

For family members who were in Vienna, Warsaw and Leipzig, there was also the fear of being recognised *as* a Jew when you walked the streets. These fears were intensified, when Jewish people were ordered to wear the yellow star, so they could be identified *at a distance* and contact could be avoided. Anti-Semitism was a political "virus" – as it has sometimes been framed, but not always helpfully – that was threatening the Jewish population in Nazi Germany, then to spread across Europe with the advance of the Nazi troops, often with the collusion of local populations. We all carry our familial legacies, and it can be difficult to anticipate *how* and *when* they might be activated in the present.

These cultural memories of fear were reactivated, in different ways, depending also on migrant and colonising histories, by the anxiety and unease around people the coronavirus virus caused. We couldn't tell whether anyone was transmitting the virus because this happened before any symptoms showed. In the case of young people, symptoms might never reveal themselves. This also helped create an *anxiety of contact* between the generations and a fear on the part of older generations that the young had *not* been taking the dangers seriously as they continue to socialise with each other in bars and clubs, even when they were advised not to visit such spaces. This led the government to give a clear instruction, on Friday 20 March 2020, that all these places where people come together to socialise should be closed.

Generations, Neoliberalism, Fears and Dis/Trust

But there was also a responsibility that the government and parts of the media carried for tending to minimise the dangers that Coronavirus presented to different generations. By initially saying it was *no* worse than the flu and that in most years thousands of people died from the flu anyway, they made it sound as if it was really no big deal and in any case the danger existed for people over 70 with pre-existing health conditions. So, it was hardly surprising that younger generations were slow to realise that not only could they transmit the disease, but they *could suffer* from it directly, sometimes in quite serious and potentially lethal ways.

Everyone needed to take precautions, but that didn't sit easily within the logic of a neoliberal common-sense that had long taught that people should look after themselves and their own achievements and *not* care about others, who also had to look after themselves. If they didn't it was their own fault and only goes to show what losers they are. The government is yet to take responsibility for the early messages that led to the unnecessary deaths of so many people who believed that Covid-19 was no worse than bad flu. The evidence was clearly there in China and then in Italy, but the government did not alert the public in time about the dangers they faced.

So many people were living with anxieties and fears because they didn't know *how* to interpret any symptoms they had and whether they had the virus or not. It is the *unknowing* and *not* being able to find out that was so threatening to people, particularly among the middle-class who are used to having a sense of control over their lives. In the early months people could not assess the threats they faced so they were careful about anything they touched. Food coming into the home was washed because of uncertainties about how the virus spread. People were constantly on their mobiles checking the latest information.

There was so much *uncertainty* not only about health, but also about economic survival and how workers might be able to cope with the schools only open to "vulnerable children" – itself a category that headteachers were often left to interpret. This could leave them as a target for angry parents unsure of how they could keep working. The self-employed, which included many in the gig economy, didn't believe they would get the 80% of their wages the chancellor offered to those who remain employed by companies.

Guardian columnist Frances Ryan reported on the shifts in Johnson's policies since his first instructions to the population. She described his premiership even before the added pressures of the crisis as seeking "power for power's sake," hiding a lack of substance behind "soundbites" and "bluster."

Reporting on protests in March 2020 that preceded the announcement of the national lockdown, she described a masked and hazmat suit-clad crowd outside Downing Street pressuring Johnson and his allies to act. Nationwide, his approval ratings plummeted: Ryan cites the lowly "36 per cent" of the population at that time who trusted Johnson to lead the country through the pandemic: a mistrust clearly shared widely by healthcare experts who were vocal in their doubts about the government's strategy (*The Guardian*, 18 March 2020, p. 5).

As Ryan noted, worried individuals and groups, frustrated with the lack of specific advice, despite the serious tones of the scientists on each side of Johnson at his initial presentation, took things into their own hands mobilising the power of social media. Ryan cites the "Stay the fuck home!" campaign: whose own website criticises: "Slow reactions, public appeasement policies, and their urge to stabilise the economy are keeping them from taking the measures it takes to protect millions from this disease."

Ryan describes social media as fulfilling a vital role, and in many cases, being a force for positive public information, counteracting the "vacuum of clear guidance" and acting as a kind of "digital triage," especially helpful for vulnerable people seeking safety advice on a range of new dilemmas.

The online world was not alone in taking unilateral action and Ryan noted the "remarkable" examples of "communities taking matters into their own hands." Finally responding to public mood following the Downing Street protests, the government acted on mass gatherings. By organising press conferences, the government put ministers in visible positions to accept responsibility for and answer questions about a situation that was changing daily.

The then-chancellor Rishi Sunak, following criticism of initial measures that were judged to do very little to protect workers and incomes, was obliged to go much further to protect workers, even if it still left the self-employed, which accounted for so many in the gig economy, relatively unprotected compared to workers employed in companies. He would be obliged to make further concessions, or he would be seen to be discriminating between different groups.

Ryan recognised the pandemic showed why trust between governments and citizens is important, and it is an irony that the very man who did so much to challenge faith in the UK establishment in recent years now requires it. Concluding her analysis, she highlighted the importance of public trust, and tasked the government "not only to keep the public safe but to convince them that it can. One of those tasks may prove as tricky as the other" (p. 5).

The levels of panic buying across the country, despite the reassurances that the government had given, showed just how little trust there was for the government. People were insisting on stocking up and making sure they had supplies in their homes, anxious about whether they might have to self-isolate for 14 days as advised if someone in their family fell ill.

New technologies offered new ways for people to support each other. A photograph of an elderly woman next to empty shelves in Mill Hill Waitrose in London was shared on a local WhatsApp group. People found out who she was and visited her to make sure she had enough food. Community support broke out across the country. People did not wait for government decisions. They created horizontal lines of trust and support. People were shaping their own ethics of care having given up on the government's advice and anticipating the moral universe they were already living in as they tried to manage their fears. They sought guidance from very different sources on the Internet but who could they trust?[6]

Risks, Anxious Bodies and Everyday Encounters

Sunday 22 March 2020. Life has changed so quickly it can be difficult to find your bearings in a transformed moral world. We are called to make choices that just a few days earlier wouldn't have arisen. What kind of risk was I taking going to Waitrose yesterday? I was careful to keep my distance, but even though the supermarket shelves were empty, that was still *not* easy as other people seemed less concerned. Some were wearing masks and I wondered whether I was showing a *lack* of consideration and should think of wearing one. Was it a matter of protecting yourself against someone coughing over you, or was the virus in the atmosphere – if not, then was there a stage we could reach soon in which it was not safe to leave your home because the virus was in the air?

That morning as I walked to Brent Park, I wondered whether the ducks and the birds resting there had noticed a difference in the atmosphere – whether they had picked up the fear? Initially I was concerned that the two swans that had settled in the park were nowhere to be seen, only to be relieved when I saw them in an unfamiliar stretch of water. Was I taking a risk in going into the newsagent to get *The Observer*? The Indian owner said I should put the money down at some distance from him and said: "I'm scared too." The encounter was charged, and we were both aware of it.

Everyone feels fearful in the uncertainties of the moments when we aren't clear about the *risks* we were taking, not only for ourselves but for others. There is a shift in the economy of risk when getting too close to someone can seem to be a risk we are taking. As I talked to the man in the park – I learnt he's called Alan and he was walking with his Scottish wife – she was constantly warning him to "stand back" – responding to my anxiety while we all acknowledged how natural it is to move forward towards someone, when you are talking and getting absorbed into the conversation – bodies move towards other bodies. But she alerted him of a potential danger.

She said she was coping because she always had a good supply of reserves at home and her children were shopping for her. One of her sons had bad asthma but didn't seem to be withdrawing from contact and was still going to the butchers. We talked about the crowds who had gone to the seaside resorts of Skegness and Brighton the previous day, the first warm spring Saturday, taking unnecessary risks with their lives. One beach in Sussex was to close, while Lincolnshire's police and crime commissioner called for caravan sites and arcades in Skegness to shut down. PCC Marc Jones said there were "hundreds of thousands of visitors." He said it was "time for everyone to be socially responsible or be made to be."

A Skegness dentist Dr Mitchell Clark, who had voluntarily shut his practice the previous week, said many local businesses were "acting like nothing is happening". In a video posted on Facebook he said: "I was appalled to see, as I drove home, Skegness looking like it does on a busy summer day. I view these actions as massively, massively socially irresponsible and I personally think those involved should be ashamed of themselves." He added: "We are a small town. We have a cottage hospital supported by two main district hospitals and this is a disaster waiting to happen" (BBC News, Saturday 21 March 2020).

But people might have felt that this was a risk worth taking – to enjoy time in the sunshine before everything closed down. They might have felt that they faced – at least at the moment – a very different level of threat than we were facing in London where people we knew were critically ill in hospital. The early government responses that minimised the condition and said it was "like a bad flu" and later warnings that stressed that it affected people in their 70s and over with underlying health conditions, shaped a difference in anticipation between generations. Young people failed to register the seriousness of the risks they faced. They had not really taken in that young people, even children, had suffered badly from the condition, even if relatively few had died.

I was unsure whether you could get the virus only if someone coughed on you or whether it was carried in the air. There was so much confusion around. She said the danger was because you don't know *if* people are carrying the virus – and it was before the symptoms showed or in the early days of symptoms that they could pass it on. This seemed to mean you were taking a risk whenever you walked the streets or in a park. You could sense in your contact with people how fears were spreading.

We were warned to stay three or four metres away from anyone we might talk to. The evidence from China also showed that people were not only wearing masks, also as a sign of respect to others, they were changing their clothes when they came indoors so keeping their outdoor clothes separate. The Chinese experience showed the dangers of people leaving home or people coming into your home who might be well but still be a transmitter of the virus. It was advised that deliveries of food and other parcels be left at the door. But essential workers, people who could not work from home, faced very different risks. It was to take time to fully recognise these structural inequalities in risks of illness and death.

We were not only taking risks for ourselves, if we were in contact with the virus, we were possibly endangering the lives of others – most specifically elderly relatives. There was a *shift* in the moral landscape. This challenged at a philosophical level the common-sense ethics of a neoliberal culture that had taught us to focus upon ourselves and our individual responsibilities and let others look after themselves. That culture had systematically undermined an ethics of care, altruism and compassion.[7]

We had learnt to be sceptical about the "nanny state" and its overreaching itself in creating forms of dependency, as Margaret Thatcher insisted. We had learnt to take for granted an enterprise culture in which individuals are locked into competitive relationships with each other over scarce resources. The grip of this common-sense was graphically evident in the panic buying and conflict between customers in supermarkets. Across the country, people in a state of fear grabbed what they could, unknowing of what the future might bring and what they could anticipate with any trust.

Global Fears, Multiple Deaths and Failed Responses

Writing at the "disastrous" start of the pandemic, Gordon Brown, the former Labour Prime Minister, warned of countries needlessly "retreating into their national silos" and "fighting their own individual battles" against the virus (*The Guardian*, 14 March 2020, Journal p. 1).

He asked tellingly: why, as the disease engulfs more than 100 countries, there has been no consistent, coordinated global approach not just in tracking, testing and travel but to openly learning from each other about the relative merits of quarantine and social distancing? He lamented the reluctance of institutions with the power to minimise the likelihood of global recession to work together.

It said something about the quality of global leadership and the impact of rising nationalisms and authoritarian populist politics across the world that, as Brown describes a "divided, leaderless world": listing the "cover up in Wuhan" followed by "delayed reporting" on the part of Chinese officials, to a subdued response from the WHO that resulted in chaos at a global level.

Brown criticised the sluggishness with which governments "absorb(ed) hard-earned lessons… from the Sars epidemic and Ebola epidemic to the financial meltdown," pointing out: "…global problems need global, not just local and national, responses", and advocated instead the kind of boldness that delivered the New Deal in response to the Great Depression.

Reporting on the state of global health at the beginning of the pandemic, a *Guardian* editorial identified a worrying trend. It noted the "low numbers in places that it could devastate" not as a cause for optimism that these areas were faring better than expected, but revealing that they were "least equipped to monitor its spread." The piece cites Afghanistan as a prime example: the country reported "22 cases" because it only had the capability to diagnose that number: not because this reflected the true number of cases.

The piece noted the devastating effect of existing poor health and living conditions on a person's susceptibility to Covid. Putting it starkly, it notes that "'Wash your hands' is great advice, but of limited use to the two-fifths of the world's population who lack access to soap and clean water at home" (*The Guardian*, 18 March 2020, Journal p. 2).

The editorial draws on Laura Spinner's *Pale Rider* about the Spanish flu pandemic of 1918, which caused the deaths of between 50 million and 100 million people. Between 13 to 15 million of those may have been from India alone. People in parts of Asia – before economic development in many countries – were 30 times more likely to die than those in parts of Europe.

Leadership and quick reactions still make a difference and as Elizabeth Hilton reported on "The World this Weekend", BBC Radio 4 Sunday 22 March 2020, with China reassured that its decisive actions had led it through the worst of the crisis, they were regretting that liberal democracies in Europe did not heed their advice and were suffering disastrous consequences for not acting earlier and more firmly. The authoritarian Chinese government saw this as proof of the superiority of their system. They also offered their expertise to the rest of the world that could benefit hard-pressed countries in the global South.

The Guardian editorial recognised the potential impact of those whose lives had already been derailed by war and conflict: displaced people and refugees already living in conditions unimaginable to the vast majority of people. It repeated the warnings from Jan Egeland of the Norwegian Refugee Council of the "carnage" likely to be felt in countries such as Syria, Yemen and Venezuela with "collapsed" healthcare systems (p. 2).

It was not only the WHO trying to help but also individuals. Jack Ma, the Chinese billionaire founder of Alibaba, donated test kits, masks and protective suits for medics to each African country. The charitable foundation of Michael Bloomberg – a Democrat presidential contender before he withdrew – said it would fund a $40m global initiative to prevent the virus's spread in low and middle-income countries, especially in Africa. This was hardly going to be enough to deal with the health catastrophes that were to come. But it might provoke governments into co-operating in a global response that would be so critical.[8]

Shifting Priorities and Failing Authorities in a Health Emergency

I first doubted the policy Johnson's government was following through reading Tony Yates, a former professor of economics at Birmingham University who questioned why the UK took such a radically different approach to lockdown measures from other countries. He questioned why the UK "eschewed social distancing measures… (opting) for behavioural 'nudges'," such as handwashing, and staying at home (*The Guardian*, 14 March 2020, p. 5).

Yates cited the chief scientific advisor Patrick Vallance's move towards "herd immunity": allowing people least likely to succumb to the virus maximum exposure to it. This is influenced by the nudge theory of American economist Richard Thaler and American legal scholar Cass Sunstein: encouraging behavioural changes by "coaxing and positive assertion... tweak(ing) the environment in which we make choices."

First introduced by David Cameron (when he was prime minister) and led by the British civil servant David Halpern (chief executive officer of the Behavioural Insights Team) the nudge unit was playing its part in shaping government policy. Yates explained that key to its success was to avoid "fatigue" setting in: instead, choosing to "reserve these measures for when we are closer to peak of the epidemic" (p. 5). The responses to the initial lockdown showed the weakness of this theory and the willingness of people to comply, a least initially, as long as they understood the logic of the demands.

This was still a neoliberal vision of human behaviour and the individual moral responsibilities people had for their lives. Yates speculates that at the "heart" of this thinking are "predictions about human behaviour based on analysing past episodes," which, as he points out, is deeply flawed. The government thought it was protecting the economy as much as it could and that its approach to the virus was well-structured and carefully planned as we would move from stage to stage.[9]

This assumed that they had control over the virus which they could not have. The UK government failed to learn about the dangers the virus presented, already evident in China and closer to home in Italy. Ultimately, the practice of 'nudge theory' promoted an uneasy division of labour that allowed the scientists to advise about the science, while the politicians did their best to ensure that the economy would not be restricted until it became necessary.

Within days, partly through the actions of the football authorities and others taking decisions into their own hands, the stages that government had set out were radically shortened. The UK became more in line with other countries and the question will no doubt be raised whether we were in fact *too slow* in closing schools knowing that children could still carry the virus and transfer it to others, even if they didn't have symptoms themselves.

The scientists proved more divided on the advice than Johnson was prepared to recognise, using the authority of science in order to legitimise the policies he was following. He presented them as sharing a singular approach, even when other countries were doing things quite differently and with much greater awareness of the dangers that people were facing. He refused to acknowledge disagreements by talking about "the best scientific advice."

The Covid Inquiry shows that the scientific advisers were being used by the government, and possibly they should have resigned. Devi Sridhar, chair of global public health at Edinburgh recalls, "I told Chris Whitty at the time that scientists were proving cover for weak leaders taking harmful decisions." She notes, "What's now clear is that Whitty and Valance were observers in a totally dysfunctional system…none of their concerns were publicly articulated" (theguardian.com, Friday 3 November 2023). Within days policies were to shift, and a different approach was taken, but this did not help the trust that people had in his government. This was further demonstrated in high levels of panic buying emptying supermarket shelves across the country.

Making Connections and Everyday Ethics

Monday 23 March. Yesterday was Mother's Day and we met for the first time as a family on Zoom and cards and gifts were offered online. At least Anna was informed that flowers were on the way because of the difficulties of logistics these days. Together we watched Johnson's daily presentation from Downing Street. It felt like a family gathering around the radio to hear the latest news about the crisis. There were some sharp questions, you were left thinking the government was making it up as they were going along. They were trying to cover their tracks by saying they *were* following scientific advice, when people had learnt how divided that could be. There was considerable pressure that the government should give clearer instructions because so many people seemed still to be ignoring the advice.

Johnson was asked at the televised press conference *how* he could expect five-year olds to maintain social distance in a playground when playing with their friends? Would it be better to close parks like other countries had done? There were no clear answers. People were increasingly aware of the very different structural situations they were in in relation to their work, everyday lives, and relationships.

They could *not* anticipate the different dangers they faced; especially emergency workers *obliged* to continue working whatever the risks. There was a widespread anxiety whether the "shielding" offered to older people with underlying health conditions would actually work on the ground. Would people volunteer in the numbers needed, given the clear instruction that people should not leave their houses.

We all felt grateful that we had an alternative means of communication. These were opportunities that people were discovering all over the world. They discovered new ways of being together while being apart. But this could also work to emphasise the distances people felt, especially if they were obliged to isolate with people they did not want to be with and were separated from family and friends at the same time.

It was as if futures had suddenly disappeared. We have been so identified with a need *to* control as a mark of achievement within a neoliberal culture that it was going to be hard to fully acknowledge that life could *no* longer be controlled. If we could surrender more fully to the present moment, could we possibly learn to place more trust in our inner relationship with ourselves?

These are thoughts a neoliberal common-sense can find *hard* to accept. So often it shapes an erasure of connections with a sense of inner life that has often been reduced to questions of individual choices within a consumerist world. Within post-structuralist theoretical traditions, we have also learnt to discount *and* devalue relationships with self, too often presented as an effect of discursive practices and so of an internalisation of social codes and cultural norms.

Often it is through knowing that we *can* learn to control our lives that we learn, across boundaries of gender, "race" and ethnicities within middle class worlds, that we are independent and autonomous moral selves. Within a neoliberal common sense this means it is not going to be easy to accept that we cannot know what the future might bring, or how long the virus will last as we are enclosed at home. With schools closing, gender divisions of labour were often reinforced as women took on more responsibilities for their children's education, often without the necessary laptops and with many schools unequipped to give the support they would need to provide for their pupils stuck at home.

Established routines of everyday life were *transformed*, almost overnight, with lockdowns. People could not think of going to see a movie or to the theatre. They could not order their lives in familiar ways they had relied upon. Regular sources of support and relationships were suddenly withdrawn as people who could, mostly the middle classes, were obliged to work from home. People felt bereft of regular contact and had little sense of how reliant they could be on their contacts at work and in the community for their wellbeing and mental health.

It was a state of *not knowing* what lay ahead – for weeks, months and even years. Control over work lives was in doubt. Suddenly, many people were without the money they relied upon to feed their children and pay their bills. Unemployment loomed for many and at this early stage of lockdown it was still unclear what financial support the government might offer and to whom. People across the country felt unnerved about what the future held for them. Too much in their lives was rendered uncertain too quickly which meant they did not know what they could anticipate.

With the growth of mindfulness practices, often encouraged by corporate logics to help people become more adaptive to the efficiency and productivity newly expected of them, people were encouraged to use these practices to deal with the pressures of lockdown. In this way they were learning to internalise responsibility, learning to blame themselves for not coping rather than the punitive demands of the corporations.

But at another level, an awareness of ourselves as vulnerable humans, more able to *name* everyday stresses and to communicate the need to take time out, could be helpful in unanticipated lockdowns at home. Those people who could work from home could feel more in control of their work. At work they might be working in settings where the rules of the game were still established by dominant white generational masculinities. Learning to take time for yourself could help support a critical consciousness, even if this was still framed in largely liberal individualistic terms. It could be supported through developing more of an inner relationship.

Taking Time and Reconnecting with Nature

Across genders questioning ethics as a matter of individual choice could still help break with the rigidity that often comes from an ethics of control as assertions of autonomy and independence. It can also be helpful in different occupational structures to be more fluid in our response to events while maintaining a sense of being grounded in ourselves. This can help in times of pandemic crisis so that we do *not* feel that we are reacting out of fear but are somehow sustaining a deeper connection with ourselves. Mindfulness teachings can be somewhat abstracted, especially when they are separated from their sources within Buddhist tradition, but they *can* still be helpful in navigating *an* uncertain and stressful lockdown.

People also discovered in a time of lockdown a renewed relationship with the natural world and a sense that life *can* be lived at a slower pace, more attuned to their bodily rhythms. Spaces of meditation could also be helpful to take in a different relationship to the world, teaching about gaining equanimity and a grounded sense of self. Rather than grabbing for knowledge that could give us a sense of control in fearful times, mindfulness suggests that we *accept* a sense of unknowing that could potentially bring a sense of inner peace and feelings of compassion to help others in greater need. We need to be in the world, rather than seeking to escape from it, able to respond to the sufferings and the deaths as they are announced with care and empathy.

A friend Terry Cooper, a formative psychotherapist, wrote about *Bird Song: The day the world stopped* – this is part of what he shared. It is an honest reflection of someone with some leisure to enjoy the pause:

> A wonderful gift of the pandemic was bird song: clear, vibrant and reassuringly confident they sang. Within the stillness, peace and quiet of a society slowing down, noise pollution was absent with no planes soaring across the skies leaving vapor scars. People began to say: 'Have you heard the birdsong?' And many of us had… It was a strange kind of freedom, beautiful but with dark edges of threat and fear of what might happen…It was a gift of relief for many people and for others stress, depression, helplessness and anger…
>
> The gift of this time was time itself…What a relief it was when the world paused and rested. People were aware of each other; they would keep their distance, some seeking connection and others fearful and avoiding it…We were together, managing overwhelm and uncertainty…Adversity can be a formative experience if we chose it to be, a challenge to growth rather than an obstacle to growth, a problem to be lived rather than just a problem to be solved…will we adapt back to the fast forward, over adrenalised, over charged competitive

world of productivity and continue with the same expectations of growth and wealth as before? What have we learned? Will we take something new from this pause? Will we shape something different and re-form our life at a personal level?

Keep the bird song and let it live in you. Remember it…"

(June 2021)

In a time of global pandemic, people felt tense anxious and insecure about their lives. Many felt they *no longer* could call on the support of their everyday relationships. We needed to shape new psychosocial theories and research methodologies to understand the nature of the crisis that so many people were going through. There was a deep and developing crisis in mental health, which was stretching across generations. Many people turned to psychotherapies and counselling online. This was often directly related to a crisis in their material circumstances. Suddenly families were obliged, often for the first time, to rely upon food banks. Desperation could connect them to unresolved deeper emotional issues, that they were barely aware of, but they needed help with. Possibly for the first time, they were risking asking for help.

With a fracturing of everyday work lives and relationships, people had become newly aware of *how* they depended on everyday routines to sustain a sense of personal value and integrity. A time of crisis can also make people question how they are haunted by a sense of lack – a sense that they could constantly do more, achieve more, be more than they were. In contrast, therapists can encourage a sense of self-acceptance *as* self-worth and a realisation that we should not withhold – hold ourselves back. Too often within a neoliberal common-sense we learn to think we have to keep our love and empathy for others, as scarce commodities, in reserve for other times.

Rather in a renewed *ethic of care* we can question why we cannot fully give ourselves in the present, but we are trapped into thinking, especially as men, that we need to be impartial and objective in reserving ourselves for a future that never really comes. We often hold ourselves back rather than committing whole heartedly to our relationships in the present. An awareness of a feminist ethic of care helped to provide an orientation in fearful times, when so many people felt a need to reach out to others, to escape the loneliness and isolation of lockdowns.[10]

In a time of crisis, when so much in our lives can *feel threatened* and the future uncertain, it can help us to live in the now in the fullest way we can, able to give love and support to others in a time of enormous need. Uncertain what a future might bring and questioning *how* time has been commodified as a scarce resource that has to be carefully curated, it can be difficult to live in the present as much as we can and not live for a future that might never come. This is a lesson with a particular relevance in a time of the plague when we cannot know who will come down with it and what awaits us.

Reflecting on a dream in the early days of lockdown, I discovered like many others that I seemed to be dreaming more deeply. Many people seemed to report this as part of a new balance between their waking lives and their sleep lives. Some people also complained about an inability to sleep, as if they could not escape the wakefulness of their everyday lives. They were too mentally alert, and their minds would be haunted by their anxieties.

In one dream I found myself in a philosophy conference with some people I knew. I felt at ease even though the famously intense philosopher Wittgenstein was there. Somehow, I got to talk to him. He was willing to listen, particularly about what could be learnt from psychotherapies, to engage with emotional lives and everyday ethics. In this way philosophy and sociology could hope to learn from each other and deepen their interrelationship.

I asked whether he knew of Etty Hillesum, the Dutch-Jewish woman who was murdered in Auschwitz, and he was interested in learning about her. I also mentioned Rowan Williams, the former Archbishop of Canterbury, and whether he knew his writings, but he didn't seem to know. I felt affirmed in the contact and somehow, through the dream, I was gaining a sense of the limits of his work in engaging moral and political experiences and conflicts in the present.

But he was willing to learn and saw the initial steps he had made in *engaging* with everyday life and relationships as part of framing philosophy as *a way of living*. This went beyond the Ancient Greek quest, too often framed in individual terms, of learning *how* to live and die well. He seemed open to the importance of transforming societies and cultures and was attuned to the dignity of manual labour, something the Greeks lacked. I then woke up, surprised, but also with a sense that something had shifted internally.

When he stressed that it was important for people *to change* the ways they were living and relating, he did *not* mean to suggest that philosophical problems would disappear, as some have interpreted his work. Philosophy *as* therapy implies the need to transform everyday lives and relationships. If the anxieties produced through a neoliberal capitalist society are *not* to continue haunting us as a pervasive sense of inadequacy, we need to imagine different visions of ourselves as ethical and vulnerable humans.

Vulnerable Humans, Crisis and Ethical Imaginations

In a time of global pandemic and under conditions of lockdown, we can *pause* and take stock and reflect upon *how* social worlds and relationships between rich and poor not only in the UK and across Europe, but between the Global North and the Global South need to be transformed. Possibly it's because of the disturbance to everyday routines and practices that philosophical questions *can* unexpectedly emerge in our dreams. Suddenly and unexpectedly, in uncertain and fearful times, we might want to think, live and act differently across the planet threatened by a deadly pandemic at a time of global climate emergency.

State and corporate power needs to be held accountable for global injustice and economic inequalities. We need to understand *how* the conditions that enabled the Covid-19 pandemic to spread globally were also produced through a European modernity shaped through a dominant white colonising masculinity that has identified progress with the control and domination of nature. It has worked to disconnect us from the natural world that is too easily treated as a resource that needs to be extracted and exploited, along with those peoples colonised by their European masters. This is why new ecological imaginations have to go hand in hand with the decolonising of the disciplines.

The pandemic allowed us to think anew and *re-vision* our existence as vulnerable humans who are part of the natural world. It also helps us shape new ethical imaginations of what the world could be. If it is to live up to the democratic ideals of liberty, equality, and social justice these need to become everyday lived realities. We need to encourage global institutions that can help shape a global ethic that is realised in the transformation of relationships between the global North and Global South in a time of climate emergency.

As I walked in Brent Park, which had become my refuge, after my dream I realised that "outside" had suddenly become a strangely hostile environment. Boris Johnson and the London Mayor, Sadiq Kahn, had now warned not to leave home *unless* it was necessary. Though the streets and the park were mainly empty, I was looking out for people in advance and measuring my pace. Each person was read as a potential danger, and we took care that we did not get too close – that two metres existed between us. Each person we passed could seem like a potential transmitter of the virus, in ways that I hadn't felt just days previously.

I noticed a bodily fear as I approached an alleyway that connects to the street where we live. I realised that if someone was coming in the other direction, I could *not* avoid them and keep the necessary distance. I saw a woman just coming out, but I took the risk of walking along it, but I was not without fear. I thought I should not take this alleyway again, since I could not know if I would not meet another person coming in the opposite direction. So it is that we are all having to learn *to navigate* through space and time in different ways as we deal with new landscapes of fear. We are suddenly living in a new economy of risk that has suddenly shaped our everyday lives and relationships.

Notes

1 Investigations into the formation and growth of neoliberal governmentality and the common-sense that it helps to form across different societies are given in, David Harvey *A Brief History of Neoliberalism* (New York: OUP 2007); James Donald and Stuart Hall *Politics and Ideology* (Milton Keynes: Open University Press 1985); Stuart Hall *The Hard Road to Renewal: Thatcherism and the Crisis of the Left* (London: Verso 2021); Wendy Brown *Undoing the Demos: Neoliberalism's Stealth Revolution* (New York: Zone Books 2017); Naomi Klein *The Rise of Disaster Capitalism* (London: Penguin 2008); Gary Gerstle *The Rise and Fall of the Neoliberal Order: America and the World in the Free Market* (New York: OUP USA 2022); Wendy Brown *In the Ruins of Neoliberalism: The Rise of Antidemocratic Politics in the West* (New York: Columbia University Press 2019); Noam Chomsky *The Precipice: Neoliberalism, the Pandemic and the Urgent Need for Radical Change* (London: Penguin 2021).

2 For an exploration of issues around the Brexit Referendum and what followed see Victor J. Seidler *Making Sense of Brexit: Democracy, Europe and Uncertain Futures* (Bristol: Policy Press 2018) and Fintan O'Toole *Heroic Failure: Brexit and the Politics of Pain* (New York: Apollo Publishers 2018) and *Three Years in Hell: The Brexit Chronicles* (New York: Apollo Publishers 2021). See also Nigel Culkin and Richard Simmons *Tales of Brexits Past and Present: Understanding the Choices, Threats and Opportunities in Our Separation from the EU* (Leeds: Emerald Publishing Ltd 2018).

3 David Edgerton *The Rise and Fall of the British Nation* (London: Penguin 2019).

4 Some reflections upon the nature of herd immunity as an initial response to the Coronavirus pandemic and the arguments between those who supported it and the speed with which the government disavowed it ever followed it, are offered in, Deborah MacKenzie *COVID-19: The Pandemic that Never Should have Happened and how to stop the Next One* (London: The Bridge Street Press 2020). She argues that it is the interaction between disease and people that matters and observes that nearly everything about its origins and spread offers lessons on how *not* to act when the next pandemic comes. She recognises that unless we repair our injured planet and address the linked issues of globalisation and the disruption of animal habitats and cautions that "hindsight helps you win the next battle, not the last one". See also the evaluation in Richard Horton *The COVID-19 Catastrophe: What's Gone Wrong and How to Stop it Happening Again* (Cambridge: Polity 2021).

5 For some reflections on autoethnography as a method see for example, Carolyn Ellis *Revision: Autoethnographic Reflections on Life and Work* (New York: Routledge 2020); Heewon Chang *Autoethnography as Method* (London: Routledge 2008); Arthur Bochner *Evocative Autoethnograpy: Writing Lives and Telling Stories* (London: Routledge 2016); Tessa Muncey *Creating Autoethnographies* (London: Sage 2010); Robin Boylon and Mark Orbe (eds) *Critical Autoethnography: Intersecting Cultural Identities in Everyday Life* (London: Routledge 2021) and Elizabeth Ettorre *Autoethnography as Feminist Method: Sensitising the feminist 'I'* (London: Routledge 2016).

6 For reflections on how social media has affected ways that people responded to the Covid-19 pandemic see, Pamela Zeiser and Berrin Beasley (eds) *Social Media Ethics and Covid-19: Well-Being, Truth, Misinformation and Authenticity* (Lanham, Maryland, USA: Lexington Books 2022). They explore how the pandemic changed our relationship with social media both for the better and for the worse. They are concerned with the ethical responsibilities of social media engagement in an era of disinformation and misinformation. Social media creates opportunities to keep people safe, informed and connected. However, the same tools also enable and amplify the current infodemic that continues to undermine the global responses and jeopardizes measures to control the pandemic.

7 Reflections on how a neoliberal capitalist culture has helped to shape an individualistic ethic that has served to undermine an ethics of care, see for instance, Victor Jeleniewski Seidler *Ethical Humans: Life, Love, Labour, Learning and Loss* (London and New York: Routledge 2022); David M. Kotz *The Rise and Fall of Neoliberal Capitalism* (Cambridge: Mass: Harvard University Press 2015); Peter Bloom *The Ethics of Neoliberalism: The Business of Making Capitalism Moral* (London and New York: Routledge 2019) and Caitlin Janzen (ed) *Unravelling Encounters: Ethics, Knowledge, and Resistance under Neoliberalism* (Waterloo, Canada: Wilfrid Laurier University Press 2015).

8 A book that challenges us to consider the global impact of the Covid-19 pandemic and how unprepared the world was, disrupting the world economy, international relations and the everyday lives of people across the planet, is Adam Tooze *Shutdown: How Covid Shook the World's Economy* (New York: Viking 2021). He explores global change and the pandemic. He argues that the crisis the virus unleashed began much earlier as the product of a much longer process of neoliberal mismanagement and selfishness.

9 For some helpful introductions to neoliberal capitalism and how it fosters a common-sense that different generations have learnt to take for granted, see David Harvey *A Brief*

History of Neoliberalism (Oxford: Oxford University Press 2007); Colin Crouch *The Strange Non-Death of Neoliberalism* (Cambridge: Polity 2011); William Davies *The Limits of Neoliberalism: Authority, Sovereignty and the Logic of Competition* (London: Sage Publications Ltd 2016); Wendy Brown *Undoing the Demos: Neoliberalism's Stealth Revolution* (New York: Zone Books 2017) and *In the Ruins of Neoliberalism: The Rise of Antidemocratic Politics in the West* (New York: Columbia University Press 2019).

10 To engage with a feminist ethics of care see, for example, Virginia Held (ed) *Justice and Care: Essential Readings in Feminist Ethics* (Boulder, Colorado: Westview Press 1995); Grace Clement *Care, Autonomy, and Justice: Feminism and the Ethic of Care* (Boulder, Colorado: Westview Press 1996); Mary Jeanne Larrabbee ed *An Ethic of Care: Feminist and Interdisciplinary Perspectives* (New York: Routledge 1993); Selma Sevenhuijsen *Citizenship and the Ethics of Care: Feminist Considerations on Justice, Morality and Politics* (London: Routledge 1998) and The Care Collective (ed.) *The Care Manifesto: The Politics of Interdependence* (London: Verso 2020) that demands that we put care at the heart of the state and the economy while questioning why we live in a world that rewards uncaring, the care-free and the care-less. It calls for an economy and society based on caring for the earth and each other.

6

HEALTH CRISIS, ECONOMIC CRISIS AND POLITICAL CRISIS

A Global Pandemic, Fractured Societies and Shifting Policies

The nature and intensity of the health crisis facing the UK was slowly to dawn. The speed with which it was to accelerate was alarming. The *Evening Standard* of 27 February 2020 pictured a woman wearing a mask with her head down, on its front page, saying in small print: "Masked city: one commuter on the tube today as the mayor prepared to call a crisis summit in London." The paper reported: "Fears of a Coronavirus pandemic hitting Britain grew today." At that point, the Italian government had just sealed off 12 towns in Lombardy with the number of cases officially put at 400 the previous night, an increase of 80 on the day before, with 12 deaths.

But what was telling was the paper also reported much worse news from Professor Neil Ferguson, director of the Centre for Global Infectious Disease Analysis at Imperial College London. Ferguson, who was to play a vital role in shifting government policy away from the initial advice that Prime Minister Boris Johnson's government had delivered, told BBC Radio 4's "Today" Programme that there were "definitely thousands" of cases in Northern Italy. He said: "The great majority of cases for this virus we think have quite mild disease and they are not being detected."

He was already arguing to "minimise social contact" if there was an outbreak in the UK and insisting: "What's been clear is that there has been transmission in Italy ongoing and not detected for at least three weeks and probably more like a month. Behind each one of those deaths lies about a thousand cases" (*Evening Standard*, 27 February 2020, p. 4).

He added that the scale of the disease meant it could not be contained by "chasing cases and isolating them", but that only "large scale community measures", as

DOI: 10.4324/9781003296874-6

happened in China, Hong Kong, and Singapore, could reduce transmission. Containment measures could buy time to push an outbreak's peak into the summer rather than the spring or the autumn. But Ferguson's colleague at Imperial, Professor Barbara Ward, told presenter Sarah Montague on Radio 4's "World at One" on Monday 23 March that the government's advice was failing and that many people were going to the parks and disregarding the two-metre social distance they had been advised to keep.[1]

Ward noted that unless restrictions were enforced by the authorities the virus was bound to spread. Hospitals were already finding it difficult to deal with the number of Coronavirus patients. There was a health emergency that was already in the making and government had to lock down so that only people from essential services were allowed to travel. People should be instructed to stay at home otherwise we would be sure to follow in Italy's footsteps. She recognised that people were assuming that they had responsibility for themselves so that it was up to them what risks they took.

But as Ward urged, we needed to shape a different moral culture and convince people in a health emergency, as part of an ethics of care, that they had responsibilities for others who would be endangered if the social distancing measures were not adhered to.

In the *Evening Standard* on Thursday 27 February, it was reported that in the US there was still a culture of denial being fostered by President Donald Trump who had put vice-president Mike Pence in charge of America's Coronavirus response. Insisting the risk remained "very low". Trump defended his handling of the crisis after being criticised for earlier lashing out at the media, accusing them of presenting the virus as a worst-case scenario.

It was still early days, but it seemed that European countries were slow to learn the lessons of the outbreak in China. On 27 February it was reported that French President Emmanuel Macron had visited a hospital in Paris treating Coronavirus patients. At that time, two people had died from the virus in France, a 60-year-old French man and an 80-year-old Chinese tourist. But as the virus was to take hold it was to develop exponentially creating a health crisis that was unprecedented for a century.

By Tuesday 17 March the UK had been obliged to shift policy mainly because of the modelling that Ferguson had reported on at Imperial College. This forced a gear change in response, though many still insisted that Johnson's government, even when it changed policies, was not taking drastic action quickly enough. At his press conference the day before, he had been obliged to shift saying the country was now "approaching the fast growth part of the upward curve" with London in the vanguard. Deaths in the UK had risen from 35 to 55 with half of the diagnosed cases in the capital. He announced stringent steps including 14 days of self-isolation for a household if anyone displayed symptoms of the disease and that everyone should work from home who could.

As Johnson said, trying to give the appearance of a carefully planned process when it was evident to all that they had been obliged to rapidly change policy:

"Now is the time for everyone to stop non-essential contact with others and to stop all unnecessary travel. You should avoid pubs, clubs, theatres and other such social venues" (*The Guardian*, 17 March 2020, p. 1).

Even though the World Health Organization's director-general Tedros Adhanom Ghebreyesus urged governments to continue tracking cases of the virus, saying "test, test, test" following the successful paths of South Korea and Singapore, the UK continued with its policy not to test suspected sufferers unless they were in hospital, even front-line health workers. This was a policy that was consistently challenged. Johnson would constantly use the phrase "following the science" when its evident that scientists across the world, including the WHO, would not reach the same conclusion. By standing alongside in daily press briefings, Valance and Whitty gave credibility and seemed aligned with the policies and direction the country was taking.

Though the government talked of scaling up testing, this was not made available to people suffering symptoms at home who were left anxious and unsure of whether they had Coronavirus. On the same day as people were advised to avoid pubs and clubs, the chief scientific advisor, Sir Patrick Vallance, said the course of Covid-19 in the UK was about three weeks behind Italy, which had seen more than 1,800 deaths.

If the government had stuck to its original plans announced only the previous week, it could have cost 260,000 lives, according to the modelling done at Imperial. Ferguson's group ran computer predictions of the impact of different interventions. The later ones took in data from the Italian outbreak that had seen a higher proportion of infected people needing ventilators – 30% needed intensive care.

Calling the original policy Scenario One – the "mitigation strategy" which allowed people to mix as usual but taking precautions to wash their hands – they modelled Scenario Two, which they called "suppression" believing that if followed intensively, it could bring the number of deaths down to 20,000 or even lower.

But Ferguson also acknowledged that they expected that on the cessation of these measures, transmission would pick up, with little herd immunity having been built up in the meantime: a strategy that the UK government thought of pursuing in the initial stages of the pandemic.

Though medical experts had advised that anything short of a lockdown as they had in Italy could leave the UK in a dangerous situation with many deaths and a National Health Service that was overwhelmed, Johnson as a libertarian Conservative was reluctant to use the force of law. He recognised that many people would think "that there is something excessive about these measures" which he himself described as "draconian" before he actually ordered the closure of pubs, theatres, bars and cinemas the following week.

Even then, it seemed many people were ignoring the advice offered and were continuing to congregate in parks and playgrounds. People well under 70 assessed for themselves the risks they might be taking as over 70 was the age repeatedly mentioned as a risk factor.

As Jonathan Freedland noted, in *The Guardian*, this shift of policy was a critical moment for Boris Johnson. By 16 March the strength of Johnson's leadership was in doubt. Freedland noted that during a press conference that day, the former Prime Minister appeared "anxious, if not overwhelmed," suggesting that he had not fully grasped the seriousness of the situation. Freeland described the chaos of the early pandemic, the "tangled messaging," and the choices made by the UK that were so out of kilter with countries further along in the contagion. For Freedland, in spite of the "gaps and contradictions" in Johnson's message, his appearances did "enough" to disarm most critics: for the moment, despite the hesitancy of a speech peppered with "should" rather than "must" (*The Guardian*, 16 March 2020, p. 3).

Freedland noted that this hesitancy extended to Johnson's responses to the questions posed by journalists. Answering for his reluctance to embrace bolder strategies, he peevishly responded: "We're a mature, grown-up liberal democracy." He stepped back on issues including schools remaining open and the question of continuous testing, allowing the experts, perhaps wisely, to take the lead. Freedland noted how his "brand" of "cheery optimism" rang hollow in front of a population unconvinced by him, and whether he was "serious enough for the task" (p. 3).

What had changed the situation and made it potentially riskier and graver, and led the prime minister to confine most of the population to their homes, was new data on the impact of Italy's out-of-control epidemic on its health sector. Ferguson's truly shocking figure of 260,000 deaths would not just be deaths from the virus, but also from other illnesses that the NHS would be too hard-pressed to treat. With his colleague Professor Azra Ghani, they likened the new measures to China's approach, which had succeeded in driving down the epidemic to very low numbers.

But as journalist Sarah Boseley reported in *The Guardian* (17 March 2020): "Unlike China, anything that happens in the UK will be voluntary. The government will need population buy-in for this to work." This was proving more difficult than expected, especially given the early messages that the virus was really no different from the flu. People had adopted a certain attitude, encouraged by the media at the time, so it was going to be difficult to change a view that had already been established for many people not directly in the threatened group.[2]

This shift in policy towards suppression dashed any hope of building up "herd immunity" in the population and meant the contagion could be more lasting with uncertainty about what any exit strategy could be, and the dangers associated with it. As Boseley reported:

> Many experts thought that this was a dangerous approach anyway. Herd immunity is normally created by vaccinating large numbers of children, safeguarding those who cannot be. Nobody has ever tried to do that by allowing infection with a disease before – and now it appears to have been recognised that it's not safe to try.
>
> *(The Guardian, 17 March 2020, p. 4)*

People would be rightfully angry when they realised that this policy had been presented to them by Johnson and his advisors as if it was the view supported by the latest science, when it was nothing of the sort and threated to risk the lives of over a quarter of a million people.

Language, New Technologies and Social Distancing

Social distancing was a key term in the lexicon of the Coronavirus, but it was a term that needed to be carefully explained. On Monday, 23 March 2020 at 8.30pm after a Cobra meeting (a crisis meeting in the UK Cabinet Office Briefing Rooms) it was announced that Johnson would address the nation. The Union Jack was placed in front and to the side of him adding to the seriousness of the moment. This was to announce a new stage when people were to be instructed to stay at home and *only* to leave it for one health walk a day or to go shopping, or to support a vulnerable person. Over the previous weekend it was clear that people were still gathering in the sunshine and on that Monday in the daytime in London it was reported that the underground was packed with people.

A step change was called for by medical researchers who were alarmed at the increasing level of the virus. With around 340 deaths the UK was exactly where Italy had been two weeks earlier and the rate seemed to be increasing at even a faster level. Decisive action was called for even if this was not a "lockdown" in that transport was still running, even if at a much-diminished level and people did not require written permission to leave their homes, as in Italy and France. The serious tone and the references to multiple deaths to come was to warn people that a boundary had been crossed and that from the next day, the UK would have to be a different country.

Tuesday 24 March. This morning, the day after the Stay-at-Home proclamation was made, there was a definite quiet on the streets. As I took my health walk, I only saw two people in the park. I noted a further shift in my walking where I was looking ahead with an embodied awareness of who might be on the horizon. I was walking with a different level of anxiety as the announcement was working its way through me.

I was keen to keep the two metres recommended and glad that it had been clarified that the virus wasn't just in the air but that you could catch it, also on your clothes, if you were close enough to someone for them to cough in your direction. I think my body had stiffened and this showed in the manner of my walking – I saw an elderly woman walking with two sticks and was careful to stay distant, only to realise with a certain sadness when she passed, that it was a neighbour. It was as if she had become a stranger in the moment and I had passed her by. She had her head down, but I still felt I had failed to acknowledge her.

My morning walk was part of a *ritual* that I had been practising for the past month or so – recognising that it is helpful to walk myself into the day and spend some time in nature, possibly doing some exercises in the park before I settled down to work. But in the past few days the ritual had shifted, and I had decided to join the morning prayers – Shachrit – organised by Leo Baeck College on zoom. I was grateful to be part of a community which was local. It felt good to have a community that stretched beyond home and family.

I gain a lot from praying and meditating as part of a community. I could usually recognise some of the voices I've taught coming together in the virtual space created through Zoom. This was very quickly being adopted as a global technology. It can be surprisingly meaningful but also hard a few years later, to realise there was a time when it did not exist at all. Moments of silence could feel full and allow connections to be made in fraught and fearful times. People tried different strategies to find out what worked for them as a daily practice when they didn't have the everyday routines of work.

There was a moment when people called out the names of people they knew, who we could offer healing to. Jeremy Schonfield, a colleague I've grown close to, was named. I had not realised he had come down with Covid. There was a shift in language as we moved from talking about Coronavirus to talking about Covid-19. We also had a special connection because his father, a Rabbi in the 1930s who was determined to rescue Jews endangered in Europe, was responsible for my mother and grandmother being able to leave Vienna. Their lives were suddenly in danger when German soldiers, after the Anschluss, marched into the city to receive an overwhelming welcome.

You didn't know what names you might hear, but there were enough to recognise how the virus was spreading at a greater intensity and you could trace its movements. I was glad my teaching had moved on-line a week earlier, so that I was not around in physical contact with people when Covid-19, as we came to identify it, was spreading. We felt that it was luck that kept us well for the virus knew *no* boundaries and seemed ready to move to *wherever* it could spread. This was a time when it was becoming clear *how* structural inequalities that meant those who could not work from home and those working in the health service, transport, and supermarkets, were at far *greater risk* of being struck down by the virus.

There was a way that people were learning to be aware of the physical distance their bodies had in relation to other bodies, especially away from the relative safety of home. It was as if "outside" had become yet more of a "hostile environment" for migrant and essential workers. But this bodily attentiveness could mean that you also saw less of things around you. Anna, my partner, felt moved as she saw some young children leaving bags of food for their grandparents who lived on Green Lane in North London. "Didn't you see?" she asked as I wondered why she was tearful. I had seen but not really taken in what had happened. I was too concerned with whether I would be able to keep a safe distance when the children were approaching us. But Anna saw what was happening and was touched by the scene.

I was gradually establishing a daily ritual giving some order to my life – it was easier for me because my life had always been pretty well organised around writing as work. But with WhatsApp messages coming in the morning and stretching through the day, time was being fragmented and at the same time stretched across space as messages arrived from family and friends across the world. Sometimes messages informed me of Zoom gatherings I could join. Initially, there was the excitement of being able to connect and communicate with people you feared losing contact with. Gradually you developed a sense of how emotionally draining time on Zoom could be.

As lectures moved on-line there were new skills that had to be developed. Those working full time could feel they were obliged to teach or attend meetings more or less full time. We were learning to live *in* virtual reality in new and imaginative ways, through much older people who didn't have access to the internet would find the enforced isolation difficult to bear. If they were lucky, they might have grandchildren who could show them how to use iPads. But many elderly people would find the break in the routine they had established to go to social clubs and meet friends for tea very difficult.

It was heartening to see community initiatives emerging all over the country where people were keen *to support* their elderly and isolated neighbours. This was part of creating new rituals and everyday ethical relationships and learning to appreciate contact so often taken for granted within the accelerated work schedules of a neoliberal capitalist culture. There was an unfamiliar quietness on the streets and very few planes in the sky, so many people were reporting a renewed relationship with nature, as they could hear birdsong for the first time, in what was turning out to be a warm spring and summer.

People who were privileged to have gardens, learnt to appreciate the space and relationships with grass and trees that so many people lacked – locked-down in crowded apartments or multi-occupied housing with very limited green spaces. People questioned the values of a neoliberal capitalist society that took this division for granted. They began to think about alternative futures and ways of restructuring societies in more equal and just ways. There was a renewed determination to question social inequalities of class, race and gender that had been *rendered visible* through these Covid times, while engaging the climate emergency and ways of living differently in relation to nature.[3]

Health Emergencies and Vulnerable Bodies

"This is going to get much, much worse, very quickly, both in terms of deaths and the economy," an anonymous cabinet minister shared with BuzzFeed News in March 2020. The minister expressed the belief that soon, the UK would share the chilling number of infections and deaths with Italy, at that time, the most Covid-ravaged country in Europe (Buzzfeed News, 21 March 2020). This partly explained the fear in Johnson's eyes and a sense of desperation to get his message across. He was already being advised that the Coronavirus was spreading faster than anticipated through the UK and too fast for the NHS to cope.

There was no consensus between the scientific advisors with some still thinking that introducing social distancing now would be unsustainable for a long period and would lead to a more disastrous second wave of infection while others pleaded with the government to change tack or face dire consequences.

As Alex Wickham wrote on BuzzFeed News on 21 March 2020, in a piece headed "10 Days that changed Britain: 'Heated' debate between scientists forced Boris Johnson to act on Coronavirus" there was fierce disagreement between the scientists. Wickham noted that the Prime Minister scrambled to find justification among "scientific advice" for his reluctance to impose strong measures.

This was something he was going to live to regret as it had become clear that the UK had not acted fast and radically enough in its policies to avoid following the disastrous sufferings and multiple deaths witnessed in Italy. There had been a time, frightening to recall, as Wickham noted when: "Political aides tacitly criticised other countries who had more dramatic steps, claiming Britain was being 'guided by the science' rather than politics." This was the government using the authority of science as the bearer of a singular truth, for its own political purposes.

Wickham recorded the intransigence of the UK government in the face of neighbouring countries pursing stricter measures, and "increasing alarm among SAGE – Scientific Advisory Group for Emergencies – experts" on their current course of suggesting "home isolation of suspected cases" in lieu of official lockdowns and quarantines. This, the UK claimed, was in line with a shared concern not to do damage to the economy or provoke an economic crisis.

Wickham portrayed Johnson's administration as struggling with the idea of prolonged social distancing, continuing to "privately defend the controversial 'herd immunity' approach (advocated by) Patrick Vallance," but never voicing this publicly.

Some scientists were calling for immediate and drastic action to transform everyday social life through enforcing social distancing and closing down almost all shops and limiting social gatherings to two people. They held the belief that the government lacked transparency. They were inquiring about Vallance's decision to refer to the contrast between the mitigation and suppression approaches as mere "semantics."

"This would all come out in the mother of public inquiries," a source told BuzzFeed News. People would surely be held responsible for the advice they gave, especially if it became clear that many lives could have been saved. The Whitehall source cited the Chancellor's own miscalculations on the severity of the crisis: "Sunak's budget gave a £30 billion stimulus to the economy, six days later he had to spend another £330 billion."

One minister told BuzzFeed that when the scientists disagreed it was up to Number 10 to decide which scientists to back, but lamented a systematic "vacuum of leadership." Describing the chief advisor Dominic Cummings and Patrick Vallance as "close allies," he claimed the government had bet the future of the country on advice from a very small group of scientists that for a long time had differed from the wider international consensus, and other members of SAGE.

The minister also noted that the government's failure to announce a full suite of economic measures simultaneously with Johnson's statement on social distancing, coupled with Sunak's statement missing out measures on wages, had likely led to thousands of layoffs across the country. There was a lack of provision for the self-employed and MPs expected Sunak to dig deeper to protect them. In the House of Commons a queue of Conservative ministers stood up, "lambast(ing) the Treasury for taking too long to announce safeguards for workers, business and those on benefits."

Even after Johnson's stern warning that people should not leave their homes unless absolutely necessary, the following day many people were left confused by the lack of coherent messaging. Matt Hancock, the health minister said that if people could not work at home they should continue going to work and stay six feet apart in order to keep the country going.

When questioned, it was little help for Hancock to insist that the advice coming out of Downing Street "was absolutely clear." Helen MacNamara, deputy cabinet secretary, told the Covid Inquiry that Hancock displaced "nuclear levels" of overconfidence and a pattern of reassuring colleagues that the pandemic was being dealt with in ways that were not true. "They bowl at me, I knock them away" he said confidently to her." He would suggest in meetings that things were under control when they "would discover that was not in fact the case" (theguardian.com, Thursday 2 November 2023). There was also conflicting advice with the Scottish government saying that construction workers should cease working unless the building was absolutely necessary, for example a hospital, a message also shared by Sadiq Khan, Mayor of London, who said it was also the cause for continued crowding on the underground.

Global Health Pandemic and Economic-Political Crisis

Writing for Discover Society, Emeritus Professor of International Relations at the University of Sussex Martin Shaw traced that Dominic Cummings, Johnson's chief of staff and his principal strategist since the days of 'Vote Leave' in 2016, had been obliged to radically shift his position on a number of issues since taking an increasingly prominent position in Johnson's administration, but particularly on Covid. Journalists Tim Shipman and Caroline Wheeler in *The Sunday Times* (22 March 2020) recorded a weekend meeting of that administration assembling to decide on course of actions for tackling Covid, and describes a moment when they sat "shellshocked," reflecting on choices that "will change Britain for the rest of our lives."

One minister said: "It took the weekend to get ourselves into the emotional position where we were comfortable taking the decisions we needed to. The decisions were massive." Ten days earlier as Shipman and Wheeler noted: "The government was slowly gearing up its response to the Coronavirus crisis, downplaying the need for drastic action. By Monday, Boris Johnson had ordered an expansion of the state not seen since the Second World War."

At the end of February 2020, Cummings was reported as saying that the government's strategy was "herd immunity, protect the economy and if that means that some pensioners die, too bad," or as summed up even more succinctly by a senior Tory: "Herd immunity and let the old people die."[4]

Shaw suggested that cynical view relied on the presumption that the younger generation would be "grateful not to have had their freedom to consume disrupted to protect the elderly." This was in line with a certain neoliberal arrogance that meant that younger men, as commented, could easily feel since it was the elderly who were threatened, what is to do with us? This showed a crisis in a political theory and an egoistic and narcissistic individualistic ethic that had long sustained a neo-liberal common sense.

As a person over the age of 70, Shaw commented that were he Covid-positive, he would be "condemned like many older Italians to take their chances at home… because the minimal supplies of critical care beds, ventilators and nurses would be dedicated to people in their 50s and younger" (*Discover Society*, 23 March 2020).

As he recalled his own fearful insight, seeing Johnson attempt to justify his actions on ITV's "This Morning" on 5 March, Shaw was struck by the "masculinist imagery" he used: that tackling the virus was a case of "taking it on the chin." By this, he meant allowing the virus free reign, avoiding "draconian measures" and pursing "balance." The interview was widely judged as having "Cummings' fingers… all over it."

In retrospect, it also helps to explain why the UK was so badly prepared and why it learnt so little from the Chinese experience, when the virus really started to hit. The government was constantly trying to catch up, promising that they had ordered 2 million test kits and they intended an exponential rise in tests, when the tests didn't exist, and it would be months before they would be available. This was hidden in the language of Matt Hancock, the health secretary, who claimed they had been ordered (*Discover Society*, 23 March 2020).

Johnson's government was falling back on its usual hype, hiding behind the authority of science whenever they were questioned. The language they used revealed a different reality – that they were doing their best to hide from the public. Given it was a crisis, they felt they didn't need to be democratically accountable.

Johnson went on from his "on the chin" exposition to attempt to reassure, when so little was actually ready or being prepared. He said:

> I think it is very important, we've got a fantastic NHS, we will give them all the support that they need, we will make sure that they have all preparations, all the kit that they need for us to get through it. But I think it would be better if we take all the measures that we can now to stop the peak of the disease being as difficult for the NHS as it might be. I think there are things that we may be able to do.
>
> *(Discover Society, 23 March 2020)*

Shaw questions what an "acceptable" number of fatalities is, when "balance(ed)… with harm to the UK economy." Research forced Cummings to face reality and embrace the "suppression" tactic that was evaluated by scientists as the most viable path towards controlling the virus. Johnson, however, "continued to vacillate."

French philosopher Michel Foucault taught in *The Will to Knowledge* that in modernity: "Power is situated at the level of life, the species, the race, and the large-scale phenomena of population." As Shaw noted: "modern epidemiology in general operates at this level (if we understand 'race' as the human race)." Foucault explained that "genocide is the dream of modern powers in this condition." Bio-politics has long been concerned with the power of life and death over the population of a nation according to Foucault.[5]

It was Downing Street's Nudge Unit, set up under Prime Minister David Cameron to apply behavioural science to public policy, which put the term "herd immunity" in the public domain. By the time Johnson held the first major conference on the Coronavirus, as Shaw noted, Vallance and Whitty, the "supposed grown-ups in the room" were on-board with this strategy, despite having seen the devastating effects of the pandemic in other countries, and being aware of systematic vulnerabilities within the NHS. In their focus on protecting the over-70s, they were already ignoring the fact that in Italy, hospitals were full of people under-60.[6]

In a helpful set of tweets Francois Balloux, director of the University College London Genetics Institute, introduced himself saying: "I should be qualified to comment on the Covid-19 pandemic. I'm a computational/systems biologist working in infectious diseases." He said:

> I believe that the pandemic is the most serious global public health threat humanity has faced since the 1918/19 influenza pandemic. There are major differences between the two events, but I suspect there will also be similarities that may emerge when we look back.

As he readily acknowledged:

> Predictions from any model are only as good as the data that parametrised it. There are two major unknowns at this stage. One: We don't know to what extent Covid-19 transmission will be seasonal. Two: We don't know if Covid-19 infection induces long-lasting immunity. Comparisons with other Coronaviridae suggests it may be relatively short (i.e., months). If this were confirmed, it would add to the challenge of managing the pandemic.

But he also noted:

> The Covid-19 pandemic is not just an epidemiological problem. It is a global health problem, which can only be tackled with an integrated and global approach. For example, there is no such thing as a choice between managing the pandemic versus protecting the economy. At the same time, health and economy are closely linked. The correlation between per-capital GDP and health (life expectancy) is essentially perfect. If the Covid-19 pandemic leads to a global

> economy collapse, many more lives will be lost than Covid-19 would ever be able to claim.
>
> *(@BallouxFrancois 14/03/2020)*

This means that when we are talking about a health crisis we are, of necessity at the same time talking about an economic and political crisis.

It can be illuminating to quote a response from Peter Palmer to this thread showing possibly how denial is so often related to unconscious fears:

> Major issue with this thread. It assumes that Covid19 is a lethal pandemic disease. It isn't that bad.
>
> It is only a serious risk to certain vulnerable groups.
>
> Those who've had it say it's not as bad as flu and doesn't last.
>
> Look at the figures. The percentages are very low.
>
> *(@peterpalmer52 14/03.2020)*

A response to this by jmatthei:

> That works wonders until your ICUs are overrun, your doctors and nurses collapse at work and your mortality goes through the roof as consequence. It is playing chicken with a blind person. That virus really doesn't care about your economy.
>
> *(@jmattheij 15/03/2020)*

Health Crisis as Moral Crisis

"Horrible decisions will be made about who lives and who dies," the chief executive of a large hospital trust told Polly Toynbee of *The Guardian*, as he recognised: "And I will be the one to make them. Liability sits with me." But it was telling that he dared not say his name – "Everyone is under a total media blackout" but he did not think that in this critical situation silence was a good policy. As he noted: "Any vacuum will get filled by Twitter or the *Daily Mail*."

As he explained, he had done the sums. Locally, he had over 130,000 over-80s and following Chris Whitty, the chief medical officer for England's high estimate of an 80% infection rate, with 10% needing a bed and 4% intensive care, even if he could extend his 15 intensive care beds, the hospital would still fall short. His staff were anxious, needing to know every detail about what was going on (*The Guardian*, 17 March 2020, Journal p. 1).

The executive expressed a belief that the NHS would not be able to handle the crest of infection rates: and knowing that these "horrible decisions" were looming, had set up a local ethics group to advise him: but being aware that "the final decisions sit with me."

Toynbee noted: "It's easy to assess medical conditions, but after that come tougher choices." She reported on Italian hospitals restricting ventilators to under

65s, pointing out that the UK "…with many fewer beds, are still a few weeks behind them." But what does this tell us about the value of a life? Are we saying that lives are of equal worth however long they have been lived or are we saying that in times of scarce medical resources, those who are young and have more years ahead of them should be given the chance to survive on ventilators?

As Toynbee recognised, these moral issues are of the moment, anticipating deeper political debates to come on why the UK was left "nakedly unprepared" with health and social care "brutally worn down by a decade of needless, ideologically driven austerity." A striking and disturbing ethical issue, emerging from Simon Stevens, the chief executive of NHS England, giving evidence to the Inquiry, as to whether the medical profession or ministers should have the final say if a worst case scenarios occurred is his report that Matt Hancock took the position that he "rather than, say, the medical profession or the public should ultimately decide who should live and who should die… Fortunately this horrible dilemma never crystallised" he added (*The Guardian,* Thursday 2 November 2023 19.29 GMT)

But more immediately, there had already been strong challenges from doctors, nurses and health workers at the lack of proper protective equipment for those working on the front line and a realisation that the government was often talking up and delivering sub-standard equipment when it finally arrived, putting so many people in danger of getting the virus.

Residents of care homes were particularly susceptible, and GP Dr Jonathan Leach said his practice was discussing how to cope with six care homes. With mortality rates high, he said that it was better not to admit these patients to hospital for their own safety: and suggested in these cases, "meaningful conversations with families" were needed (*The Guardian*, 17 March 2020, Journal p. 2).

Dr Leach noted actions that were being encouraged among NHS staff in various branches: paramedics doing their best to avoid transporting patients to hospitals, GPs encouraging end-of-life care, implementing DNR (do not resuscitate) protocols, and increasing the availability and access to pain medication. He lamented the lack of information being shared at official levels, and sharing that services needed to prepare themselves for the reality that there are "few good alternatives" to these responses.

Meanwhile Dr Leach prepared for substantial rates of staff illness, hearing from his colleagues that their only option for childcare when schools inevitably closed was "grandparents." He explained that he was trying to encourage shared childcare among colleagues, blanching at the idea of the country being tens of millions of pounds in debt. He expressed worry about the legal protections and immunity available to him, and to others in a similar position, making mortal decisions. He said: "Families will be within their rights to call us to inquests."[7]

Warnings and Failures to Anticipate

As Anthony Costello, professor of global health at University College London and a former World Health Organization director, anxiously wondered whether the WHO planned to "keep things damped down until drugs and a vaccine are available," questioning the wisdom and ethics of pursing a course of action all but guaranteeing "immediate casualties on the basis of uncertain future benefits."

Citing the Singaporean approach to phased school closures, Costello recognised the importance of local data collection to drive such decisions, but maintained that "testing and sharing of information on-line" was key to making them. It did not help trust in the government that they did not seem to have planned for the testing that was needed and had acted uniformly across the nation when people knew that the risks in London were so much higher, and that London was possibly two weeks ahead of the rest of the country.

As Costello noted, after the initial three weeks of denials and inaction were broken, the Chinese authorities listened to the WHO and tested intensively with mobile centres. They got the test result time down from four days to four hours. They cut the time from onset of symptoms to lab results from 12 to three days. They identified family clusters and arranged isolation centres. Above all they mobilised communities. As he said: "This was not a terrorised population but one passionate about tackling an existential threat."

Costello explained that having a population increasingly comfortable using smartphones and apps was powerful in containing the virus: in Wuhan, its 11-million-strong population ordered their shopping on-line. The result? "In seven weeks, China stopped the epidemic in its tracks… (reporting) 10 to 20 new cases a day in a population of nearly 1.4 billion." Other neighbouring countries embracing the potential of online behaviours such as South Korea, Japan, Singapore and Taiwan did the same, and similarly experienced a huge decline in fatalities and new cases (*The Guardian*, 17 March 2020, Journal p. 3).

Reflecting on the success of this, Costello was disappointed that the UK squandered the opportunity to follow this model from the beginning by integrating "nationwide testing, contact tracing, quarantine and a progress policy of social distancing" into the pandemic response plan, instead favouring the disastrous exposure plan to build herd immunity, for which Costello saw little research evidence. He questioned the cessation of track and trace outside the hospital setting, as I too noted with increasing anger and desperation, only for severe cases of the virus to surge, and without a test being available to medical staff on the front line.

Fears, Disturbances and Shocking Deaths

Friday 27 March 2020. Yesterday I heard that my brother, Tony, had come down with the virus. I was upset to hear the news, but he assured me it was not too bad and was taking it lightly. He said on the phone, if he died, he would have had a good life. He had a high temperature and could not sleep easily at night with cold sweats. He had caught it on Sunday and previously had taken some care, but had somehow absorbed the early messages from Johnson that it was like bad flu.

Part of him was saying that it was possibly better for him to get over with it now and then he would have some immunity, he at least hoped. I was disturbed by the news and as Anna and I took a walk in Brent Park in North London, we both felt anxious and fraught, aware of each body that was approaching, as if they were zombies that needed to be carefully avoided.

Walking had become a different and disturbed experience when you felt you had to be constantly on guard and aware of the possibilities of social distancing whenever someone appeared on the horizon. You looked in a different way and your eyes moved ahead of you, wary of what they might see. As we approached a bridge towards the end of our walk, there was warning waiting for us that was chilling and reminded us that this was "a time of the plague" – *Corona Virus on this estate – Bridge closed. Turn Back.*

It was a wonderful relief on Thursday evening at 8pm and against anticipation in this orthodox Jewish community, that almost everyone opened their doors and windows and shouted support for the NHS in response to the national call. I hadn't expected the sound to carry so well, and the strength of support people were showing for the NHS in this moment of health crisis. Apparently, it was a call that was responded to throughout the city, and I imagined throughout the country. A mark of a deep sense of appreciation for the risks that NHS workers in hospitals and social care were taking on our behalf. The country seemed to have *come together* in this time of crisis and the numbers that had already volunteered to help those in need was approaching half a million people.

There were definite signs of a renewed sense of appreciation for the value of community and the ethic of mutual aid. At this stage in the lockdown people were willingly looking out for their neighbours and there was an atmosphere of empathy and compassion. People were gradually taking in how, though we were in this together, the virus was clearly discriminating, and some people were in much *more* vulnerable situations than others, most evidently workers on the front line in hospitals and care homes and those obliged to work as essential workers and living in precarious and overcrowded housing.

I had a disturbed dream that night, about the dangers of movement and planned to take an earlier walk when there were fewer people around. I realised that Green Lane was a wider street which was so welcome even though there was hardly anyone I passed. In the park I was taking a photo when someone jogged past and said "good morning" – I felt shocked and as if I had jumped out of my skin. Later I avoided another man walking his white bulldog. As I sought to move on the grass to avoid him, he said "You should be at home friend. Don't you have a garden?"

I replied: "'I need to have my exercise," but it was clear that in this encounter – which also had elements of class as well as age – there was a sense that older people in their 70s shouldn't be walking around in the park. They should be at home *so* that the rest of the world could walk their dogs as usual without having to worry. It seemed as if the government warning to be at home specifically applied to those defined as at risk. This was possibly *why* even then far fewer young people seemed to be observing a two-metre social distance. In the park they were more likely to gather and assume in their styles of walking that they were keeping their distance only as an act of altruism to those defined as more vulnerable.

The Guardian's view on the government's response to Covid published on 16 March feared an "exceptionally difficult period" to come, likely to be "far harder to manage for those already struggling with health or family difficulties, or to make ends meet." The editorial noted the danger of people "turning inward…. (but) we must do everything in our power – including through public policy – to reach beyond our family circles and ensure the poorest and loneliest do not bear the brunt" (*The Guardian*, 17 March 2020, Journal p. 2).

In what they continually talked of as 'unprecedented times' the government took steps to support those workers who were on a payroll, guaranteeing them 80% of their wages. On Thursday 26 March, after considerable public pressure, the chancellor Rishi Sunak offered similar terms to many self-employed but there would be many poorer workers forced to stay home who would inevitably *not* be covered, including many of those in the gig economy and part-time employees. There had already been a reported rise in incidents of domestic violence as many people struggled with children at home with schools closed and the responsibility for education passed to parents already stressed out with the demands of lockdown.

For people living in limited space it could be impossible to maintain distance and for many it was hard to know how to stay safe and put bread on the table. These were testing times made so much harder because there was no anticipated exit strategy and no future that people could plan for. This was disturbing for generations brought up to shape their experience within a neoliberal culture and common-sense.

It was as if anticipated futures had suddenly disappeared. People were exhausted listening to news and social media, often offering contradictory advice. It was hard to know whether they could *trust* government guidance since it had to shift its policies over a weekend – when the prediction of a truly catastrophic health emergency, which should have been foreseen, was at last taken seriously. It was easy for people to take out their anger and frustration on those around them, uncertain of what the future would bring and no longer able to believe that a summer holiday could offer some relief.

There was *no* real conviction that the lockdown would be effective or what would come afterwards. The future had suddenly disappeared, and people feared living in an endless present, often unsure of how they could keep themselves safe and fearful of losing their jobs and a future of unemployment. Many people on low salaries felt obliged to use food banks, often for the first time. Deprived of traditional means of support, it was hard to know who they could turn to and how they were going to get through a pandemic that few anticipated or took seriously. Even the government *had ignored* its own reports and been unprepared and left the NHS and the care sector in an unprepared state after years of cuts and neoliberal austerity.

Notes

1 To explore the social and political responses to Covid-19 and the role played by social distancing in virus mitigation and the comparative effect of social proximity and distance on national anti-viral behaviour see Peter Murphey *Covid-19: Proportionality, Public Policy and Social Distancing* (London: Palgrave Pivot 2020). He explores how contemporary societies think about risk, threat and harm and how social mood has also affected responses to the pandemic. See also for an insider's account of how the government into disaster and tried to cover its role in the tragedy that cost so many unnecessary deaths, Jonathan Calvert and George Arbuthnott *Failures of State: The Inside Story of Britain's Battle with Coronavirus* (London: Mudlark 2021).

2 For a deeply analysed case study of the intersection between science and politics that warns us to beware of politicians claiming to be following the science and offers a searing indictment of the government's serial failures to follow the science and their attempts to cover their tracks afterwards see Jeremy Farrar and Anjana Ahuja *Spike: The Virus vs. the People – the Inside Story* (London: Profile Books 2022).

3 For a deeper cultural and historical frame for living in lockdown as a result of the Covid-19 pandemic and for reflections upon how human beings have experienced confinement across history see, Paul Crawford and Jamie Orion Crawford *Cabin Fever: Surviving Lockdown in the Coronavirus Pandemic* (London: Emerald Publishing Ltd 2021). See also Ken Menon *Lockdown 2020: Covid-19* (London: Author House 2020) who argues that the fear is not only about health but also about the future, employment and quality of life. There is a fear of the present and concern for the future.

4 *Discover Society*, 23 March 2020. *Discover Society* was established in October 2013 by John Holmwood and Sue Scott and is published by Social Research Publications in collaboration with *The Sociological Review*.

5 Michel Foucault's *Archaeology of Knowledge* (London: Routledge Classics 2002) and *The Order of Things: An Archaeology of the Human Sciences* (London: Routledge Classics 2020) as his methodological reflections before he shifted his attention to engaging with the voices of prisoners themselves that questioned the discourses through which they were disciplinary framed in *Discipline and Punish: The Birth of the Prison* (London: Penguin Modern Classics 2020). For some helpful historical context see, for instance, *Foucault Live: Collected Interviews, 1961–1984* (London: Penguin Random House Semiotext(e) / Foreign Agents 1996); David Macey *The Lives of Michel Foucault* (London: Vintage Books 1995) and Stuart Elden *Foucault's Last Decade* (Cambridge: Polity 2016).

6 For an understanding of how David Cameron's learnt about nudging people to adopt different policies and everyday ways of behaving so embedding behavioural insights into the fabric of organisation see, David Halpern *Inside the Nudge Unit: How Small Changes Can Make a Big Difference* (London: WH Allen 2016). To grasp the theoretical principles underling this shift in policies which seek by knowing how people think to nudge us in the right directions without ever restricting our freedom of choice, see Richard A. Thaler and Cass R. Susstein *Nudge: Improving Decisions about Health, Wealth and Happiness* (London: Penguin 2022).

7 The life and death decisions that medical staff find themselves suddenly involved in making without having anticipated the ethical judgments they are being expected to make are explored in Dr Roopa Farooki *Everything is Trye: A Junior Doctor's story of Life, Death and Grief in a Time of Pandemic* (London: Bloomsbury Publishing 2022). He gives an eloquent testimonial of grief and fury through the first forty days of the Covid crisis conveying the fear, confusion and uncertainties. See also Kelly Critcher *A Matter of Life and Death: Courage, Compassion and the Fight against Coronavirus – a palliative care nurse's story* (London: John Blake 2021). She weaves together he raw

emotional diaries with a broader reflection on the truths about a life spent struggling for her patients' lives and helping them to face death with compassion. See also Louise Curtis *A Nurses Story: My Life in A&E During the Covid Crisis* (London: Pan 2020). She traces how she also saw an increase in domestic abuse cases and suicide cases loneliness hit people hard. There are also the reflections of Anthea Allen *Life, Death and Biscuits* (London: Harper Element, 2022) that catches some of the experiences of those working in critical care which already in 2023 everyone now tries to forget all about and pretend it isn't happening anymore.

7

GLOBAL CRISIS, LOCKDOWNS, DEATHS AND DISTURBANCES

Global Crisis

On Tuesday 10 March 2020, *The Guardian* front page announced, "Stock markets in biggest fall since 2008 as virus fears trigger panic selling," prompting widespread panic about the "soaring economic cost of the coronavirus outbreak" and fears of another financial crash, at a point at which many countries took the decisions to impose restrictions on movement (*The Guardian*, 10 March 2020).

Reporting on the prospect of economic woes, columnists Richard Partington and Graeme Wearden anticipated that the worst was still to come:

> Trading on Wall Street was frozen within minutes of the market opening as the system to buy and sell shares failed to keep pace with events. The Dow Jones closed down by more than 2,000 points for the first time ever, a decline of 7.8 per cent.

We were genuinely in unprecedented waters, and it was hard to anticipate what measures would be needed to respond to the speed this global crisis was accelerating. There was widespread fear about the deaths that would inevitably follow as the virus moved across borders in the Global South.

Columnist Larry Elliot in *The Guardian* acknowledged:

> For the past decade, the underlying fragility of the global economy has been masked by low interest rates. Cheap money has fuelled asset price rises but has done little to boost investment and historically weak productivity growth.
>
> *(The Guardian, 10 March 2020, p. 4)*

DOI: 10.4324/9781003296874-7

Elliot pointed out that this disconnect was exposed when markets dismissed Covid as a trivial concern, believing that it would pass swiftly like past global health scares, including SARS in the early 2000s. However, as the severity of Covid-19 became evident, deluded speculation held that that central banks would intervene and support the value of financial assets. In this way global capitalism would ride the storm to come in relative safety. "Crash Monday" was a wake-up call for financial bodies, as they were forced to acknowledge the "giant wave of debt" on which the market had been floating.

Elliot posits this as the largest threat to the world's economy since the 2008 crash when total collapse was narrowly avoided by the "international community (coming) together to prevent a second Great Depression." He noted that large institutions, including the International Monetary Fund, favoured a collaborative approach between large world economies to "settle their differences and unite behind an action plan that would boost consumer and business spending and support for businesses, and tax cuts" (p. 5).

In the G7 virtual meeting, governments were realising how far they would have to go to give financial support to businesses and workers as their economies were forced to close down. There was a need to reimagine the social contract between citizens and states, as people were ordered to stay at home. There were uncertain futures that could *not* be planned for as governments, even in relatively prosperous countries, had to face the reality that their health services would be overwhelmed by the number of patients needing intensive care and ventilators in short supply.[1]

Fragilities, Disturbances and Shutting Down

Things were going to have to radically change in the UK. Italy was to prove to many that the threat of the coronavirus was far more deadly than early government reports.

As self-confessed hypochondriac and *Guardian* columnist John Crace said, he was, perhaps surprisingly "relatively unbothered by the coronavirus", citing a focus "on conditions with a far higher fatality rate than about two per cent. Or, to put it brutally selfishly, people not like me." Things rather shifted for him, though not as quickly as for some others. He said:

> But this week, as the virus rapidly approaches pandemic proportions, and it became clear that the WHO has no idea how to stop it and the UK government has almost no contingency plans in place…I've had a few wobbles. Not enough to go out and buy face masks and hand sanitisers, but enough to make me think that I could possibly be dead by the end of next month.
>
> *(The Guardian, 28 February 2020)*

As he intimated lightly:

> I also did vaguely wonder if this was all a government plot. For more than six months now, Boris Johnson has insisted that he has a fully thought out and

> costed plan for social care but has so far refused to share with the country. Maybe Covid-19 was the secret plan all along. (*The Guardian*, 28 February 2020, p. 23)

By Saturday 21 March everything was to be different as *The Guardian* reported under a frontpage headline: "Britain shuts down". Columnists Heather Stewart and Peter Walker reported on the moment that the order came to close drinking and dining establishments nationwide, and an "unprecedented wage-support scheme" was announced by the government to minimise the potential of a "tsunami of job losses." Johnson said it went against what he called "the inalienable freeborn right of people born in England to go the pub." Many people seemed to have agreed. Even if ordering of places to close had been a response to increasing pressure to take stringent action, at that point, "social distancing measures avoiding all unnecessary social contact" were being routinely flouted (*The Guardian*, 21 March 2020).

After the restrictions were ignored on a beautiful sunny spring weekend when people flocked to beaches and gathered in parks, pressure on Johnson increased. The following Monday the country moved into a lockdown, and were told to stay at home. It was enforced by criminal law and the police were ordered to break up gatherings of more than two people. At first, it was hard for people to take the danger seriously. On 3 March Johnson boasted to journalists of visiting a hospital, and shaking hands with every Covid patient there.

At the Birds Pub in Leytonstone, northeast London, after that lockdown announcement, it did not fill up with drinkers hoping for last pints as happened in other places, it was actually less busy than usual. Caitlin Morgan and her colleague Nick Slotnick, from Woodford, said: "It's sad but inevitable. It had to happen." Chris Henry, manager of a pub in Manchester said at least the announcement brought an end to their "limbo". "We got put in the position where it wasn't in the best interests for our customers' health to be open, but no one said we should be closed… It's been a horrible week" (*The Guardian*, 21 March 2020, p. 5).

On 11 March in Rishi Sunak's first budget, he set aside £12 billion for dealing with the coronavirus, but this was never going to be enough, and events were to move so quickly that as Larry Elliot pithily put it: "Having waited more than a year for a budget, Britain has now had three in the space of nine days" (*The Guardian*, 21 March 2020, p. 7). Under further public pressure there had effectively to be a fourth. This was to deal with the self-employed, initially excluded from the job subsidy scheme, paying out 80% of an employee's wage up to a limit of £2,500 a month.

The self-employed were eventually to be offered something like parity, but it was going to take till June for the policies to be in place and delivering. According to Elliot, these were timely measures from the treasury and from the chancellor, for whom winning plaudits from the Trades Union Congress (TUC) was an indication of how much progress had been made to meet workers' expectations, despite a more gloomy long-term forecast.

But Elliot was also clear that the government was open to the charge, initially levied by George Osborne against Gordon Brown in the 2008 global financial crisis, that it "had failed to mend the roof while the sun was shining": trying to fight the epidemic with a critically underfunded health and social care infrastructure and rampant precarity and insecurity for millions "one pay packet away from penury."

There was terrible anxiety across the land when so many workers had been left unsure of whether the financial support would come in time given that so many families were left with no income. People were under extreme stress with children at home and pressure for someone in the family to continue with a job that brought money in. Already a week into the lockdown with people ordered not to leave home unless it was absolutely necessary, there was a rise in reports of domestic violence. People took out their anxieties within the limited space of home. They felt locked-in, unsure of the threats outside and often angry at those around them.

Shock as a New Moral Landscape Takes Shape

The speed with which changes were introduced, and the lack of preparation since the virus first showed its devastating effects in China, added a sense of unreality where people felt confronted by an *unknown.* Schools were closed and families found themselves living together as if in new spaces. People were working at home, if they could reorganise their domestic space. For professional workers this had been familiar for a while, under the advent of new technologies.

But the fact that adults were left with the responsibility for educating their children, or at least keeping them occupied, added an extra pressure, especially having to explain to young children why they could not play with their friends. Puzzling, when for a time you might have been encouraging them to play more. Why do they have to stay two metres apart? What are the invisible dangers carried by the virus? What *is* a virus, and a child might fear: do I have it anyway?

We were at the end of the first week of school closure. Only children whose parents were working in the NHS and social care or who were particularly vulnerable were still in class. Headteachers talked of the pressure they faced from parents who insisted that their children *should* be at school because they could not cope with them being at home. They might not have access to the technologies that schools were relying upon to stay in contact with their pupils.

Stressed parents might be angry at headteachers who they felt had the power to decide who to keep at school and who had to go home. Their frustrations at the impossibilities of the new situation meant they needed someone *to blame* for *how* the world had changed so dramatically. When they felt anxious about the invisible threats they faced, unsure of how to protect themselves and endlessly washing their hands in desperation and getting their children to do the same, when for children they already feel clean for there was no dirt to be seen, they desperately wanted to hold someone responsible.

Guardian columnist Jonathan Freedland noted the eerily transformative power of the pandemic, reflecting on "deserted" streets, empty schools, and an ever-accelerating news cycle bringing missives that "in normal times, would constitute an epochal, ground-shaking development… struggle(ing) for airtime." This, he observes, sent the Conservative government into disarray, on the realisation that "as there are no atheists on a sinking ship, there are no free marketeers in a pandemic."

Part of this transformation, Freedland notes, is whole new vocabulary: "social distancing," "self-isolation," and "WFH (working from home)" being just some of the phrases that became "near-universal." All areas of etiquette and social cues were touched by the virus: with the "rejected handshake," "elbow bump," and virtual drinks rapidly taking their place in our collective behaviour (*The Guardian*, 20 March 2020, pp. 8–9).

Meeting places, even for families living apart, became virtual. There have been attempts on the part of universities to deny the long-term consequences of what was happening by attempting to shift lectures and seminars on-line. They are still behaving as if course work can replace examinations and be handed in later if need be. It was as if people were still relying upon things being able to return to "normal" once the virus had passed over the land and we came out from our homes and returned to business as usual. It seems as if many people are dealing with their fears and gaining a sense of balance by being able to tell themselves that the future will look very much like the past, with a few months abandoned along the way.

So often in times of fear and anxiety we take refuge in myths. We don't want to be reminded of historical truths that question the nostalgic "creation myth of modern Britain" that we have drawn upon to offer comfort – of what actually happened in the Blitz. Freedland reminds us of the reality: crowds in impoverished parts of the capital booing passing royalty, the resentment of a nation against a booming black market profiting from people's desperation

But this hasn't meant that stoicism in the face of danger has been our national look. Freedland wryly notes that footage and reports of shoppers fighting over toilet roll in particular may fail to "inspire our grandchildren." So much for our national self-mythology. The truth is that for years we have lived in a very different neoliberal world in which the winner takes all and the weak are defined as losers who have failed to achieve and look after themselves. They only have themselves to blame for their failures and the difficulties they are having in supporting their families. They can feel obliged to turn their anger in and against themselves or against the partners they are closest to.

Freedland recognised that national patience wore thin quickly with lightweight measures, when citizens were moved to ask questions like "…Why are all doctors and nurses not being routinely tested, or given the right protective equipment? Why were more ventilators not ordered weeks ago?"

It was also a chilling reminder that questioned us all, in relation to our moral responsibilities to others, to see the video go viral of a nurse, Dawn Billborough, sobbing into the camera after coming off a 48-hour shift only to discover there was no food was left in the shops. She warned those picking the shelves clean they would need nurses like her to look after then "when you're at your lowest."

But Freedland also recognises that it was fear – something which has been spoken about less in this week of transformation – that was driving responses. As he noted: "When people see that Britain is on an even steeper death curve than Italy, they become terrified. Arguing about policy on Twitter is a good displacement activity for people petrified of dying a horrible death."

Fearful Memories and Bodily Anxieties

As Freedland shared some of his own fear, he recognised:

> Even before it has killed Britons in huge number, it's already got under our skin – reminding us that we are not masters of nature, but as humans vulnerable to a tiny, microscopic virus; that even the mighty civilisation that we have built on these islands hangs by a thread.
>
> *(The Guardian, 20 March 2020, p. 9)*

Suddenly people were also increasingly aware that nature had taken *its* revenge for the ways it has been mistreated. European modernities have been too quick to identify progress with the control and domination of nature. They have rendered nature mute, as its suffering *cannot* be heard. It is as if nature exists within the capitalist imagination as a resource to be exploited for human needs and capitalist profit.[2]

Simon Armitage, the poet laureate, has addressed some of these fears in his poem *Lockdown* that draws contemporary resonances from the small Derbyshire village, Eyam, that placed itself in quarantine to save others when the bubonic plague hit in the 17th century (*The Guardian*, 21 March 2020, p. 3).

His poem touched on the doomed romance between a girl, Emmot Syddall who lived in Eyam, and the boy Rowland Torre, who lived outside the village but would visit to talk to her at a distance, until she stopped appearing. These lines in the poem refer to them:

> star-crossed lovers on either side
> of the quarantine line
> whose wordless courtship spanned the river
> till she came no longer.

Armitage told journalist Alison Flood that he felt a message was to be drawn about "being patient and trusting to the earth" and embracing slowness as a corrective to our "hectic lives," which, as he points out, was a major factor in the spread of the virus.

For Armitage the "contemplative" nature of poetry was "by definition consoling", by finding the "sacramental in the ordinary descriptions of everyday life," and being "considerate" and "thoughtful" of the language we use, especially around others.

Breathing and Gasping for Air

Sunday 29 March. There was a shift in atmosphere yesterday and I felt haunted in a different way by listening in to "Any Answers" on BBC Radio 4 and hearing people talk about the difficult life and death decisions many of us, particularly those who are over 70, are going to face. A doctor had thought carefully about his situation if he caught the virus, and he wanted to be able to stay at home *if* he got the virus and so to be *with* people who loved and cared for him. He didn't want to go to hospital, knowing that given his age and health condition he was unlikely to survive on a ventilator when they were in demand for people possibly with more years of life to look forward to.

He wanted the chance not to be separated from family and friends and he said he had written to the prime minister to say that people should be given the option to have oxygen and nursing at home. He felt that the health authorities had a moral responsibility to provide this *if* people wanted to die in their own homes. He knew *how* stretched the hospitals were already becoming. He knew that things were expected to get a lot worse as they become overwhelmed with the demands of very sick people who are having difficulties breathing without the aid of ventilators. They are already in short supply.

There was also talk about requests *not* to be resuscitated and the help available to make living wills that set out clearly people's decisions about end-of-life care. It was moving to hear people talk about the need to have conversations with families about these issues. I felt a need *to talk* about these things with Anna and our children Daniel and Lily. There was talk about the difficulties of dying when you are gasping for breath, especially if ventilators were *not* available. Some people would prefer to have morphine and other drugs available to them at home.

I've talked to my brother each day since he told me that he had the virus and on Friday I could *hear* his shortness of breath and was concerned that he could not sleep. I was fearful about ringing him up but knew that I would. I wanted to say how much I loved him and talk about some of the questions that had just been raised about life and death, and what he wanted for himself. I phoned him and felt relieved that his voice was clearer and though he felt he had no energy at all, he had a good night sleep and I think his temperature was not so high.

We talked and he said he had a good life and that *if* this was his time, he was ready to go and had no regrets of how he had lived his life. I said how he was loved but somehow could not say, "I love you Tony" though I did say that I had been feeling worried and concerned. He was happy that others in the family had contacted him and said he didn't really need anything, and that people were looking after him well, though he couldn't really eat anything.

It was Tony who told me in the same conversation that Rabbi Kraft had died. He was a lovely and caring man who Tony had got to know better when he went to synagogue for Rosh Hashana and Yom Kippur. He wondered whether I already knew. He was sad but also accepting, which is his way as a realist. I remember him talking about what a warm and supportive human being Kraft was and how he would talk to anyone. This was the first death from the virus of someone we knew. Later in the same afternoon we were to meet for a Zoom family call to celebrate Lily's husband Rich's birthday. It was to be a call in which Tony requested we were *not* going to talk about the virus.

Before that call I got an email from my men's group that said that my friend Paul and his partner Oriel had both been admitted to Barnet Hospital. This was the news that people were hearing across the country as the rates of infection increased and people were finding themselves needing hospital care because of their difficulties in breathing. I was shocked because I knew *how* vulnerable Paul was and that he had been waiting for an operation on his lungs. He had so little energy and couldn't walk easily for a while, as he often said in his broad Yorkshire tones – "I take one step at a time".

I also soon learnt that other dear friends were also suffering with the virus. I felt for them knowing their underlying health conditions and suddenly it felt that the virus had moved very close. It was *no longer* about distant others but was affecting family and close friends. It was serious and very real, especially for our generation. Younger friends would still say that it was a distant fear as they did not know anyone directly affected, even if they had heard of people. But people across age groups were still worried what the next weeks might bring – what unknown and uncertain futures we were all living with.

The clocks had changed last night. As I walked along Green Lanes in North London, there was not a soul I could see. As I approached Brent Park, I could see Alan, the man I had befriended, just walk into the park ahead of me. He did not wave. I wondered whether this was a sign of the shift on atmosphere. We were all locked into ourselves in a firmer way, making it *harde*r to reach out and so, almost automatically, withdrawing from contact. People we were not living with had suddenly become other. They had somehow become objectified. As the philosopher Martin Buber understood, we seemed caught in instrumental I–It relationships. We were losing the capacity to shape I–Thou relationships. Others were being transformed into strangers who were already suspect because they could unknowingly be asymptomatic carriers of the virus. We could no longer relate in human terms.

It was as if the trust we had for others was being attacked and undermined as the streets were empty. But it was *not* to be so harsh, at least with Alan, for our paths were to cross in the park and we were to talk keeping a safe two meters apart. We noted *how* the world had become a different place in the last seven days.

He talked about knowing friends of friends who had the virus. He also shared how they had made living wills before the present crisis had broken. He was relieved it was something they had already talked about with family. They already had the difficult conversations that many families were still finding it hard to approach. What would happen if they got Covid-19? How would people live safely with each other and provide the care that would be needed? There was a sense of the *vulnerability* of human life as ethical humans and a sense that life was suddenly rendered precarious in new and unexpectedly fearful ways.[3]

As I walked the phrase "gasping for breath" walked along with me and I wondered whether it was a fear I was carrying, that was forming itself into these words. Possibly it echoed my reading about Tara Jane Langston a 39-year-old fit and healthy mother of two who started feeling unwell and went to hospital after calling 111. The hospital staff told her that she had a chest infection. She was prescribed antibiotics and sent home.

Possibly this response was related to her age and the desire to believe that it was *only* people who were much older that were in danger of the virus. When they called 111 again, desperate that her condition had significantly worsened, an ambulance was sent to take her back to hospital – which her husband described as "a horrific and terrifying ordeal."

After being diagnosed with Covid-19 she sent a video to her WhatsApp group with her colleagues, which has been viewed tens of thousands of times. She warned others of "taking any chances," lest they also end up in intensive care. Her husband Richard Langston told Aamna Mohdin of *The Guardian* that he was glad he packed his wife's phone when the ambulance arrived to take her to hospital: the only method he had of staying in touch with her and receiving updates (*The Guardian*, 21 March 2020, p. 23).

But there were images that people did not want to see and voices they did not want to hear. So many people had invested emotionally in the notion that it was only those over-70s who were in any real danger of getting the virus. This meant that what has happened to her could *not* be true because it threatened the emotional denial they were shaping their lives around. This was a way of minimising the risks they felt, as many people did in the early weeks of the virus. The government was insisting that it was really no different to the flu, especially if you are not old. There has been a generational divide that is still working itself through.

The family's trauma, as Mohdin was augmented by being subjected to cruel trolling online, with some taking to social media to harass them, and dismiss Langston's ordeal as a "hoax." Unfounded online claims that her widely shared video was bogus made the experience even more upsetting. "It made me question humanity," Langston said from his home in Middlesex, where he was self-isolating with his children. "How could people be that negative? It just doesn't make sense" (*The Guardian*, 21 March 2020, p. 23).

But making sense of the pandemic as it was spreading involved so many unanticipated anxieties that people *projected* onto others. There were conflicts around what people could believe and social media messages that offered very different stories about the dangers people were facing. It's not easy shaping psychosocial imaginations that can engage with everyday fears and denials. Often these can be projected as anger and hatred of others who are blamed for spreading messages and videos people aren't ready to see. We need to shape psychosocial imaginations that can help us understand *different* forms of self-protection.[4]

Covid patient Karen Mannering similarly posted footage of herself on Facebook, imploring people to stay home, after being hospitalised with the virus while in her third trimester of pregnancy. As Jessica Murray reported in *The Guardian*, the video showed her "struggling to breathe" and speaking from her hospital bed with an oxygen tube in her nose. She warned people tempted by the prospect of meeting people, saying: "you are going to kill someone…it's not worth it." The beauty therapist from Herne Bay, Kent, later posted a video update to say she had come off oxygen for the first time in five days, and was still struggling to breathe: "So this is me managing to sit up, only for a minute but it's a start…" (*The Guardian*, 27 March 2020, p. 7).

Sharing his experience, columnist John Crace in *The Guardian* said:

> …the coronavirus is playing havoc with my mental health. I'd thought I had been doing OK at keeping my anxiety levels manageable, but over the weekend I completely collapsed. It was all I could do to get out of bed around lunchtime and even taking the dog for a walk felt horribly scary. Mostly I just lay curled up in a sustained panic attack, obsessing about an increasingly uncertain future.
>
> *(The Guardian, 21 March 2020, p. 34)*

As he also explained:

> My mother's care home is in lockdown, so I have no idea when I will next see her. My daughter and her husband are in an increasingly quarantined Minneapolis with all flights cancelled. My son and his girlfriend are holed up in Brighton. Often work provides an excellent distraction but now I was stuck in a catch-22 as what I was writing about was the very thing I was anxious about, … I couldn't bring myself to follow the news.
>
> *(p. 34)*

Crisis, Broken Futures and Tense Adaptations

The etymology of "crisis" is Greek: "krisis" means decision or judgement, political writer William Davis reminded us in *The Guardian*, as he described feeling a sense of "(inhabiting) a world that is temporarily up for grabs," or presenting possibilities of multiple actions all at once. Acknowledging the Imperial College predictions that the one "guaranteed exit route" from the pandemic, the Covid vaccine, was at that point a year away from readiness, Davis couldn't imagine a set of policies that could successfully navigate such a lengthy hiatus, and it would be harder still to implement them.

Referencing the "inevitable…deep global recession" to come, Davis painted a dark picture of seemingly indefinite chaos: "a breakdown of labour markets and the evaporation of consumer spending." In contrast to Brexit where there was an outside not drawn into the negotiations, this was a global health crisis in which a third of the world's population had already been locked down.

It was also a crisis *within* us all, haunting our inner lives and making us feel often at sea with ourselves, unable to tell where our fears and anxieties were coming from and how we might be able to discover more balance in our lives. Many people were turning to spiritual teachers and mindfulness practitioners. It was a crisis that crossed the boundaries of inner and outer life, as if suddenly life had become unknown and unknowing.

Davis said our contemporary view of crisis had been the 1970s, which in Britain set an economy and a society on a new path. It was this period that marked the collapse of the post war system of fixed exchange rates, capital controls and wage policies, which were thought to have led to uncontrollable inflation. This *also* created the conditions in which the new right of Margaret Thatcher and Ronald Reagan could rise to the rescue, offering a novel medicine of tax cuts, interest rate rises and attacks on organised labour. As Davis notes, "The 1970s inspired a vision of crisis as a wide-ranging shift in ideology, which has retained its hold over much of the left ever since" (*The Guardian*, 24 March 2020).

Reflecting on the aftermath of the 2008 global financial crisis, Davis notes that despite significant upheaval, the crisis did not meaningfully change policy. Instead, the "free-market Thatcherite" perspective gained even more prominence after initial public spending to rescue banks. The 2016 political upheavals aimed to challenge the "status quo" but lacked a "coherent alternative." However, the emergence of a "globalised capitalism" during the Wuhan health crisis caused huge disruptions worldwide through airline and transport routes. Davis points out that the coronavirus is not a distant "spectacle" but a *shared*, intense experience, making the present feel "closer to a war than a recession." Ultimately, Davis concludes, government policymakers will be judged based on the human cost.

But, reflecting upon the impact of the Lisbon earthquake in 1755 that killed as many as 75,000 people and the ways it eventually helped shape secular European life through the influence it had on Voltaire and Kant's Enlightenment thought, Davis anticipates: "It will take years or decades for the significance of 2020 to be fully understood." He also noted:

> …it is also a global turning point. There is a great deal of emotional, physical and financial pain in the immediate future. But a crisis of this scale will never be truly resolved until many of the fundamentals of our social and economic life have been remade.
>
> *(The Guardian, 24 March 2020)*

Anxieties, Missings and Fears

Monday 30 March 2020. I miss *not* being able to go over to sit with my brother Tony who is suffering with the virus. I have been able to talk on the phone but hearing him gasp for breath is upsetting and I feel helpless. But it is still good to hear him. We are doing whatever we can to support him. Anna has prepared some chicken soup – the "Jewish penicillin" – to be picked up by his friend.

I've also been in contact with another close friend of his. It's good to know that he is being held in the thoughts of friends and family who love him. Like so many friends and families across the country and around the world, we are hoping for a good outcome, but *fearful* that the virus might take a tight grip because, as people have reported, it seems to go for your weakest points.

Last night, as a family in different spaces, we gathered to listen to a home concert by Richard Thompson, the guitarist from Fairport Convention who has a global following. Many gathered on Facebook to hear him sing songs from different times in his long career. Our son-in-law Richard said how he missed the audience response that helped shape the atmosphere and his playing. With a light and humorous touch, Thompson reached out in sounds to all those who had gathered with him in his living room in New Jersey.

Zoom as a new technology was spreading fast, transforming global possibilities as people could gather online. So many people wrote in the chat how the songs brought light and a *sense of relief*, in dark and fearful times. Thompson promising to try to do a concert in two weeks gave people a sense of future. They expressed deep gratitude.

More generally, I miss just going out in the city and seeing people around. The streets round here are empty. When I went to Brent Park, I only saw another friend – an East End Afro-Caribbean ex-boxer who was walking a neighbour's dog. We have become close over the year but neither of us wanted to stand and walk. Something had shifted in our contact, and it could *not* be the same. I miss the contact but feel grateful I can still walk in the park every day. I could see a swan preparing her nest where she will soon sit for two months before giving birth. I wonder whether the swans and the ducks have realised a shift in atmosphere and the fear people now approach them with their bread offerings.

I feel grateful for the contact I can still have with nature. I also appreciate the technology that has allowed me to join the Leo Baeck College community for prayers. It is *not* the same as being assembled in the special prayer space at the college but listening to familiar voices was reassuring. I had woken up later than intended from a deep sleep and a dream where I was visiting the house I once lived in, in Tredegar Terrace, Mile End, with a friend, Jo Ryan.

The present owners were there as we looked at how the house had been transformed, walls taken down and light let in. I was missing a certain relationship to the past – wanting somehow to feel a connection with earlier times and places that carried meaning, as this part of the dream suggested. It was also good to finally receive a text from my friend Terry saying 'Still in the thick of Covid-19!! Too exhausted yet to be social…" We were all finding our own ways to navigate a crisis that none of us had anticipated or prepared for.

At the morning gathering a prayer, especially written for this time of Covid-19, helped to shape language that expressed what so many people wanted to say.

People seemed involved in a search for narratives that could help to *give voice* to what they were living through and the dark places they could feel trapped in. I'll frame it so it potentially talks across different secular and spiritual traditions in words that can resonate:

Living God,

In our hour of need we turn again to you, for we have nowhere else to turn.

We put our faith in you because you have proved your faithfulness time and again.

We affirm our love for you because you have never let us go.

We thank that you are not distant from us…

We pray as this pandemic spreads across our world, remembering all who have lost loved ones and pray for all those seriously ill at this time.

We uphold the National Health Service as it responds to this added pressure on its already overstretched services.

We pray for doctors and nurses and all in the caring professions, who work to help and support people as best as they can.

We remember those working behind the scenes testing samples, confirming results, giving information to patients….

May this crisis bring out the best in us, not the worst.

Help us to live by faith and not by fear; to build bridges not barriers, and to resist all who would speak ill of any other group.

May we not forget our responsibility to one another, not least to the vulnerable and the voiceless in our communities.

Help us to find ways of keeping in touch and offering reassurance…

We pray in the midst of the disruption it causes to normal life, bringing new fears and anxieties:

We pray for those who have been laid off as their work disappears; in light of the financial hardship for individuals and businesses; for the impact on the economy and pensions, when austerity has already left its mark….

We remember those who cannot visit loved ones in locked-down care homes; for the elderly whose social contacts have been severely curtailed; help us to find creative ways of keeping in touch, of assuring them they are not forgotten or ignored.

May congregations find new ways of living through this time. May we not forget our faith but draw strength from it. So may our worship be heartfelt…

Questioning Neo-Liberal Moral and Political Legacies

Under a headline "Coronavirus means we really are, finally, all in this together", John Harris in *The Guardian* recalled how in January just as China's Covid-19 story was turning critical, the story broke of Errol Graham, a grandfather of two and lover of football, who had died aged 57 in June 2018. Bailiffs pursuing him for non-payment of his rent had found Graham's body which weighed just four and a half stone. A coroner's report said he suffered from severe social anxiety and had isolated himself from even family and friends. Graham had had his benefits paused less than a year before his death when he failed to show for a "fitness for work" assessment. Upon his death, a letter written by Graham was found that pleaded with "welfare officials," to "judge me fairly" (*The Guardian*, 29 March 2020).

Graham was a particularly tragic victim of the "nasty, punitive benefits system" that has been in place for over a decade, and "inhuman rhetoric" it espouses, Harris suggests. People knew about it, but they *didn't* want to see, and they had grown so accustomed to a neoliberal common-sense that it was hard for them to break with it. Harris sees this exemplified in a narrative of the "skivers" versus "strivers," which takes aim at chronically ill and disabled people and fails to acknowledge myriad reasons preventing people from finding work. The benefits system, Harris makes clear, is dangerous: as he notes, in one month, "the National Audit office linked at least 69 suicides to the workings of the benefit system."

Yet six weeks later, a Conservative government in the face of the Covid-19 crisis was suddenly speaking the language of solidarity, compassion and responsibility for others. They seemed to be accepting that unemployment was a consequence of economics rather than a character failure. The chancellor Rishi Sunak was talking about people "not being able to pay the rent or the mortgage" and "not having enough set by for food and bills," so undermining that basic logic of the benefits machine.

As *Guardian* columnist Polly Toynbee noted there would be a shock for those new to the benefits system but somehow obliged to rely upon it. They would be trapped between the communitarian words of politicians and the help this might lead them to anticipate, and the *reality* they would have to face. They would discover how that supposed "welfare" falls far short of what is required to avoid debt, bad housing and ill health.

Toynbee said: "Millions of people are about to discover something they didn't know about Britain. There is no longer a safety net." She also noted:

> The incapacity of the HMRC (Her Majesty's Revenue and Customs) workforce, with 15,600 staff cut and 157 local offices closed: can they pay the wage subsidy to companies in time to save them? Many firms could still close, sending millions into unemployment.
>
> *(The Guardian, 24 March 2020)*

As Harris noted, the everyday cruelties and inhumanities might well return when politics returned to normal, evidence of how "deeply entrenched" in society they are, "which even this international tragedy might not shift." In 2018, as Harris reported, 43% of British people agreed that a generous welfare system generates "dependence" and 56% of respondents agreed that "most" jobseekers "could find a job if they really wanted one," compared with just 17% who disagreed.

Harris recognised how neoliberal common-sense can *shape* the thinking of working-class people, those whose everyday experience could show how misplaced it is. He recalled an interview with a 27-year-old man in Warrington who said he averaged 25 to 30 job applications a week, most of which had not even got a reply. The interviewee claimed he could have made more applications, but at your most dejected, it is easy to "feel the world owes you. And it doesn't." This is a sentiment that echoes a view held by politicians across political parties chasing votes and which Harris characterises as "a manic belief in personal responsibility" and a British character that encourages individuals "to focus your furies on people down the street."

George Osborne as editor of the *Evening Standard*, London's free newspaper, championed the slogan "London stands together." But Harris recalled Osborne's infamous speech in 2012, as Chancellor of the Exchequer when he thundered: "Where is the fairness… for the shift worker, leaving home in the dark … (looking) up at the closed blinds of their next-door neighbour sleeping off a life on benefits?" In response to this attitude, Harris noted in the time of coronavirus, individuals should "(embrace) their common humanity" by "checking on each other's welfare." Polly Toynbee in response to Osborne's appearance at the Covid Inquiry asked, "How did they get away with it?" with his evidence being a useful reminder of how cleverly he persuaded voters that his state-shrinking austerity was not an ideology, but an economic necessity, "essential to rebuild fiscal space to respond to future economic shocks". He even claimed he tried to "ring fence" the NHS, despite cutting its funding per capita (theguardian.com, Thursday 22 June 2023).

As Toynbee notes:

> He simply rejected the evidence of Dame Sally Davies, the former chief medical officer, who was close to tears as she said the UK did not have enough resilience to cope with the epidemic, with fewer doctors, nurses or hospital beds than similar countries, echoing Sir Michael Marmot's damning testimony on the impact of inequality.

She remarks, "Osborne began with a little homily on his 'heartfelt sympathy' for the bereaved, sounding about as sincere as the wolf grieving over eating up Little Red Riding Hood's granny." Toynbee also points out, "Even if you accept his economic analysis that cuts were necessary, there was no excuse for piling them on to children, while protecting old people and wealthy people."

Though it had been widely conceded by authorities in the NHS and public health that austerity worsened the pandemic, neither Cameron nor Osborne was ready to concede this. As Andy Beckett notes, they are still in denial about the damage they inflicted on Britain: "'they both claimed that it had made the pandemic bailouts possible, by rescuing the government's finances. It was just the kind of move that Johnson would have made: presenting a contentious or discredited policy as a triumph" (theguardian.com, Friday 23 June 2023).

Notes

1 Governments were slow to respond to the threats of the unprecedented challenges of the global pandemic. To trace how governments and people responded see, for instance, Ellen Rodger *Pandemic Strategies and the Global Economy* (Crabtree Publishing Company 2021) and Adam Tooze *Shutdown: How Covid Shook the World's Economy* (New York: Viking 2021) who compares the global coronavirus shutdown to the global financial crisis of 2008–2009. Few previous economic or health disasters can match the scale and global reach of the pandemic when the entire world economy contracted by 20% in a matter of weeks; nor in the historic record of modern capitalism had 95% of the world's economies suffered all at the same time.

2 How notions of progress identified with the control and domination of nature help to shape the colonising ambitions of European modernities and how these are tied into dominant white Christian masculinities are investigated in Victor J.J. Seidler *Unreasonable Men: Masculinity and Social Theory* (London and New York: Routledge 1993). More recently it has also been a theme in *Ethical Humans: Life, Love, Labour, Learning and Loss* (London and New York: Routledge 2022).

3 For some reflections upon trust and vulnerability as we learn to think of ourselves as ethical humans and re-imagine the terms of moral philosophy and social theory as we confront the workings of structural inequalities and painful histories of oppression, displacement and grief, see Victor Jeleniewski Seidler *Ethical Humans: Life, Love, Labour, Learning and Loss* (London and New York: Routledge 2022).

4 For helpful discussions in the shaping of psychosocial imaginations that can help in the revisioning of sociology and social theory see, for example, Stephen Frosh *Psychoanalysis Outside the Clinic: Interventions in Psychosocial Studies* (Red Globe Press 2010); Victor J.J. Seidler *Transforming Masculinities: Men, Cultures, Bodies, Power, Sex and Love* (London and New York: Routledge 2005) and *Embodying Identities: Culture, Differences and Social Theory* (Bristol: Policy Press 2010); Neil Cooper and Sandra Kielty *Psychosocial Theory and Self and Society* (London: Pearson Education Ltd 2007); Stephen Frosh *New Voices in Psychosocial Studies* (London: Palgrave Macmillan 2019) and Stephen Frosh (ed) *Psychosocial Imaginaries: Perspectives on Temporality, Subjectivities and Activism* (London: AIAA 2015); Wendy Holloway and Tony Jefferson *Doing Qualitative Research Differently: Free Association, Narrative and the Interview Method* (London: Sage 2000); Wendy Holloway *The Capacity to Care: Gender and Ethical Subjectivity* (London: Routledge 2006) and *Knowing Mothers: Researching Maternal Identity* (London: Palgrave 2015).

8

SUFFERINGS, ILLNESS, FEARS, BREATH AND RESTRICTIONS

Different Worlds

There was a striking interview on the BBC Radio 4's "World at One" programme on 17 March 2020 by presenter Sarah Montague with the contemporary historian Peter Hennessy. He believed the coronavirus was a watershed moment in British history. The programme started with a clip of him saying: "What is being flung at us is of such a magnitude that future historians will divide post-war Britain between BC and AC – before Corona and after Corona."

He saw this as a pivotal point. That must have surprised people slowly coming to terms with the suffering that coronavirus was bringing. They were shocked to be part of a global health emergency which no authority seemed to have anticipated. The WHO would eventually announce a pandemic that could affect almost the whole planet.

Sarah Montague acknowledged:

> We are living in extraordinary times. Our whole way of life, our sophisticated fast-moving world, has been brought to a halt by a tiny particle and though it might be one of the simplest organisms on the planet, it has proved to be one of the most devastating. We don't know how to fight it and stop its spread. It has led to borders going up around the world….it is not just countries sealing themselves off, now families are doing the same.

She said:

> Like millions of others, I am working from home, the World at One studio is now my kitchen table…Everything we took for granted seems under threat at the moment. Our advanced technology and medicines seem powerless. The best

DOI: 10.4324/9781003296874-8

> we can do is wash our hands and stay inside waiting, hoping that human ingenuity will find a solution and restore the life that we knew.

Lord Hennessy thought we were entering the dawn of a new era.

> It shows that even the most advanced technological societies are vulnerable to forces of nature. We are rediscovering those old virtues of altruism, stoicism and social solidarity. What we are going through is a stress testing of our cherished public services and our health service.

He said the atmosphere was already so different from the atmosphere of the Brexit debate. "The whole tone and pitch of our national conversation has changed."

He said:

> A new politics might come out of this with a new political language. This will be very different from the one we have been living through. The Corona question doesn't take spin. It is entirely different from the questions we have been used to… This virus could be a great unifier for this virus is blind to national boundaries, local boundaries, class, status, income distinctions between us in our society. It is silent and it is spreading, and it is making us look at things in new very different ways.

Hennessy thought it might be unifying, even if at that moment it was dividing us and making us afraid of other humans because of it. He said:

> It is reaching into every household in the land, even if we are atomising as a society with the need for social distancing. It is bringing us together because it is a shared experience of a kind that we haven't had since the Second World War.

He also thought we were learning about the values of community and solidarity that we had lost sight of in these neoliberal times, but which are necessary for decent and just human societies.[1]

He had little doubt that something had changed forever:

> This will leave a level of anxiety lingering in all our minds at what could happen in a matter of days and weeks. This will be edged deep into the consciousness and the memory, and it will be a benchmark against which we test future developments. This will be known as the Corona year and the sequence of the divide between AC and BC will be there ever more.

The ways people had grown used to organising their time and giving a structure to their lives through leaving home to go to work, were gone. Freedoms taken for granted were no longer there. We could not even leave our homes without a sense of an invisible threat presented by any other human being we met on the streets or in the park.

People were going to feel restricted, trapped and even imprisoned at home, sometimes with people they found difficult to live with in the first place. Unable to take refuge in a different life, the world and relationships at work, people felt obliged to stay in a home that could be tense, even fearful and violent, with no possibility of escape.

Cultures, Risks and Differences

Within days, suburban streets felt dead with hardly anybody around. I took my morning walk in more or less empty roads. Anyone walking in my direction was suddenly reduced to an object to be avoided. Different communities responded in different ways. There were certain hot spots where fear of social isolation, for example in the West Midlands, explained a sharp rise in coronavirus cases and where, as Nazia Parveen reported for *The Guardian*, 28 deaths had been recorded by the 21 March.

The Birmingham MP Khalid Mahmood told her that elderly Muslim and Sikh people in the area were struggling with the social distancing guidelines and that despite most religious services having been cancelled, some older people were continuing to attend mosques and gurdwaras. “Part of it is because they feel religious observance is more important now than ever – they feel they may die and lose loved ones – so they need to pray. These are people who have incredibly strong religious convictions and it’s hard for them to stay away” (*The Guardian*, 21 March 2020, p. 6).

Mahmood added: “For some of these elderly people the gurdwara and mosque is where they’ve always met their friends and they are finding it hard to give that up because they are scared of becoming socially isolated.” He was encouraging people to set up FaceTime chats so they could keep in touch with friends and help them with praying at home. This was *not* easy where people’s identities were framed by being part of a community. Saidul Saeed, a charity worker, said that panic buying was a particular problem. “You’ve got all these people standing next to each other for hours in queues trying to pay, which is not going to be helpful with infections” (p. 6).

London hospitals by the 21 March were seeing a 15-fold rise in cases of patients seriously ill with Covid-19. Hospitals across the capital were dealing with rising numbers of patients, many of whom were being ventilated to try to keep them alive. Medics said numbers were doubling every three or four days and that the city’s NHS would be treating thousands of people with the disease within a fortnight.

The Guardian reported that the number of people confirmed or suspected of having Covid-19 being treated in an intensive care unit (ICU) in hospitals in South London rose from seven on 6 March to 93 on 17 March – a 15-fold increase according to unpublished NHS figures. “There’s been an explosion in the numbers that began last weekend and that continued all week, with more and more cases every day,” said one London intensive care specialist (*The Guardian,* 21 March 2020, p. 6).

ICU doctors in south London worried that 86 out of 93 cases required ventilators, highlighting a high demand for critical medical attention. None of the cases were level-one critical care (occasional oxygen) and only seven were categorised as level two, with patients receiving non-invasive ventilation through face masks. One doctor explained that for the most part, patients needed more interventionist "level three care, in which they are anaesthetised and have a tube put down their throat and the ventilator takes over the work of their lungs while they are unconscious."

These figures were the first to underline the steep surge in cases over a weekend in London. The capital was facing more stringent social distancing measures after accounting for a third of the coronavirus deaths. An ICU consultant at one London hospital described the "panic stations" setup that was failing to deal with the volume of patients. Doctors also raised concerns about widespread shortages of personal protective equipment needed, including face coverings, to treat Covid-19 patients.

Northwick Park in North-West London the previous Thursday evening was forced to declare a critical incident after running out of critical care beds. It meant other hospitals were asked to help look after patients because they could no longer cope. A senior manager at another London trust said it raised serious concerns about the ability of London's hospitals to deal with the surge of patients. "Given we're in the low foothills of this virus, this is fucking petrifying," the official told the *Health Service Journal* (*The Guardian*, 20 March 2020, p. 6).

Wordless, Fearful and Breathless

Wednesday 1 April 2020. When I went on my walk to Brent Park on Tuesday, I was already wordless and feeling mute when I saw my new friend walking with his wife. I waved and realised that I was waving as I passed people in the street. Since I was keeping my distance and often swerving around them, I wanted the wave to acknowledge their human presence.

But on Tuesday, I was also fearful and turned in on myself as my brother Tony had been taken to Barnet hospital at 3.30am. He had waited for six hours for the ambulance to arrive to test his oxygen levels. There was fear across his face, as his friend Rhys was to tell me later. They passed the time waiting for the ambulance, watching TV. It was a difficult and anxious time. Tony had not wanted to go to the hospital. He wanted to get through the Covid-19 on his own.

That afternoon he had agreed for me to ring his GP and put him in the picture about what was going on. I spoke to the doctor who knew that Tony was over 70 and had high-blood pressure. I mentioned that he was breathless, and I knew that when he spoke to Tony, he would tell him that he needed to go to hospital. I was grateful that he would be there before the NHS became overwhelmed with the sheer number of Covid-19 cases so that he might not get access to a ventilator. It was only later we realised that this was actually at the height of the first wave and that many London hospitals were already working at over full capacity.

I could not speak. I felt frozen. It was as if Tony was already dead in some way for me. This was amplified by hearing that he had not been able to take his mobile phone with him because it could be infected. This was a myth that I had readily absorbed because it emphasised the *separation* I felt – as if he had been transferred into *a different world* and I would never see him or hear from him again.

It turned out that he had taken another phone and a laptop and that he had been able to message some of his friends in the afternoon. I wondered how he had been able to do this. It felt it was a kind of miracle, as if the boundary that separated Barnet hospital from the rest of the world had somehow been breached. He was not imprisoned after all or if he was, he could still communicate and get messages from the outside world.

Tony's first text to a friend read: "At Barnet General, sleeping and resting" to be followed up at 4pm saying: "Let's live in hope. At 70 no regrets. Loved the journey." Later in the evening he was able to talk to Rhys who told us: "This was the worst 24 hours of Tony's life." This just intensified my fear. I realised that I had turned in on myself all day and had been able to communicate with hardly anyone. This was a pattern I think many men will be familiar with, at least of my generation. It can seem easier to reach out to others when we feel good but hard to reach out to people when we are feeling down or depressed.

I realised that Anna, my partner, responded to crisis in a really different way. She had spent most of the day speaking to a friend, telling her what had been going on with Tony and allowing herself to feel loved and nourished by the support she was receiving. Often as men, we can still feel that in a time of crisis we can *only* really rely upon ourselves, as if this is a sign of strength.

Personal Trauma and Emotional Histories

I realised that I was reliving fears of my older brother Johnny's sudden hospitalisation in 1982 and later diagnosis of cancer. Memories were surfacing. We *carry* embodied emotional memories that can be triggered. Events in the present somehow make the past present to us. I had been able to visit Johnny in hospital, but he was only to live for seven weeks – exactly the 49 days counted in the Omer in the Jewish calendar between Passover when he got ill and taken to hospital and the eve of Shavuot – the receiving of the law at Sinai.

References to the Jewish dates makes me aware that, even living in a secular world, I have always at some level, like so many people carrying migrant and refugee histories, learnt to live between different worlds. People from ethnic and non-Christian backgrounds live their lives across different calendars. They learn, tacitly and privately, to negotiate between separate civilisations.

This becomes second nature. Often it is only at moments of crisis when these different worlds come together, and references are made. Unless you are studying religious and ethnic minorities, these differences remain unspoken. They can be a sign of embarrassment and unease in a culture that focusses upon assimilation and often teaches us to be silence about sources of difference, even as it acknowledges multicultural and multi-faith traditions.

Somehow the timing of Johnny's death has always felt significant. Griefs are so often connected and *blend* with each other. Loss *is* personal while at the same time being lived communally around the globe. Covid-19 was causing suffering that was never anticipated. People are making connections with past losses. For me, the time of year of Johnny's illness and death was being uneasily echoed through Tony being in hospital with Covid-19, at a similar time. Part of me can't really believe that people go into hospital and can come out alive.

The echoes of Johnny – my older brother's death – when he was just 38 – shaped a fearful anticipation that I *was* somehow destined to relive this experience again with Tony. But I had learnt through years of psychotherapy that I could learn to respond differently. There was a moment when I realised that I *could interrupt* my own pattern of withdrawal into an inner space *so* making myself inaccessible to those around. I could listen and be open to learning from my wife Anna. Possibly I could also attempt to reach out to friends and tell them *how fearful* I was feeling about Tony's reported breathlessness in hospital.

In Jewish tradition there is a connection between breath and soul. There is the vision that you *receive* life through God's breathing a soul into you. This means the experience of being breathless carries a particular cultural fear. The experience can be quite terrifying even to hear about. When I heard that Tony had said the last 24 hours were the worst in his life, I was shocked. I found it hard to trust that feeling this way, especially on your first day in hospital when you've always hated hospitals, could be part of the process of illness. I remembered that the last time he was in hospital, years back with pneumonia, he had signed himself out against the doctor's wishes.

I felt terribly fearful and found it hard to trust that he was in good hands. I had learnt from Anna to shift my habitual insular pattern. I spent the afternoon writing texts and emails to people to let them know what was going on and *how* scared I was feeling. I felt really supported by the responses and promises that others would send healing and prayers. If there was a time for prayers, whatever tradition you could call upon, this seemed to be one. I had to also support others in the family. We were separated physically and could be together only intermittently through Zoom and social media. Like people around the world, we were grateful for these new technologies.

Somehow hearing that people with Covid-19 had survived, even though it had been a very gruelling experience, gave me hope. Possibly I could interrupt my family's emotional legacies, tracing back to the multiple family deaths in the Holocaust – the Shoah – that often left me with catastrophic fears – that something terrible *is* about to happen, even if there is no rational cause for feeling this way.

I think it's a pattern hard to dislodge because of the traumatic histories we carry *as* a family. It also traces back to my father's early death when I was just five. Many people with migrant histories of loss and displacement seem to carry similar experiences. They can share a sense, as children, that they were often left *alone* to deal with the different griefs of migration, loss and displacement. Adults can assume that as children we were *too* young to understand – so they didn't have to help us through our mourning. I learnt, from an early age, that when terrible things happen you are often left on your own to sort them out.

We are more conditioned by the embodied histories and cultural memories we carry than we like to suppose. As second generation of Holocaust refugees and survivors, these can be difficult to discern when we grew up with tense silences and few words to help us navigate. It was as *if* Tony had already died as soon as he was in hospital, and I felt I could *not* make any connection with him when this was *not* the reality. This was a mythical structure I had locked myself into. It took a couple of days to realise I could actually phone the hospital, and speak to one of the nurses on his ward and find out how he was doing. This had *not* really occurred to me. I had accepted that he had no phone, when the next day I learnt he had been able to send a few texts out.

Somehow, I had learnt to deal with feelings of feared loss by behaving *as if* the person has already died, so that I did *not need* to fear a loss that could come. I expected the worst to happen, as a way of dealing with my fears in the present. Other people in the family across generations responded differently, but given the physical separations in lockdown, we were not together to see how others reacted. Like other people in lockdown, even in very different material and class circumstances, it was *harder to check* our senses of reality in relation to others, as we might have traditionally learnt to rely upon. We were left more vulnerable to our own instincts.

What had also limited my contact with people was my response – because of defences created by my own histories of loss – that if I'm no longer connecting to people in everyday life, then it is *as if* they are gone – that at some level they cease to exist. This has been an issue I've had to *work through* in my friendships and over time I've learnt to shift this pattern, but in moments of crisis it can return.

But I've also learnt to shape a language that can explain *why* I don't contact people, especially when I feel down, a trait that I think is gendered but can also move across genders and sexualities. But even when people recognise this emotional pattern, it isn't easy to change. Hopefully this pattern *is* ending, as I learn *how* to deepen my connection with myself and others but there are times of regression to habitual patterns.

Unless we can soften boundaries between sociology and psychology, in the shaping for formative sociologies, these issues will *not* be given serious attention but only be appreciated as of personal concern. They call for a deepening of understanding of ourselves as vulnerable humans across differences of class, race, ethnicities, genders and sexualities. Across generations, we are subject to colonial histories of violence and displacement and scarred by structural relations of power, discipline and abuse. Somehow all these features of life need to be engaged in renewing the relationships between philosophy and social theory.

Rituals, Spirituality and Everyday Practices

As part of creating an everyday structure during the isolation of Covid times, I've found it helpful to connect through Zoom to the morning Shachrit prayers even though some days I can't take any words in. I need to just sit quietly and listen. It was wonderful to see Debs, a fifth-year rabbinic student leading the prayers with such feeling. Somehow it helped me, knowing she had just recovered from Covid-19, so breaking a fear that I was still in the grip of. She gave evidence that people could return from the dead. I was touched by the slowness with which she read in Hebrew –

> My God, the soul
> You have given me is pure, for You created it,
> You formed it and You made it live within me…

She repeated this a couple of times with a voice that had been softened through her recent experience of the Coronavirus.

She talked about her own experience of a restriction of breath and the difficulties of breathlessness. This had brought a change which meant she read this prayer in a much slower way, connecting to her own in-breath and out-breath. She maintained a similar slowness as she read other prayers. She stressed *how* the restrictions in the human body are reflected in the organisation of social institutions. She read a passage written by the revolutionary Rosa Luxembourg from prison. She described hearing the footsteps of her guards as a mark of her restriction, but *also* how she could feel – in a way she could not explain – joy at being alive.

Rosa Luxembourg's connection between her inner feelings and the power structure within capitalist societies *is* reflected generations later in feminisms that recognises how the personal *is* political. This gives recognition to *voice* and the ways it reflects experiences and connections we have with ourselves. As heterosexual men, we can also learn *how* estranged and distanced, we are from ourselves as we face tendencies to rationalise and intellectualise experience.

These structures can be hidden within post-structuralist anti-humanisms that can present themselves as more theoretically driven. Insights into *how* the personal *is* political, without reducing the significance of voicing personal experience or minimising the difficulties of engaging in truth with others, can also be learnt from LGBT communities and non-gender binary people. As vulnerable humans it takes time to value and honour our differences and to voice experiences that otherwise remain hidden and shamed.

But there was a danger in the turn towards post-structuralisms, whatever insights they offered, since the philosophers Foucault, Derrida and Deleuze were *so* different in their approaches. In different ways, within traditions of secular rationalism, ethics could be treated as one discursive practice amongst others. This could make it difficult to recognise ourselves as ethical humans within discrete social, historical and cultural contexts. They could leave people in an *externalised* relationship with their own lived experience so making it difficult to appreciate the long-term effects of abuse, violence and emotional neglect. It can so easily be reductive to treat inner experiences as if they were an effect of discursive practices. The very category of "experience" becomes suspect, and people can be left muted, unable to really find words to express what they are living through.

This can be distressing in the time of Coronavirus when so many feel abandoned and bereft in unfamiliar emotional spaces. Many are searching for their own voices and new theoretical narratives that engage language and experience, rather than assuming in post-structuralist terms, that there is no experience that is *not* discursive. They don't want their experiences to be dismissed as ethical and vulnerable humans and their confidence in voicing themselves undermined.

Often, they are keen to find words that *can* help express what they are living through in an unanticipated global pandemic and the personal and cultural memories it has brought to the surface. There is a way that Wittgenstein's later philosophy can help offer a counter-tradition, that is Hebraic in inspiration as he frames it and keeps alive tensions between language and experience but also invite different ways of understanding ourselves as ethical and vulnerable humans, as I've tried to show in *Ethical Humans: Life, Love, Labour, Learning and Loss.* Post-structuralisms can, despite their explicit intentions, help produce an externalised relationship with self, where even the languages of "self" and "experience" are deemed to be "embarrassing", as the novelist Iris Murdoch suggests in her discussions of Derrida.[2]

There was another prayer that felt universal in its aspiration. It seemed particularly timely in its appeal to an ethics of care and compassion, when so many people were suffering from illness or were fearful of the deaths of those who they loved and felt close to:

> With deep love You have loved us, and with great and overflowing tenderness. You have taken pity on us. Source of our life… show us compassion... because of our ancestors who trusted in You, for You taught them rules to live by, to do Your will with their whole heart. Let our eyes see the light of Your teaching and our hearts embrace Your commands. Give us integrity to love You and to fear You. So shall we never lose our self-respect, not be put to shame….

When people we love are in hospital struggling with breathlessness and trying to heal, they often appreciate healing energies we send them through prayer. Of course, prayer will often be dismissed within a rationalist culture that has little time for it. But within post-secular philosophy and social theory we can still understand the place healing thoughts have in many people's lives, even those who don't regard themselves as religious, but have possibly been influenced by new age spiritual traditions. These are rendered as personal and private concerns that, as yet, have no place within academic disciplines, too often set within the taken for granted terms of secular rationalism.

Often it is a resource that people draw upon in a time of crisis, whatever religious or spiritual traditions they have grown up with as children. They seek ways to give strength to those in desperate need. It provides a language that seems indispensable in the moment, even if it is *not* related to any sense of belief as faith. There is a materiality of energy at work in prayer and in spiritual traditions which is affirmed through the evidence of neuroscience that has also often confirmed findings from psychoanalysis and post-analytic psychotherapies. Energies can work in mysterious ways *in* a reductive world where science is a central form of knowledge.

But as Iris Murdoch insisted in her philosophy and often acknowledged within eco-feminist movements, there are other aesthetic, moral and spiritual ways of knowing. The human sciences have often been too dismissive in the attention they are willing to give traditions that fall outside a secular rationalism and too narrow in their readings of Marx and Freud, especially when they had been read through Althusser and Lacan.

I was struck how friends in these difficult times eventually admitted they had been practising mindfulness and listening to spiritual teachers, though they would *not* mention this to their colleagues or students, out of a fear of embarrassment. It says a lot about a neoliberal culture or form of life that we have learnt to be *embarrassed* about *lived experiences*.

Within a neoliberal common sense, life is often, across intersectional differences, carefully compartmentalised. At work we might feel obliged to think and feel in particular ways but at home, especially in post-secular times, we might find space *to* explore what has been rendered *unspeakable* within the academy and wider secular culture. We might turn to fiction to explore realms that would be closed down within a culture of secular rationalism. We might be searching to make sense of experiences that fall outside of a secular common-sense. We learn to share more of our emotional and spiritual lives with those we care about, as we live through times of crisis that have challenged traditional rationalist certainties and brought us face to face with the deaths of those close to us and so also with our own mortalities.

Personal Hauntings and Public Health

If sociology deals with questions of spirituality, it very much seeks to explain belief through social factors, at some level to explain them away. Even the sociology of religion as traditionally imagined has found it difficult *to engage* with religious and spiritual beliefs *as* shaping everyday experience and relationships. This is something that Ludwig Wittgenstein explores, at least in his notebooks, where he talks about *how* beliefs matter in transforming everyday lives. He has learnt from American philosopher William James's theory in *The Varieties of Religious Experience.* He investigates what energies religious beliefs help release and whether they can help to deepen a person's relationships with themselves and with others.[3]

These are also questions that Iris Murdoch engages in her difficult but insightful *Metaphysics as a Guide to Morals*. She questions a certain aspect of the way

Wittgenstein talks about language games and forms of life in linguistic terms. According to her, this makes it difficult to fully acknowledge inner lived experiences and what it means for people to give voice to different levels of their lived experience or different levels of consciousness.

Murdoch, in her later writings, influenced by Simone Weil, largely relies upon Plato to make sense of ascending levels of consciousness and the depths of connection people *can* develop with themselves and others. As they learn to be more *truthful* and *honest* in their relationships, so they can gain more *access* to their emotional and spiritual selves. But it is harder for Murdoch in her later writings to stay in touch with the moral and political understandings that informed her identification with the left, especially in her earlier writings. We need a vision of ourselves as ethical and vulnerable humans that *can* move easily between the personal and the political. This means learning *how* to engages intersectionally with the workings of structural inequalities that means people are facing very different risks and uncertainties in struggling to survive and put food on the table in the time of Covid.

In a piece written for the *Boston Review*, Michael Bronski in an article entitled "Fighting for Public Health" recognises that "The HIV/AIDS and Covid-19 pandemics are very different," but both show that the USA has always failed to make "the connection between community and personal well-being" (*Boston Review*, 1 April 2020). This struck me as referring to the feminist insight that the "personal is political" – even though the language was framed through the terms of feminist post-structuralism. As Bronski notes: "For queer people over the age of 30, a spectre haunts the Covid-19 pandemic. A disease that threatens all of our loved ones and upends our world? Since the early 1980s, we have lived through it with HIV/AIDS."

Framing the strong "cultural and political parallels" of the viruses, Bronski laments that the USA "learned almost nothing from HIV about how to deal forthrightly and honestly with a major health crisis," and that the nationwide underestimation of the importance of supporting public health on the "understanding that the health of each group and person is fully dependent on the health of all" was to the country's detriment.

We have long been aware of the interdependent connection between the health of the community and the health of the individual, advocated by health and social care pioneers such as the American nurse Lillian Wald, who saw examples of this daily in her work with New York immigrants in the late 19th century. We also need to recover social and political theories that appreciate the interrelation *between* individual lives and collective and community lives, framed through the institutions and moral cultures of late capitalism.

The notion of the "public" seems to be at odds with US traditions of "individualism, competition, and capitalism," bearing "the taint of association with the lower classes" and "being a drain on society." Bronski notes that: "Culture shapes not only how we view disease, but how we experience it," and in his example, disease is something for the individual to strive against.

He said this can help appreciate how: "Because of our cultural biases, the *concept* of risk tends to play out as a logic of blame: Who is responsible for this disease? Who should be avoided? Who should be contained?" He recalls how William F. Buckley, a conservative spokesperson proposed in a *New York Times* op-ed on 18 March 1986: "Everyone detected with AIDS should be tattooed in the upper forearm, to protect common-needle users, and on the buttocks, to prevent the victimization of other homosexuals."

Bronski notes that in the age of Covid-19, the Trump administration (with the President acting as "ringmaster") sought to "(characterise) Chinese people as agents of disease," having the effect that a surging number of hate crimes were reported against Asian Americans in the wake of Covid's arrival in the USA. Following the research of thinkers such as British anthropologist Mary Douglas, who in her book *Purity and Danger* warned that disease and concepts of contamination always give rise to othering, Bronski notes that viruses tend to produce narratives that promote division and separate the "pure" from the "impure."[4]

Many people advised to stay at home across the world could easily fear the outside as a space of danger. There can be antagonism within relationships as one partner, often men in heterosexual relationships, might insist on going out for walks while their partners might fear that they are threatening to bring the virus back into the home and so put them in danger. Often these antagonistic relationships can, at an extreme, provoke domestic violence as people feel locked away with their children and desperate as to *how* they are going to cope with limited incomes in limited spaces.

Speaking on the rise of the religious Right in *The New York Times*, Katherine Stewart made a compelling case that: "denial of science and critical thinking among religious ultraconservatives now haunts the American response to the coronavirus crisis" saying Donald Trump's reliance on that base had worsened, if not caused, the virus's spread.

As Bronski recognised, HIV and Covid are contracted in radically different ways, with the former having "limited" conditions for transmission, and the latter transmitting "easily, efficiently, even casually." It is easy to contract Covid without knowing who passed it on to you, which, Bronski notes, in theory at least, "should reduce the miasma of blame: we might all be someone's Patient Zero." This did not stop state departments encouraging federal agencies "to blame China for a coverup that had caused the pandemic," and politicians, such as Mike Pompeo, the then-Secretary of State using the phrase "Wuhan virus" in his briefings to further encourage this agenda of blame.

In a postscript to the article, Bronski claimed that "separateness" and "isolation" were the "hallmarks" of the Covid pandemic, sadly dwelling on the prohibition of even the "most casual intimacies" and the halting of vital social and behavioural rituals that bond us: that things that were "public (had) now become private."

This he sees as in stark contrast to the crest of the HIV and Aids crisis of the 1980s and 1990s; although those years were "horrifying, confusing and grief-filled,"

Bronski "experienced them as being about "closeness…(c)ommunity was what defined both the grief and the shared devastation …and the resistance."

Isolation, Bodies and Loneliness

"The only person I have touched in a week is my two-year old daughter," wrote Leslie Jamison in *Since I Became Symptomatic* (nybooks.com). "Every selfie I take of us is a photograph of me trying to inhale her."

When she contracted the virus, she described a sense of "shame" over its "intimate" nature. She paid attention to it closely: "what does it feel like in my body today? Shivering under blankets. A hot itch behind the eyes." She dwells on the strangeness of losing intimacy with other people: "First, I lose the touch of other bodies; then I lost the air." This was particularly challenging for her as a single mother, sharing that it felt like "inside of your mind has become an insane asylum echoing with the sound of your own voice reading the same picture books over and over again."

Sharing an experience that still reminds many people of what they lived through:

> When I wake with my heart pounding in the middle of the night, my sheets are soaked with sweat that must be full of virus. The virus is my new partner, our third companion in the apartment, wetly draped across my body in the night. When I get up for water I have to sit on the floor, halfway to the sink, so I don't faint.

My brother Tony said something similar – he had fainted a couple of times on the way to the toilet in the middle of the night. But he was much older, in his early 70s.

Jamison dwelt on her pre-pandemic intimate life: "I can remember sex before quarantine: the opposite of distancing, the opposite of illness, the opposite of restraint." The pandemic changed the relationship that so many had with their bodies, perceiving what had been normal before as the remotest possibility, at a time when physical touch became hazardous, and the most prosaic physical actions took on new challenges and resonances.

Shock and Impossibilities of Trust

Friday 3 April 2020. I had wanted to believe that although my brother had had a really hard day on Tuesday he had turned a kind of corner by Wednesday midday when he seemed able to send messages to people. I dared to trust and to breathe more easily, even though I had felt unable to speak on Tuesday just taking in the gravity of the situation if he was moved onto a ventilator. I also felt relieved that he had arrived in time for that to be available knowing that in two weeks' time, because of his age and high blood pressure, he might not have even been given the option. In this regard, at least, he had been lucky.

By mid-afternoon on Wednesday when we were scheduled to have a Skype meeting with friends in Oxford, I felt I was able to breathe a little more easily and was prepared to talk about the anxieties of the past few days. I would have been quite unable to speak just a day earlier.

But when we ended the Skype meeting, Anna received a text that silenced her and brought immediate tears to her eyes. She was in shock and could barely speak. Gradually she read it out and said it was from Tony – it was a stark text saying that he was dying and asking for forgiveness from anyone he had wronged in the family. It was an ending, and he was saying goodbye. My body went rigid, and I felt shocked. I just cried and felt a terrible longing for Tony – to be near him and to be there with him, while knowing that we could not even visit the hospital and that he would be dying alone.

We felt desperate. Gradually able to speak through tears and a sense of horror, we decided to call Rhys who was in closest contact. He was shocked and said that the Tony had sent a similar message to two other people close to him. He was preparing for an ending of his life. But somehow Rhys had been in contact with the hospital a little earlier and knew that they had adjusted his oxygen levels down. It was such a relief that a medical procedure might have affected Tony's mind, though we knew that could have been a false hope we were creating for ourselves.

I recalled that when in 1982 I first visited my older brother Johnny in Westminster hospital, he was completely out of it and hallucinating. I spoke to nurses who said that it takes time for them to get the right level of pain relief and that I should *not* be shocked. I remembered this years later, but still I was finding it hard to trust – I felt in the moment my faith had been shattered and my talk of "turning corners" had been a sham. It was possibly a way of comforting myself and others but a failure *to really face* the reality of the situation which was far grimmer.

We tried to believe that his goodbye message – his ending of life text – was an outcome of his confusion created by his oxygen levels – but at the same time it was hard to trust this. On another level we felt this *could* be the end and we had to prepare ourselves for his death. As we talked to Rhys, we talked about the need to prepare for his death – that he might well die and that so many people were *not* getting through at his age, that this was a real possibility we *still* had to face. All I could do was to meditate and send healing to him that night.

Trusting Ourselves and Fearful Anticipations

I've been thinking about *how* we learn to rely on others or whether as the Danish philosopher and theologian Knud Ejler Logstrup recognised, we come into the world trusting that others will be there for us, but then relationships disappoint or events happen, that lead us to distrust people. The first paper I published was about Marx and it was entitled "Trusting Ourselves" – a title that would still be met with ambivalence. I know it has been a life process for me *to believe* that others *can* really be there for me. It was a significant moment in my relationship with Anna when I could really take this in – and somehow embody with trust – that she was *really there* for me, when I was in need.

As I've mentioned, the still haunting pattern stretches back to my early childhood, and my father's early death, when he was on a business trip to New York when I was just five. Somehow, I learnt that the only way of staying *in* connection with him was to *allow* part of me to die at the same time – and it has been years of helpful psychotherapy to retrieve these aspects of myself. It is strange *how* we still learn to hide large areas of our lives that are deemed too personal and out place, even within a discipline like sociology that hopes to include the whole of life.

So often we still seem to hide so much of what goes on in our lives, even though, at some level, we recognise its social significance and how much we can learn from it. The personal is never just personal. Even if in Emile Durkheim's hands, sociology sought to radically separate itself from psychology as a discipline that supposedly dealt with individuals, within the terms of a positivist tradition of scientific rationalism, this was never the whole story.

What is difficult in relation to illness – which is why we so often avoid thinking about its possibility – is to accept that you do *not* have the control over your life, decisions, and actions that you usually take for granted. It is easy to feel angry at your body for letting you down when you get ill. But there was also a danger that you minimised the threats of coronavirus. You got on with work as long as possible and somehow continued to think, as Tony did, that it would be *no* bad thing if you got the virus because, as Johnson and Trump were insisting, in those early days, it was no worse than the flu and you would have immunity. It meant Tony did *not* isolate himself when he should have. He also took risks both with his own health and those he was in contact with when he should not have done.

To talk about *losing* contact with aspects of yourself or reconnecting to core aspects of self, as you live out the aspirations of a neoliberal culture, has become embarrassing in much post-structuralist social theory. But in the Covid-19, we needed a new psychosocial ecopolitical imagination because it had become vital *to find words* for the fears and anxieties people were living with. People felt at a loss, disoriented and out of touch but if the self, as a notion had been disappeared, how were these embodied experiences to be traced.

This called for a renewed language of the self and its vulnerabilities to relationships of power and oppression. This meant understanding ourselves as vulnerable humans and reclaiming sociology as an ethical practice, connecting to philosophy as a way of living. But these issues could *not* be engaged with if languages of the self, along with notions of 'experience' had been already rapidly discounted as "essentialist". Nor did a language of "strategic essentialism" really get us where we needed to be, to make sense of the everyday predicaments people faced in a time of Covid. Often it wasn't a matter of searching for reasons for actions, as philosophers often frame it, but of facing difficult and often impossible moral choices in everyday lives.

In these unreal and anxious times, we can recall the title of Werner Fassbinder's movie *Fear eats the soul.* It's a story about Turkish immigrants to Germany and the impact of displacement and precarious wage-labour. It explores different ways fear *can* eat away at a person's very sense of identity, as they feel driven to do things in their lives that they consider humiliating. It traces lines of anxiety in class and racial relationships, as it opens a new vocabulary to explore the predicaments of displacement and poverty. In the present Covid-19 situation, so many people, across the world, had suddenly found themselves without enough money to put bread on the table. They couldn't afford *not* to work, whatever dangers it presented them with.

Adewale Maja-Pearce, the Anglo-Nigerian writer, wrote about a "Rich Man's Disease" on the LRB Blog (*London Review of Books*, 31 March 2020). He described Nigeria and the move he decided to make from Lagos to Bwari, even though at that time the figures of those infected with the virus were still low – 51 in all, including 32 in Lagos. As he noted:

> Not that people were panicking. In Bwari, as in Lagos, the few who went about wearing masks were looked on with bemusement. The idea had firmly taken hold that the virus disliked high heat and humidity and was, besides, only dangerous for the elderly with an underling medical condition.

My brother might have thought something similar before he was infected. Even though people he was close to had it, he somehow felt he would *not* get it and even if he did, it would be no bad thing. He thought very differently after being admitted to Barnet Hospital and warned us *to* keep a safe distance from others. There had been fake news and myths spread about the virus also in the global North where governments were unprepared to act in time. In the UK, the testing programme failed to keep up with the need for tests even among front line health and social care workers.

As Maja-Pearce reflected, in Bwari that "telling the majority poor to stay indoors may prove impossible." He pointed out that many relied on being paid on a daily basis to buy their essentials: that being outside and mobile is an existential necessity. Observing people going about their usual activities, between "churches and the mosques, and beer parlours," he summarises that it is "hunger, that people here fear, not a virus they can't even see."

Notes

1 To be reminded of the solidarity that people felt in the early post-war years that was partly produced through the experiences of the Blitz see the documentary film by Ken Loach *The Spirit of 45* which celebrates the radical changes in post-war Britain under the Labour government of Clement Atlee which came to power in 1945 which introduced the Welfare State, nationalised key industries and guaranteed full employment. In a time when the free market is dominant, Loach says, "It's time to put back on the agenda the importance of public ownership and public good, the value of working together collaboratively, not in competition."

2 For some illuminating discussions of Iris Murdoch's critical engagements with Derrida, see Sylvia C. Panizza and Mark Hopwood eds *The Murdochian Mind* (London: Routledge 2022).

3 William James *The Varieties of Religious Experience: A Study in Human Nature* (London: Penguin Books 1982). As Wittgenstein recognises James' work tells us not just about religious experience but about features of human nature that we are too easily missed. For an understanding of Wittgenstein's life and philosophy, see Ray Monk Ludwig *Wittgenstein: The Duty of Genius* (New York: Viking 1991). For a helpful general introduction see Ray Monk *How to Read Wittgenstein* (London: Granta Books 2005).

4 Mary Douglas broke important new ground in her writing of her influential *Purity and Danger* (London: Routledge 2002) which helped to reflect critically on resonances between Hebraic Biblical cultures and ways that people are still learning through their formative religious experiences to relate to their bodies, sexualities and emotional lives, even when they insist to have broken with their faith years ago. Douglas identifies the concern for purity as a theme at the heart of different societies. Is cleanliness close to godliness? What then are the implications for those considered unclean?

9

DENIALS, LANGUAGE, ETHICS AND RESPONSIBILITIES

Valuing Life and Counting Deaths

There is a biblical story around the Tower of Babel told by Andre Neher that finds echoes in our time of Covid-19 that records:

> According to a rabbinic commentary on the building of the Tower of Babel (Genesis 11), if somebody fell and died, nobody paid any attention to it. However, if a brick fell, they would sit and cry and say, "whenever shall we erect another in its place" (*Pirke de Rabbi Eliezer* 24). The Tower of Babel instantly demonstrates…the crushing of the individual by the collectivity; mass civilisation…depersonalisation: the work does not stop when a worker gets crushed, but the entire project fails when by accident a brick is dropped.

As Neher teaches we have "to remember always the limit and the tragic consequence of the limit – between a charter and its practice, between a Declaration of the Rights of human beings and its actualisation" (MRJ Forms of Prayer p. 556).[1]

Reflecting on the nature of social responsibility, Abraham Joshua Heschel also shares:

> The more deeply immersed I became in the thinking of the prophets, the more powerfully it became clear to me what the lives of the prophets sought to convey: that morally speaking there is no limit to the concern one must feel for the suffering of human beings. It also became clear to me that in regard to cruelties committed in the name of a free society, some are guilty, but all are responsible.
> *(p. 554)*[2]

DOI: 10.4324/9781003296874-9

There is also a telling comment on changing times and ways we learn within a liberal moral culture *to forget* and to put the past *behind* us, by Joseph Roth, the Austrian Jewish writer. Roth, whose family saga *Radetzky March* in 1932 was about the decline and fall of the Austro-Hungarian Empire, recalled:

> In the years before the Great War…it was not yet a matter of indifference whether a person lived or died. When someone was expunged from the lists of the living, someone else did not immediately step up to take his place, but a gap was left to show where he had been, and those who knew the man who had died or disappeared, well or even less well, fell silent whenever they saw the gap… everything that ended took a long time to be forgotten. Everything that existed left behind traces of itself, and people then lived by their memories, just as we nowadays live by our capacity to forget, quickly and comprehensively.
>
> *(p. 557)*

Within the utilitarian ethics that helps shape the common-sense of a liberal moral culture, it becomes so easy to take individual lives for granted and to assume that they can be sacrificed for the greater good. The government was slow to acknowledge that some individuals would inevitably die as a result of their reactions to the vaccines, but they preferred *not* to talk about the risks, knowing that so many more lives would be saved. They also found it hard to talk about different ways of treating Covid, by supporting the immune system through alternative medical practices. They were mesmerised by the numbers as they mentioned, almost in passing, that "every death was a tragedy". This is also what makes it hard to grieve and to shape public narratives of loss in a time of Covid.[3]

It can also be helpful in these times of plague to recall the insight of the liberal philosopher Isaiah Berlin's that:

> Injustice, poverty, slavery, ignorance – these may be cured by reform and revolution. But human beings do not live only by fighting evils. They live by positive goals, individual and collective, a vast variety of them, seldom predictable, at times incompatible. It is from intense preoccupation with these ends…that the best moments come in the lives of individuals and people.
>
> *(p. 555)*[4]

Shannon Pufahl in her reflections on "Numbering the Dead" in *The New York Review of Books*, 21 April 2020 (nybooks.com) helps to engage a historical consciousness, showing how vital this in shaping a sociological imagination in the present. Her analysis begins around 150 years ago when a peculiar idea emerged that the deceased could be quantified. During the Civil War, Americans in the South began envisioning death in numerical terms, a concept previously uncommon in the mid-19th century.

Civil War officials, Pufahl argues, hesitated to assign numbers or names to the deceased, as military leaders worried it might empower their foes. However, as she notes, our cultural landscape has changed, as has our perception of time and loss. In this "world of measurement," statistics have come to dictate our emotional response to loss and help us assess the magnitude of tragic events. She indicates that it was around the 19th century that people began to "give our counting meaning beyond numerical designation."

After the Battle Appomattox, in April 1865, one of the last battles of the American Civil War, Pufahl argued, "compiling a definitive statistical record of human loss became a preoccupation of the post-war recovery," a tool for reckoning with loss. With Covid-19 the daily numbers of the dead *also* seem to assume a meaning of their own, as if a situation that *is* tragically out of control is thereby communicated *as* somehow being in control.

Pufahl speculates that with more than 620,000 casualties, the American Civil War catalysed a "cultural need for numbers": that a "statistics of death" made "every individual meaningful," reshaping the philosophy of tragedy for the era. She notes the power of counting to render fatalities "bearable," and they appeared "specific and contained, rather than abstract," when quantified.

She herself reflects on "watch(ing) the numbers" during the pandemic to assess her own feelings about it. The "epidemiological models" cited by news outlets of the time became "not just projections of a possible or likely future" but "the metric" dictating policy and response, and filtering down to real outcomes, even as modest as when a family might next eat in a restaurant together.

As Pufahl noted, analysts "have warned" about the dangers of creating a statistical class based on immunity: for example, historian Kathryn Olivarius highlighted how immunity was used as a "weapon" against marginalised groups in the antebellum Deep South. Incomplete numbers of Covid-19 cases, recoveries, and deaths ultimately impact hospital resources and necessities.[5]

She believes that the future will be shaped by the "strange irony of our present." While physically separated, we are bound by a global shared experience. However, there is no avoiding that this common experience is influenced by numerous inequalities: presenting a challenge so large that it threatens to "(overwhelm) our capacity for empathy" and turning tragedy into an empty algorithm. In the post-Covid-19 era, she concludes, we'll need to seek new ways to express collective grief beyond mere numbers (*The New York Review of Books*, 21 April 2020).

As people wish for Covid times *to become* history, so they often *want* to put it behind them, not wanting to be reminded of their losses and vulnerabilities. Despite the desire to commemorate the dead of the First World War, there was no official memorialisation for the other major death event of the early 20th century – the influenza epidemic of 1918–19. Though it killed approximately 228,000 Britons there was no national memorial to the memory of the influenza dead. In the USA it has been suggested that this was because the majority of deaths were of marginalised working-class women.[6]

Language, Power and Deception

Writing from lockdown in the city of Parma in Italy journalist and author Tobias Jones shows the everyday racism that circulated, often as a form of denial and self-protection, as he expressed his feelings of being "offended at the latest international media coverage. There was a discernible glee in some quarters that the "silly Eye-ties" had messed things up again. "They'll never follow the rules," some said." As he recalls, "Prejudices about Italy – assuming that the problem was the country itself, and not the virus – meant that few people took note when, for weeks, Italian leaders, epidemiologists and journalists urged similarly decisive action across Europe" (*The Observer*, 15 March 2020, p. 38).

He informs us that:

> …actually Italians are very well-informed (some might say obsessive) about personal health. They learn about plague and contagion at school because two of the classics of Italy's literary canon – Alessandro Manzoni's *The Betrothed* and Giovanni Boccaccio's *The Decameron*, deal with precisely those themes.

Jones notes, "Now that so many other countries are following Italy's lead – closing schools, universities and sports events – we feel, at least, somewhat vindicated" (*The Observer*, 15 March 2020, p. 39).

Taking Jones's cue citing this foundational text of plague, medievalist Kathryn McKinley recalls how Boccaccio's *The Decameron* gave us a window into the workings of the Black Death and how similar fissures opened up between the rich and the poor, where the urban poor are packed into small apartments and compelled to keep showing up at work.

It begins with a vivid depiction of the Black Death: a "virulent" and fast-acting disease that claimed the lives of 40% to 50% of the European population in under five years in the mid-14th century: including many members of Boccaccio's family. He tells of how the "ruthless" wealthy abandoned their neighbourhoods in favour of remote countryside estates, "as though the plague was meant to harry only those remaining within their city walls."[7] The rural poor died "like brute beasts" without medical attention (*The Conversation*, 16 April 2020).

McKinley traces the influence on Boccaccio's writing of the dreadful inequalities of society, amplified by the plague, describing that *The Decameron* dwells on "how wealth and advantage can impair people's abilities of empathise with the hardships of others." Noting the Proverb used to open the tome ("It is inherently human to show pity to those who are afflicted"), McKinley notes the irony to follow in the tales, with a cast of protagonists "sharply indifferent to the pain of others, blinded by their own drives and ambition."

Boccaccio shows a deep understanding of the inherent hypocrisy of humanity: that an individual can regard themselves as "upstanding and moral" but act with "indifference to others," as his narrators show: indulging in displays of "brutality, betrayal and exploitation."

He wanted *to challenge* his readers through his stories and make them reflect upon *how* they think and feel about their responsibilities to others. *The Decameron* poses questions of how different lives are valued: deeply relevant to conversations around the Covid-19 pandemic.

A conversation between Joe Humphreys and Kantian scholar Katy Dineen in *The Irish Times* reflects on the "shock" of the pandemic that gave a "jump start to moral consciences," noting that in-built inequalities "tolerated" in normal times, such as stagnant wages for essential workers or healthcare barriers inflicted on low-income patients, seemed "abominable." Discussing these inequalities through a moral lens informed by Kant's challenges "to avoid privileging oneself in moral deliberations," Dineen makes the case for learning from the Enlightenment figure, in assessing "what values we would rationally choose if we could stand back from our own circumstances and judge rationally."

But on the question of whether Kant's position really engages the injustices of social inequalities, Dineen reminds us of Kant's description of human deception and ability to launder "self-serving actions as motivated by duty and virtue" as "the foul stain of our species," and particularly poisonous at times of social turbulence.

As a Kantian, Dineen more easily recognises the value of individual lives and Kant's moral injunction that we should never treat others as a means to our ends, but always as ends in themselves. She argues that "egalitarianism based on reasonableness" has being never more "pertinent" than during the pandemic. As an indiscriminate crisis, Covid touches "prime ministers and paupers and doesn't care one whit for our special interests." Dineen points out that vulnerabilities in one quarter have ripple effects, using the concrete example:

> If workers are more at risk because they are not isolating or they are not provided with adequate PPE, then they are more likely to pass on the virus… they are now using a precious ICU bed. That's one less bed available for everyone else.
>
> *(The Irish Times, 23 April 2020).*

Politics, Denial and Avoiding Responsibility

The Sunday Times's Insight team published an article on Sunday 19 April 2020 under the headline: "Coronavirus: 38 days when Britain sleepwalked into disaster" that laid bare the incompetence and irresponsibility of the Johnson's government in the face of what was to become a national emergency that was to prove the greatest since the Second World War. It was an article that was to send shock waves through the government and the media that had failed to hold the government to account in much of its reporting.

As they noted "Boris Johnson skipped five Cobra meetings on the virus, calls to order protective gear were ignored and scientists' warnings fell on deaf ears. Failings in February may have costs thousands of lives." The indictment was clearly made and revealed shocking and widespread denial on the part of Johnson's government. I recall reading it late on Saturday night on my iPhone and feeling it was tantamount to a call for the government to resign, for how could it continue when such failings had been identified.

As the article opened:

> On the fourth Friday of January, a silent and stealthy killer was creeping across the world. Passing from person to person and borne on ships and planes, the coronavirus was already leaving a trail of bodies. The virus had spread from China to six countries and was almost certainly in many others. Sensing the coming danger, the British government briefly went into wartime mode that day, holding a meeting of Cobra, its national crisis committee.

But as they also report:

> …it took just an hour that January 24 lunchtime to brush aside the coronavirus threat. Matt Hancock, the health secretary, bounced out of Whitehall after chairing the meeting and breezily told reporters the risk to the UK public was "low".

No doubt he was to live to regret those words and would pretend they were never said. In a message sent by Cummings, the senior advisor at No.10 to Johnson, in May 2020, shown to the Covid Inquiry, he said, "You need to think through timing of binning Hancock. There's no way the guy can stay. He's lied his way through this and killed people and dozens and dozens of people have seen it" (theguardian.com, 2 November 2023).

Responding to the claims made in the *Times* piece, Polly Toynbee of *The Guardian* described it as "confirm(ing) all our worst fears: the prime minister's handling of coronavirus has been shockingly complacent," highlighting the then-Prime Minister's poor work ethic and lack of "urgent crisis planning."

Johnson apparently took two weeks' holiday at Chevening as the virus began to spread in the UK: a dereliction of duty that Toynbee speculated would "surely stick in the public memory," alongside images of him attending Twickenham matches and shaking hands with Covid patients early on in the crisis (theGuardian.com, 20 April 2020).

Toynbee pinpoints Johnson's "natural antipathy towards the state" as making him "supremely unsuited" to the task of tackling Covid. In February 2020, he attacked the lockdowns in Wuhan, criticising "bizarre autarkic rhetoric," and claiming, "Humanity needs some government somewhere that is willing at least to make the case powerfully for freedom of exchange."

At this level of free-market ideology he was in line with Trump and it added to their shared conviction that, like other threats before, this would die away and that in any case it was like a getting bad flu that anyone man enough should be able to take in his stride and that if he got it, it would be no bad thing. These were the deadly messages that had their consequences and would lead to many possibly unnecessary deaths.

With *The Sunday Times*'s report revealing so many failures, including that the UK moved protective equipment to China in February thereby helping to create the very shortages that were to lead to deaths of NHS workers on the front line who were working with Covid-19 patients, it's hardly surprising that Labour has accused Johnson of having been "missing in action," as they did earlier of being a "part-time prime minister."

Labour's health spokesperson John Ashworth told the Ridge show on Sky that Labour was aware that "frontline NHS staff don't have the PPE" and that "testing capacity is not at the level that is needed" (*The Guardian*, 19 April 2020).

Writer Caitlin Moran @caitlinmoran tweeted:

> This report from the Sunday Times reads like the obituary of Boris Johnson's government. An absolutely extraordinary catalogue of complacency, error and long weekend holidays even as departments were sounding the alarm.

But as Damon Evans @damocrat tweeted "To be honest, if you needed a Sunday Times article to tell you Boris Johnson is a tosser, you haven't been paying attention." By late January the seriousness of the virus was clear, as was the fact that it was imminently going to arrive on British shores.

The government *has* consistently said it was "led by the science" – a phrase that conceals so much more than it reveals, and a cover for many mistakes made. Government advisor Professor Neil Ferguson, who headed the Imperial College Covid-19 Response team, warned there needed to be a lockdown, but the government dismissed this as something out of a post-apocalyptic movie. On 22 January he had warned that coronavirus could be more infectious than Spanish flu, which killed tens of millions. The scientists had pleaded with the government that mass casualties were coming, and they needed to obtain emergency supplies of protective gowns and masks.

As they reported, we carried on *pretending* that a pandemic was the number one threat facing Britain, in practice preparations for the pandemic had been destroyed by austerity that allowed stocks to fall to unsafe levels. We knew we didn't have enough PPE and intensive care ventilators because a pandemic rehearsal was conducted in 2016 but the recommendations weren't implemented.

The Insight team noted that this was partly because government energies were focussed upon a no-deal Brexit, pandemic planning was repeatedly bumped off the diary, and the government advisory group on pandemics were left desperately joking among themselves about the possibility of the pandemic. They knew what a disaster it would be and how unprepared the country was for the loss of lives that could result.

Even in February when a nightmarish scenario looked even more likely, there was little real urgency. The government pursued a policy of herd immunity, though this was essentially a policy that meant they were treating the virus *as if* it were essentially a flu which it was *not*, as they were soon to learn and change policy. It was already very late in the day and had allowed the virus to spread, which helps to explain why they abandoned a testing and contact tracing strategy, which they were later going to have to reinvent to escape the lockdown measures they were forced into once aware of the catastrophic health crisis they were facing.

The laissez-faire ideology, a mindset that government should not interfere in people's lives – and that capitalism should be allowed to run free – helps to explain why they felt they had to do so little. It fitted in with Trumps' inaction in the United States. Singapore copied the UK pandemic plan and has been successful in combating the virus, but the difference is that they implemented it and in the UK we didn't.

As has become evident, government complacency has killed, not only in the actions it failed to take, but *also* in the messages they were giving out, that everything was under control and that there was *no* real danger offered by the virus, that people could handle it if they were man enough. It is striking how Covid-19 seems to have had a more devastating impact on men who have had to learn a terrible lesson, often too late to save their lives. The threat level was kept at "moderate."

The prime minister, like Trump was telling everyone to be "confident and calm". As one senior department of health insider told the Insight team, "We could have been Germany but instead we were doomed by our incompetence, our hubris and our austerity." And many people were to die for this, and the government should still be *held accountable* for its actions and responsible for level of deaths that followed that could evidently have been avoided if Johnson's government had acted earlier and decisively. As Owen Jones has noted, 'Thousands and thousands of people have died, and will die, because of what this government had done" (@OwenJones84, 18/04/2020). My brother Tony was one of them and he died on 6 April at Barnet Hospital.

The editor of the medical journal *The Lancet* accused the government of "rewriting history" after Downing Street issue a furious and detailed rebuttal of a *Sunday Times* article that claimed that Johnson's administration had "just watched" as the death toll mounted in China in January and February and "missed the boat" on securing sufficient supplies of tests and PPE. As Andrew Woodcock, political editor of *The Independent,* writes "The move suggests deep concern at the centre of government over the danger of losing control of the narrative about its handling of the crisis" (*The Independent*, 20 April 2020,).

That characterised the government's *misuse* of scientific controversy in its insistence that they were following the best scientific advice, as if there was a singular truth agreed by all. They had used a tweet from Richard Horton, the *Lancet* editor on 23 January, urging "caution" on suggestions that a killer virus was coming as proof that there was no scientific consensus at that point that coronavirus was a threat. He accused the government of "deliberately rewriting history in its ongoing Covid-19 disinformation campaign" and insisted his message related to the need for caution in media reporting and was "followed by a series of tweets drawing attention to the dangers of this new disease" (Richard Horton, 23 January).

On 23 January he had accused the media of "escalating anxiety by talking of a 'killer virus' and 'growing fears'.'" As *The Sunday Times* reported, the dangers were clear at the time and that:

> Imperial's Ferguson was already working on his own estimates – putting infectivity at 2.6 and possibly as high as 3.5 – when he sent to ministers and officials in a report on the day of the Cobra meeting on January 24. The Spanish flu had an estimated infectivity of between 2.0 and 3.0 so Ferguson's findings were shocking.

But there was still little government response to the dangers evident to so many medical scientists who had long warned of the dangers of a pandemic. As they report by the time Johnson chaired a COBRA meeting on 2 March: "The virus had sneaked into our airports, our trains, our workplaces, and our homes. Britain was on course for one of the worst infections of the most insidious virus to have hit the world in a century."

As a *Guardian* editorial noted in the wake of more than ten years of austerity, a more "proactive government mindset" was required to intervene and properly pursue a course of testing. Instead, "voluntarism remains the creed of the current government" (*The Guardian*, 27 April 2020).

The editorial speculated that in the upcoming weeks, a debate will unfold on whether the "shutdown" would be "deadlier than the virus." Advocates for lifting restrictions emphasise personal responsibility. However, evidence suggests that the elderly and low-income individuals are more susceptible to the disease. Given the highly communicable nature of the virus, the health of the wealthy relies on the health of the poor. Therefore, according to the article, sending "at-risk" adults back to high social contacts was illogical, even by Conservative standards. As the editorial concludes: "Having emptied Covid hospital wards, would this not just risk filling them up again?"

Threats, Warnings and Denials

As Chris Tyler, UCL, and Peter Gluckman, University of Auckland, acknowledge, although Bill Gates had been talking for a long time about the dangers of a pandemic, those in government were slow to grasp the "magnitude of the problem," perhaps owing to previous pandemics happening outside living memory, such as Spanish flu, or viruses that, although severe, did not spread as widely as feared, such as SARS, resulting in scepticism in some political quarters over "risk analysts and scientists (crying) wolf over past viral threats." They indicated that in "modern medicine, at least in advanced countries," there was a complacency that led to a belief that they "could cope with anything the microbiotic world threw at it" (*The Conversation*, 27 April 2020).

The market ideology of many neoliberal politicians also means that they are *less likely* to take warnings seriously and to assume that that the market will have its own solutions if a threat arises.

This leads politicians to "focus more on the short term" and on their election chances: assuming that "the public does not know about the risks or that they do not care." In contrast, in areas with experience in dealing with a population living with these risks where these viruses took a stronger hold, they note that the politicians "have handled the current pandemic with more urgency and success."

From 2012 to 2019 Ian Boyd was chief scientific adviser to the British government. He insists in March 2020 that planning should have been done for a pandemic the size and scale of Covid, no matter how difficult the task of preparing for such as unknown quantity. Referring to a flu pandemic practice run commissioned by the UK government, he claimed that the "assessment, in many sectors… was that the resulting medicine was so strong that it would be spat out. Nobody likes living under a fortress mentality."

In the Covid crisis the behaviour scientists too readily assumed, in ways that echoed Tory ideology, that people would *not* respect a lockdown that went on too long which is why they delayed introducing it early enough, even though Italy had done it successfully with wide public support when people recognised the dangers they faced.

Boyd acknowledged that after the first outbreak, "there is no manual to follow," but underscored that lessons could be learned from past epidemics to enable the best response, even if this "provide(s) only a template" requiring a "highly fluid" execution.

He acknowledges the importance of values at this stage, in order to ensure that "we are less likely to continue with our unsustainable rates of resource consumption." He sees the pandemic as an opportunity to "rebuild our systems into something more resilient" (*Nature*, 30 March 2020).[8]

Contemplating the response of the Right to the pandemic, journalist Jason Wilson noted the "seductive" power of denial in responding to outbreak, but like Boyd, notes the "sinister" path this can take in presenting fast-acting dangers to the path. Those choosing this in the US, "the denialists and minimisers – including the President," according to Wilson, were soon to be "confronted with the grim reality of the coronavirus death toll," but warned that not even this would deter them. He cites Candace Owens, a right-wing media personality "forestalling her own reckoning by putting about the idea that the deaths themselves are hoaxes" (*The Guardian*, 7 April 2020).

He describes the approach of right-wing figures operating in liberal democracies, such as Boris Johnson and Australia's Scott Morrison, as "reluctant realism", required to "abandon habits of thought developed over a lifetime." As Wilson puts it, in times when crises are likely to increase, "the neoliberal, managerial state simply doesn't cut the mustard."

He posits that Wilson progressives need to be more assertive in the face of this: to foreground "social solidarity, equity justice and peace." Otherwise, he suggests, we risk enshrining a "western chauvinism (undermining) anyone who claims to be on the left."[9]

Risk, Neoliberal Capitalism and Denial

Jonathan Watts, *The Guardian*'s global environmental editor, identified the distribution of risk as the "defining political question of our age" and expressed doubt over the stronghold that neoliberal capitalism has on our politics to tackle this. He points out that the pandemic revealed how a "government's propensity to acknowledge risk, act rapidly to contain it, and share the consequences" was a life or death matter: identifying the most successful Covid response came from those investing and acting promptly: decidedly not "laissez-faire capitalists" (The Guardian, 24 March 2020).

Watts noted that the relationship between a government's place on the political spectrum and its response was closely entwined: a far-right government, such as Trump's administration was "more inclined… to delay action and offload blame elsewhere." Trump's plan was to "downplay early warnings," mindful of the election cycle, with dire consequences: the USA was ravaged by the disease, with new infection rates some of the worst in the world.

Watts therefore made a case for the "importance of assessing and controlling risk before it gets out of hand." In the cases of "deny and delay" strategies employed by Trump and Bolsonaro, the people were punished with appalling infection rates. This, Watts points out, for the Right poses "a greater political threat than the climate crisis has ever been," speculating that the pandemic could be one of the most "catastrophic failures of free-market capitalism."

The Left could use these lessons to inform future decisions: that "the same principles should be applied more aggressively towards the still more apocalyptic threats of climate disruption." Put simply, Watts argues, "delays are deadly and expensive": messages that anyone, regardless of their politics, can understand.

Questioning the precedence that has for too long been given *to* economic growth, we have to think of *well-being* of communities in a radically different way as we come to terms with the painful truth that older people, especially in care homes, have been largely sacrificed and their lives deemed of less value because they have less time to live. Watts, prescribes that going forward, governments "transform risks into responsibilities we all bear." Hesitation merely breeds risk.

The Indian writer, Amitav Ghosh in *The Great Derangement* also reminds us about the risks and threats to human life on the planet of neoliberal capitalism:

> What we have learned from this experiment is that the pattern of life that modernity engenders can only be practiced by a small minority of the world's population. Asia's historical experience demonstrates that our planet will not allow these patterns of living to be adopted by every human being. Every family in the world cannot have two cars, a washing machine, and a refrigerator – not because of technical or economic limitations but because humanity would asphyxiate in the process.
>
> *(p. 91)*[10]

He also recognises a way that speaks *to the dangers* of Covid-19:

> Yet now our gaze seems to be turning again; the uncanny and improbable events that are beating at our doors seem to have stirred a sense of recognition, an awareness that humans were never alone, that we have always been surrounded by beings of all sorts who share elements of that which we had thought to be distinctly our own: the concepts of will, thought and consciousness…could it also be said that the earth has itself intervened to revise those habits of thought that are based on the Cartesian dualism that arrogates all intelligence and agency to the human while denying them to every other kind of being?
>
> *(pp. 30–31)*

Ecologies, Climate Breakdown and Ethics

"We have been living in a bubble," columnist George Monbiot claimed, "…of false comfort and denial… wealth we've accumulated… has shielded us from reality." This reality he cites is that we are all vulnerable to natural disaster and hazards: an uncomfortable fact we would prefer not to face (*The Guardian*, 25 March 2020).

This opens up a conversation with Ghosh's insights in *The Great Derangement* that:

> It is not impossible, for instance, that in dealing with situations of extraordinary stress the very factors that are considered advantages in coping with extreme weather – education, wealth, and a high degree of social organisation – may actually become vulnerabilities…
>
> In many parts of the global south, breakdowns are a way of life, and everybody is used to improvisations and work-arounds. In poor countries, even the middle classes are accustomed to coping with shortages and discomforts of all sorts; in the West, wealth, and habits based on efficient infrastructures, may have narrowed the threshold of bearable pain to a point where climatic impacts could quickly lead to systemic stress.
>
> *(p. 147)*

As the pandemic has burst some urban middle-class bubbles, Monbiot warns us not to "succumb" to the "temptation" to replace them, instead calling on people to face "the painful realities we have denied for too long."

He is concerned, for example, with how climate breakdown is likely to affect food supply: with daily realities of conditions that would previously be described as "biblical." He notes that despite a surplus of food, "hundreds of millions are malnourished" as a result of inequality. "Hoarding will happen," he notes, as a sad reality.[11] This "illusion of security" is dangerous, and it leads to a culture of complacency: "Every food-producing sector claims that its own current practices are sustainable and don't need to change."

So many corporations and institutions are trapped into *short-term market thinking*, as they were around the dangers of a virus. We learnt in post-war generations to assume that progress was still to be defined within the terms of an Enlightenment rationalism *as* the control and domination of nature. We have denied our existence as vulnerable humans and traditions in moral philosophy often fail to provide alternative visions and vocabularies. So it was that nature was reduced to silence and people could no longer imagine ways it could kick back with such intensity and human devastation.

There are two ways this could go, according to Monbiot. The first: total paralysis and denial. The right-wing authoritarian populist leader of Brazil, Jair Bolsonaro, claimed the coronavirus is nothing more than "a little flu". The media and opposition politicians who *are* in favour of maintaining a lockdown are, apparently, part of a conspiracy against him.

Bolsonaro dismissed what he called media "hysteria" and attacked governors of key states, including Rio de Janeiro and Sao Paulo who had ordered residents to stay at home while they imposed quarantines. As his own health officials reported 25 deaths and 1,546 cases of coronavirus in Brazil, Bolsonaro in a television interview insisted that his people were being "tricked" about the severity of the pandemic. He claimed the pot-banging protests that took to the streets, were part of a media-backed plot to topple him.

Citing research from Imperial College London, Brazilian journalist Eliane Brum reported: that "the difference between adopting total isolation and not doing so equals one million lost lives in Brazil." She pointed out that as the crisis was raging, Bolsonaro embarked on a campaign of not just "post-truth but self-truth. He goes live on Facebook to discredit scientific research." He insisted on shaking hands with his supporters, even after more than 20 people who travelled with him to see Trump came down with the virus. He insisted he never had it. At no point when he held his supporters' mobile phones for selfies did he stop to think he might infect others.

With the death toll rising, he was obliged to change tune, as did his mentor Trump, calling the pandemic "the biggest challenge of our generation" at the same time as street protesters in major cities clanged pots and pans and shouted: "Bolsonaro out!" for the fifteenth consecutive night.

But this, journalist Elaine Brum notes: "doesn't represent a meaningful U-Turn. It just adds to the chaos" (*The Guardian*, 2 April 2020).

But as Monbiot argues, this could, as the deaths rise across the world, help *question* the truths that have served to legitimate a globalised neoliberal capitalism. By recognising that we are "governed by biology and physics," and that we "belong to the material world," we will no longer need to seek refuge in falsehoods.

Listening to Nature, Fears and Memories

The UN's environment chief Inger Anderson also recognises *how* nature is sending us a message with the coronavirus pandemic, if only we could hear it. She says humanity was placing too many pressures on the natural world with damaging consequences and warned, as Damian Carrington reports, "that failing to take care of the planet meant not taking care of ourselves" (*The Guardian*, 25 March 2020).

She notes, along with leading scientists, that Covid-19 was a "clear warning shot" about how human behaviours impact the planet, continuing that the "continued erosion of wild spaces has brought us uncomfortably close to animals and plants that harbour diseases that can jump to humans… At the end of the day, (with) all of these events, nature is sending us a message." Contemplating a future with significantly depleted resources and tougher living conditions, she makes the case that "we need to go into this future with nature as our strongest ally."

Carrington cites Andrew Cunningham, of the Zoological Society of London, who noted that diseases from wildlife have much higher fatality rates in people: 50% for Ebola and 60%–75% for Nipah virus, transmitted from bats in South Asia. In the case of diseases of this nature, Cunningham suggested: "It's almost always a human behaviour that causes it."

A wet market in China is still believed by some to have been the source of Covid-19. On this, Cunningham notes the terrible transport conditions used for animals, who become "stressed and immuno-suppressed… excreting whatever pathogens they have in them," creating a prime environment for the emergence of virus and disease, and a "a scenario to maximise chances of (transmission)."

Cunningham is sceptical about what will really change, citing the "sigh of relief" that followed the end of the SARS contagion that marked the end of vigilance. He warns: "We cannot go back to business as usual" (*The Guardian*, 25 March 2020).

Revisiting Boccaccio as a powerful chronicler of plague, historian Paula Findlen in *The Boston Review* ponders what he would make of Covid, as the creator of "one of the most thoughtful and critical accounts of a society living under a pandemic." In his native Florence, a third of the population were lost to plague, including his father and stepmother, leaving him to deal with the chaos and grief of interrupted lives. Returning to the city in the aftermath, he noted how quickly society had broken down. In the introduction to *The Decameron*, he recalls the "painful memory of the deadly havoc wrought by the recent plague."

Findlen sets out how he painted the portrait of a deeply changed world: he "documented changes in burial practices… (and how) ordinary activities became a source of enormous anxiety." Florence as a "corporate body" fought for the "integrity" of the hitherto strong "social fabric of the city" (*The Boston Review*, 24 April 2020).

As Boccaccio recognised, widespread *fear* became the basis for further mistreatment of the poor, foreign and disenfranchised sectors of society that did not have the luxury of flight. The understanding of the transmission of disease was minimal at that time, Findlen explains, so medics relied primarily on their proficiency in "recognising the symptoms" of various diseases, which informed Boccaccio's writing, as he "describes in gruesome and precise detail" the physical "manifestations" of the plague. This was a time when medicine was rudimentary: "cures" were ineffective, so experience and recognition were the most valued medical commodities.

Boccaccio's "critical" writing on responses to the plague was evidence not only of his "scepticism" about the research and limits of knowledge of the day, but also of his concern about his city. Findlen perceives in the writer a yearning to restore "the collective sense of well-being that had made the city prosper." As a proud Florentine, Boccaccio worried for the effects of "society under quarantine, with strained social relations and a fractured economy."

Boccaccio realised that plague arrived in a city *not* because of the constellation of the planets had aligned badly, *nor* because it was God's will and a punishment for bad deeds in the past, but at the inevitable consequence of a restless and consuming society ever on the move. As Findlen concludes: "Whether the values of society would ever change, especially after a moment of such profound disruption, became his enduring question. It has now once again become ours."

Notes

1 "The Challenge of Civilisation" in *The Movement for Reform Judaism (MRJ)* (London: The Movement for Reform Judaism 2008). Andre Neher was a French Jewish scholar and philosopher who writes in *The Exile of the World: From the Silence of the Bible to the Silence of Auschwitz* (Philadelphia: Jewish Publication Society of America 1981) about biblical silence and God's silence after the Shoah. He draws on the image of a suspension bridge to describe human "ontological insecurity and pain" noting how human freedom is characterised by a "radical factor of uncertainty." This is why it is necessary to concentrate our attention not on ideas of redemption or salvation, but on "being here in our life."

2 For an understanding of the background of Abraham Joshua Heschel and the different sources of his theology, spirituality and politics, see Edward K. Kaplan and Samuel H. Dresner *Prophetic Witness* (New Haven CT: Yale University Press 1998) and *Spiritual Radical: Abraham Joshua Heschel in America 1940–1972* (New Haven CT: Yale University Press 2007); Julian E. Zelizer *Abraham Joshua Heschel: A Life of Radical Amazement* (New Haven: Yale University Press 2021). For his own writings see *The Prophets* (New York: Harper Perennial 2001) and *Moral Grandeur and Spiritual Audacity* (New York: Farrar Straus and Giroux 1996).

3 To understand the historical and cultural context of Joseph Roth's writings see Keiron Pim *Endless Flight: The Life of Joseph Roth* (London: Granta 2022). His novel in prose of dark foreboding that brought him recognition was *The Radetzky March* (London: Granta 2013).

4 Shannon Pufahl writing on "Numbering the Dead" in *The New York Review of Books*, 21 April 2020, traces a shift in how we now speak easily in the statistics of absence while 150 years ago it was a strange notion that the dead could be counted.

5 Kathryn Olivarius *Necropolis: Disease, Power and Capitalism in the Cotton Kingdom* (Cambridge MA: Harvard University Press 2022) She notes, "In this system of class rule, people who claimed to be immune used their immunity and vulnerability of others to consolidate their power...I came to think about yellow fever less as background noise and more as dark matter".

6 An epidemic is not merely a medical crisis but always has sociological, psychological and political dimensions. What made the influenza epidemic of 1918 which took close to 30 million lives worldwide, including more than 500,000 in the United States, even more frightening was the fact that it occurred when death rates from most common infectious diseases were diminishing. Patricia J. Flanning in *Influenza and Inequality* (Boston MA: University of Massachusetts Press 2010) traces the epidemic through the

town of Norwood a small, ethnically diverse, industrialised town in Massachusetts that relied upon ink, printing and tanning factories. When the epidemic struck, the immigrant neighbourhoods were most affected with tragic results. Well-intentioned elite groups implemented strategies that exacerbated rather than relieved the medical crisis.

7 Giovanni Boccaccio wrote about the ravages of the Black Death as it ravaged Florence in 1348 in *The Decameron* (London: Penguin Classics 2003).

8 For discussions about what was already planned for, if not enacted and what was learnt through the Covid pandemic see, Lawrence O. Gostin *Global Health Security: A Blueprint for the Future* (Cambridge MA: Harvard University Press 2021) which charts a better course through global solidarity and enlightened self-interest. He shows lessons from Covid-19 that can help remake society to be better prepared for future health threats.

9 For arguments that help to advance the human right to health, as enshrined in the Universal Declaration of Human Rights and engage with the complex clinical, ethical, legal and socio-cultural questions raised by injury, disease, and deeper determinants of health, such as poverty so engaging with profound inequalities in health see, Jose M. Zuniga, Stephen P. Marks and Lawrence O. Gostin (eds) *Advancing the Human Right to Health* (Oxford: Oxford University Press 2013).

10 Amitav Ghosh in *The Great Derangement: Climate Change and the Unthinkable* (Chicago: University of Chicago Press 2016) offers a non-fiction work that engages with climate change by reflecting on our deranged modes of political and socio-economic thinking and organisational structures.

11 The concerns about the climate emergency and ways they interrelate to a crisis in the political, economic and cultural worlds of a globalised neoliberalism that still insists that progress is to be measured through the control and domination of nature are explored by George Monbiot *Out of the Wreckage: A New Politics for an Age of Crisis* (London: Verso Books 2017), *How Did We Get into this Mess?* (London: Verso Books 2016) and *Regenesis* (London: Penguin 2022).

10

HOSPITAL VOICES, RISKS, GRIEF AND EVERYDAY ETHICS

Trusting Voices

As I write in real time, I am very aware that in Jewish tradition today marks the *Shloshim* – the 30th day since my younger brother Tony was buried in Rishon-le-Zion in Israel, very close to our father and within walking distance of our stepfather, who are both buried in the same cemetery. This was his wish, though it was not one I could easily understand, but came to appreciate and honour and as a family at the time of Covid-19, it felt like a miracle to have been able to ensure that his bones were laid to rest where he wanted to be.

I joined the morning Shachrit prayers at Leo Baeck College – given with so much feeling and thought by Elena, a first-year rabbinic student. As I joined the morning prayers on zoom, I was struck by the words she was sharing. I was able to trace them to "Reflections" in the Movement for Reform Judaism's *Forms of Prayer for the Sabbath and Daily Prayer*. It seemed to reflect a voice that spoke to the moment – an awareness that my younger brother Tony's journey after death takes another step today.[1]

The words I heard came from a reflection on the question, "What are we?"

> Body and mind, feelings and spirit. This is where we start. One life, our life, here and now. As blood pulses through our veins, our heart beats out the hours and the days. And our bodies speak the mundane majesty of human life on earth. As neurones fire through the myriad pathways of our brain, a maze of thoughts spark in our skulls. And our minds declare the baffling glory of human life on earth. As the fabric of feelings spins on the loom of our lives, we sense a pattern emerging: love and loss, hurt and healing, sadness, joy, pain and pleasure…

DOI: 10.4324/9781003296874-10

> As we contemplate our own unique physical, mental and emotional life, do we not glimpse another truth about ourselves? Something we cannot grasp, cannot name, though names we have aplenty? Soul, spirit, Self, the spark of God within – how can mere words reveal the essence of ourselves? We are more than we can ever know, a mystery through and through.
>
> *(p. 333)*

My eye catches a reflection that follows on "What is our life?" – each echoing a prayer said in Hebrew and says:

> We are one link in the great chain of being. Carbon atoms from the very beginning of time are in our every breath – the universe is imprinted without our flesh and blood. Strangely and wondrously wrought, we reflect the image of God, or so it is said. What meaning does this have? What meaning can we make? Adrift within the unyielding flow of time we struggle to understand our lives, our own small place in the larger scheme of things. Yet nobody like us has ever been or will ever be again. The mystery of creation is mirrored in ourselves.
>
> *(p. 333)*

There was another reflection that seemed apt to the moment, and it was about truth – it seemed to reflect where we were at that moment in time, in our knowledge of Covid-19. It is a new virus that medical scientists and researchers are still learning about as they experiment with different ways of treating, aware that there is no treatment as yet, for a virus that seems to work in very different ways in different bodies.

We are learning a great deal very quickly, but it feels also important to acknowledge how unknowing we are about very basic questions: about how it spreads asymptomatically and whether children can pass it on to their parents if schools return? It can be hard to reflect back to acknowledge what our questions were and how pressing and urgent they felt at the time. Years later we are still constantly having to learn from our experience about the truth of this virus. In the spring of 2020 doctors in hospitals had to be very adept at learning from each other, as they tried out different possibilities. They had to trust what they witness and learn to acknowledge how unknowing they still were.

> Emet, "truth", is not an abstract truth, a theoretical ordering of the universe, a system of belief that explains it all, that demands our loyalty and consent.
>
> Emet, "truth", and "emunah", "trust", belong to the world of experience, affirmed by generations past, but to be tested in our own lives. Both derive from the word "amen", that which is "firm", "secure", on which we can rely, which we "affirm" when we say the word aloud.
>
> *(p. 339)*

As this philosophical reflection on the Hebrew notion, Emet – truth – goes, it relates to a time of Covid-19 and the time it has taken us to take the threats seriously, when we thought that medical science would be able to protect us from any viral threats:

> Every generation has its doubts when faced with its own challenges and pain, and our liturgy invites such questions. The assurances of the past give us hope, but do not remove the task of seeking our own answers in our time and place.

They go on to quote:

> Religion offers answers without obliterating the questions. They become blunted and will not attack you with the same ferocity. But without them the answer would dry up and wither away. The question is a great religious act; it helps you live great religious truth.
>
> *(p.339)*

Before I move on, I just want to recall a final reflection on the Kaddish, the Jewish prayer for the dead. I've said it most mornings since Tony has died. This morning his Shloshim was acknowledged by the community, marking a shift in the mourning process that is publicly acknowledged in moving his name to a different list, but still in an uncanny way joined with the name of Rabbi Neil Kraft who is also being remembered by the Leo Baeck College community. In a time of Covid there is much to learn:

> Yitgadal, v'yitkadash sh'mei rabba … The old words stir memories: of those now long gone, or those more recently departed. So many have left us. Parents… friends… family… community… those we loved and those we could never love enough. And we, the survivors, reflect awhile as the ancient text is read anew. This is the prayer for those no longer with us. And as we pause, we hear the euphemisms we use: "gone", "departed", "left us", "no longer with us."
>
> We hesitate to name the unavoidable truth that underpins our life. Yet the end of life is a destination all must one day reach, a fate we can never overcome, a destiny not to be denied. Now we recall another truth, that often slips from view: this Kaddish prayer never mentions death. Instead defying our fears, it extols life…It overwhelms our doubts, persuades us – if only for a moment – that every day is holy, that all of life is precious….
>
> *(pp. 347–348)*

Different Christian, Islamic, Hindu and Buddhist traditions will each also have their own way of marking these changes in living and dying. In largely secular times we might surprise ourselves by a need to recall and remember spiritual traditions we left behind in childhood and had broken with intellectually. Having learnt so much from Marx and Freud, there are times when experience can take us beyond the terms of secular rationalism, while still engaging with critiques of racial patriarchal capitalism, as author bell hooks often showed.[2] Lived experiences might echo in the present, as we seek for language in which to make sense of the shocks, fears, and losses that we are living with in a time of Covid that we never anticipated. We might feel a need to find words beyond the secular traditions that have shaped our everyday ethics of care.

Hospital Voices, Lockdown and Covid-19

In a BBC Radio 4 File on Four on "Coronavirus – stories from behind the mask" it is noted that when we see intensive care staff on the TV news they are usually in their protective equipment, so we can't see their expressions – even their own colleagues can find it hard to recognise them behind these masks. They can be trapped in feelings of isolation and loneliness as they come together in a sense of community when their shifts end.[3]

The broadcast said, "We can't read their faces, but we can hear their thoughts." The programme recorded, as an ethnography in real time, a series of diaries as the weeks in the grip of the virus go by. Featuring doctors, nurses and other health care practitioners, the stories document the "private emotions and professional fears" reflectively, as well as showing the "emotional toll" of being on the frontline. They are challenged philosophically to make sense of situations they had never anticipated but now feel firmly in the grip of, without really knowing what they can offer.

As we listen to their voices both in the hospital and when they are at home, we hear ethnographic moments that also raise philosophical questions and ethical concerns. I was not sure how to write about them, knowing that readers cannot hear the anguish in their tones of voice or the fears and sadness they might be sharing on their sound recorders. The recordings were made in mid-March 2020 as the coronavirus pandemic was reaching panic proportions and a group of doctors and nurses from around the country had agreed to keep diaries for the programme.

At moments of pause, when they can leave the immediate demands of their work, they record their thoughts and feelings without much sense of how these might be put together by the programme makers. They share their concerns but also the difficult ethical choices they face as they work on the front line of what some persist to think of as "a war against the virus."

Monday 16 March 2020. The day that "social distancing" has been set to start across the UK as an instruction by the government. "A virus that seems to have come out of nowhere seems to have changed our life completely," Jane Deith, the narrator acknowledges that at that point, the vaccine is a remote possibility, and reflects on the uncertain and fearful environment as the virus begins making an impact on healthcare workers.

We hear testimony from Rupert Pierce, a consultant in intensive care at the Royal London Hospital in Whitechapel, in the East End. He shares how he is with a local Bangladeshi man in his 50s who is on a ventilator. He has a nurse, Anna, by his bedside all the time. Although she is not a trained intensive care nurse, she has relevant experience and has been given this task during the Covid pandemic.

Already hospitals have become unrecognisable as routine surgery wards have been turned into Covid-19 wards.

Monday 23 March 2020. Week 1 of lockdown, an unimaginable measure, until it happened, put it in place to keep the NHS from being overwhelmed.

Larrisa Thorn, an intensive care nurse, lives in Aylesbury with her husband Graham and two children and she has been working as an intensive care nurse for 19 years. While they are staying home to save the NHS, she is going to work to save lives. She describes her fear of what is to come: mentioning how warm the previous weekend was, and speculates on the impact this socialising may have had, and what her and her colleagues at Stoke Mandeville hospital may expect. She worries that people will fail to listen to the advice being given to stay home.

Anita, a midwife and nurse lives on the south coast with her little girl. She's been looking after people with suspected coronavirus but is worried she needs better quality protective equipment and says she is not convinced that the basic equipment she has is good enough. She anxiously reflects on the possibility that she could transmit the virus before being aware that she is herself infected. She is left feeling unsafe even though she is assured by those in authority about what she should be wearing.

She knew there is a lack of the necessary PPE equipment and that the issues have been all over the media but is somehow left in an impossible situation because she wants to work but also feels worried about bringing the virus home as a single parent. When sometime later people started clapping for the NHS it brought tears to her eyes and she said, "it meant a great deal."

While the country was considering the new realities of life under lockdown 336 people have already died of Covid-19, more than 6,000 have caught the virus and infections are doubling every few days. As intensive care consultant Massiah Sandri acknowledges, not being able to "cure" his patients is deeply frustrating: "it breaks you into pieces." He is responsible for life and death decisions in his London hospital. On 23 March, he despairs of having to turn away patients, and restricting the use of ventilators, because of their frailty and underling diseases. He recalls one man who strikingly reminded him of his own father, which made the decision not to put him on a ventilator all the more painful.

He demonstrated the importance of being impartial in the allocation of what are still scarce resources but also the difficulty of decisions he has to make because he is dealing with human lives and with people he has developed a relationship with. Being impartial does not mean being impersonal or imagining that you can make a choice from a neutral place because it is in a particular time and place, in the midst of an emergency that decisions are being made.[4]

Spreading Virus and Fearful Times

Nearing the end of March it was clear the virus was spreading and picking up speed outside of London. In the West Midlands 32 people have died. Ron Daniels is a consultant in Birmingham who reports that the intensive care unit is at capacity due to the crisis. He expresses concern in the lag of their collective understanding of the virus.

He readily acknowledges that this is a new virus and that they are in a position of unknowing, gradually learning from their everyday experience with patients but also learning that it seems hard to generalise across patients because people seem to be hit by the virus in such different ways, even if there are similarities between some patients. Daniels describes the situation as a "waiting game" in this respect, trying to trace the virus's progress and how patients are likely to respond to treatment.

Saturday 28 March 2020. Rupert Pierce's team at the Royal London has been hit really hard. He records how he has been called into work to cover a colleague who is poorly, with symptoms of Covid-19. At this point, less than half of his team remain healthy enough to continue to work, and he highlights how "frightened" they are for their health, for their families and for the decisions to come.

As the ventilator carries its own risks, they try alternative ways of healing with breathing and providing oxygen to patients first. Even though the nurses want to do their best for their patients it can be hard to even smile when you are behind a mask. It can be stressful for nurses who feel they cannot provide the standard and quality of care they would want to give and are used to giving in normal times, when the hospital feels literally overwhelmed with Covid-19 patients.

Larissa worried about the care she can give to her patients, knowing she has a family at home but also a father who is self-isolating as a cancer patient. She also feels overwhelmed by the kindness of strangers who have left food for her as a means of supporting the work she does as a nurse. When she comes home, she feels dirty because she's had to wear the PPE all day and needs to clean herself before she comes into contact with the family.

She's also concerned with how her father is doing so her mind is full, though work can take her mind away from worrying about him. She's not sleeping well as she's anxious about getting a phone call about her dad and at the same time feels she cannot support her mother through this difficult time. If she feels hot at night, suddenly she wakes up and thinks "Covid!". She describes this as "such a bizarre feeling," and it is a fear that seems to be almost always with her, that working where she does, she is vulnerable to the virus. It's a feeling she hopes "she will be able to learn to live with and get over."

1 April 2020. In London consultant Massia Sadri has worked ten days strait. Normally there is enough protective equipment but this week it's been an issue. He reflects on the previous day as being particularly hard, and that he "was getting medical emergency calls every hour." He notes that the PPE situation is becoming more acute.

In Birmingham where the pandemic is still intensifying Ron Daniels records his distress at witnessing the last hours of a young Covid patient, who is only able to see one of their family members: "to watch a teenage girl saying good-bye to her mum on Facetime and saying, 'I'm going to make you proud'… it's hard."

Severe Illness, Intensive Care and Dying

Monday 6 April. Week three of Lockdown and the day my brother Tony was to die. Across town Sadri was having a hard time working in intensive care, after returning to work after a few days off, and recorded a high number of deaths in the unit. He describes the situation as "hopeless" in elderly Covid patients, and reflects on "finish(ing) the day signing a lot of 'do not attempt CPR' forms," and struggling with this.

At the Royal London Rupert Pierce is worried and is putting as many people as he can on ventilators, but more patients are dying than he expected, showing how much is still unknown about the different ways Covid-19 takes over different bodies and renders them breathless. He would expect to be able to save two out of three lives, but in the pandemic, it seems like one out of two are surviving on ventilators and then often with considerable damage to their bodies.

He wondered whether Covid-19 might have been a more severe disease than typically seen, as the most critical patients were primarily placed in intensive care, while less severe cases were treated in standard hospital wards. He expressed the self-doubt experienced by NHS staff on the adequacy of patient care, due to this severity He expressed worry regarding the possible rise in ventilator usage without enough trained nurses, potentially resulting in increased mortality rates.

Anita is one of the intensive care nurses who is being spread more thinly over many more patients than normal in an ICU, but her PPE won't stretch. She records on Wednesday 8 April wearing the same mask for the whole day, even when seeing different patients, an unsafe practice. As the narrator Jane Deith says on the same day that Anita recorded, the surgeon Abdul Choudry died from Covid-19 – now more than 20 health workers have lost their lives.

When Choudry fell ill, he warned Boris Johnson on social media that there wasn't enough PPE. His son Intasar says he was desperate that others should be safe and protecting, describing him as a "grand soul", noting how ill his father was when he took to social media to issue this warning.

Intasar felt proud of what his father did and will never let others forget his name. He was able to read a prayer to him as he said goodbye to him, asking him to forgive him for anything he had done wrong as a son. His mother was also able to visit to say good-by in hospital. These moments of saying good-bye are so important for the grief that is to follow and can be invaluable within a mourning process. In lockdown it is hard to realise that there are families and friends across the country and the world being torn apart in grief.

Abdul Choudry had worked at the same NHS trust as Masia Sadri and his former colleague was to die in his hospital. Sadri described that seeing Choudry's wife "broke me to pieces." He described having seen many people pass away in his professional life, but reflected on how his personal connection to the family was particularly "disturbing", and his "sense of failure" was "overwhelming."[5]

It is the Easter weekend and the weather is good and the government is insisting people to stay indoors, making no allowances for the different situations people find themselves in and the particular risks they might be under. Hospitals and care homes are still reporting the highest levels of deaths since the outbreak and doctors and nurses are still asking for more PPE. Matt Hancock the health secretary has suggested that some staff are using more than they need, so attempting to shift responsibility away from government incompetence and lack of preparation towards the nurses and doctors themselves.

I remember feeling intense anger when I heard the announcement as an abuse of government power in relation to the media. Hancock criticised people for overusing PPE, but claimed he understood why they did. But this is exactly what he was doing in his double-speak, shifting responsibility to those who had consistently questioned the shortage of necessary PPE.

Anita was not impressed by Hancock's statement on PPE "misuse", stating that she "(felt) like screaming." At that time, the guidelines stated that PPE should not be used with patients not showing symptoms, but as Anita pointed out, the nature of the virus was that people could be contagious whilst being asymptomatic. To Hancock, she issued the challenge: "I dare you to come and do my job in such close proximity to so many patients who are so vulnerable and not to wear a mask."

Caring, Frustrations and Deaths

Monday 13 April 2020. Week 4 of lockdown. Boris Johnson is out of hospital and says the NHS saved his life, but 10,000 people now have died. The news is that we are staying in lockdown for at least the next three weeks. Larissa feels it is so difficult because her father is really ill and she cannot support her mother who is also self-isolating with him. She delivers food but feel the intense pain of separation – "I know that I cannot touch my dad."

She was on a night shift, and it has been a tough one. She leaves the hospital at 9.00 in the morning after a really busy night. She had a cry, feeling that she would not be able to cope with the pressure she was under, and give the kind of care her patients deserved: reflecting on the challenge of dedicating time and attention to vulnerable people whilst all the while wishing she could go home to her children and partner.

Monday 20 April 2020. Week 5 of lockdown. At the Royal London hospital Rupert Pierce wants to break the isolation of the ICU to manage the risk and to allow family in *to say good-bye* to their loved ones. He has witnessed the pain of people who have died alone away from family and the limits of the video-phone call. He recognises that they should do everything possible to allow people to die with dignity, even if this meant making changes to their procedures, as long as family were aware of their risks. He noted that these circumstances were "really sad" as providing the best possible palliative care is so important to his team and is "something we take such pride in."

He acknowledges that this means the family member is going to be really upset at witnessing and being with someone as they die at a time when their nurses are really stretched and will find it hard to give the care and quality of support that they are used to giving in more normal circumstances. It's complicated as they also need help to take off the PPE and that is a critical moment because it is when you can infect yourself.

At the weekend the number of people who have died in hospitals passes 20,000– 51 days after the first death was announced. Larissa intends to "stay strong" for her patients and her family. This proves hard in the environment both at work, and in the spaces she has to enter. At the supermarket, she is disgusted by a man who deliberately "coughed in (her) face and started to laugh," having clearly spotted her NHS ID. The encounter left her shaken and in tears, bewildered by his "cruel(ty)." She notes that this is particularly hard when she thinks of her colleagues, and the sacrifices they are making in order to do an "amazing job under such hard circumstances."

Monday 27 April 2020. Week 6 of lockdown. Overall hospitals are starting to see fewer people with coronavirus and fewer deaths. In Birmingham Ron Daniels is feeling the first bit of hope in a long time. He is seeing more patients stabilise and beginning to get better and four of them are getting ready to return to the ward and soon possibly another two. Across the county people have seen thousands of people in intensive care – and giving that care has never been that intensive. They've lost nearly as many critically ill patients as they have saved.

Adrenaline has got people this far, but as Sadri acknowledges, "I'm completely drained. The experience of Covid was a very hard experience for all NHS staff. They all put their lives in danger at the same time they always had worries at the back of their minds that they could take a deadly virus home and expose their families to illnesses. I really hope the NHS has some reserves so that when we are stretched, we can cope with the difficult times."

The narrator Jane Deith notes that the hospital system has been forever changed by the challenge presented by the pandemic, and the horrendous toll it has taken on the NHS staff confronted with an unprecedented level of crisis, and witnessing so many people dying in their care, and "not being able to do anything about it."

Rupert Pierce in Birmingham and his colleagues make it clear that they will have to live with the effects of coronavirus for a long time. He considers the news at that time that the government are entertaining a softening of regulations, and even then, sees an increase of traffic on the roads. This is unnerving for him and his team, still fighting for extremely ill patients. He speculates that for them, the pandemic will continue in all likelihood for the next year. Considering the state of the NHS, he sounds despairing and exhausted: "we are just a little bit broken."

Covid-19 and the Hard Path to Recovery

As Haroon Siddique reports: "It is a general rule that the sicker you are, the longer it will take to recover," indicating that patients unwell enough to be put on ventilators would "face the toughest convalescence." Those who respond successfully to intensive care treatment and able to be discharged from hospital *still* faced a long road to recovery.

Faiz Ilyas from Clayton near Bradford spent eight days in Bradford Royal Infirmary, including five days in ICU but was not put on a ventilator. He describes being "really breathless" doing lightweight tasks such as going to the bathroom when he was ill, and described being discharged from hospital having been instructed to do "exercises to utilise the whole of my lungs," but having no sense of when he might fully recover. He was 24 years old at the time (*The Guardian*, 7 April 2020).

David Hepburn, an intensive care consultant at the Royal Gwent hospital in Newport described the experience of being a patient in an ITU (intensive therapy unit) as "life-changing," noting the significant physical weakness of patients when they are awake again: "they can't sit up unaided, many can't life their arms off the bed due to profound weakness. They need to be taught to walk again, breath again, and have problems with speech and swallowing."

Recovery from this is a long road: Hepburn called time spent on a ventilator in this proves as a "small footnote." He emphasises the impact on former ITU patients' mental health, with PTSD and depression as common side-effects.

Hylton Murray-Philipson was in intensive care and on a ventilator for five days and expressed his struggle with understanding why he survived, and others didn't. Speaking to Sarah Johnson for *The Guardian*, he described being ill for just under a fortnight before being admitted to hospital: a period in which his nonagenarian father passed away, and his mother and sister fell ill with the virus. Despite listening to the constant coronavirus coverage on the radio, he found it difficult to think it was actually happening to him. He had a persistent temperature of 40 degrees. When he finally got through to NHS 111 the advice was quite general.

As he recalls a couple of days later, despite wanting to "push through" and maintaining a "stiff-upper-lip", his illness overwhelmed him: he not only had a temperature and a cough, but he also suddenly felt quite faint and dropped to the floor and vomited. Shortly afterwards, he was admitted to Leicester Royal Infirmary.

He was under observation for one night. The next day they said they were taking him to the ICU where he was attached to oxygen, a drip feed, a catheter, antibiotics and morphine. He had a device in his mouth to stop him choking and tube down his throat into his lungs. He shares his experience of "drift(ing) in and out consciousness," the "panic" he felt when he "had this sense of drowning and dying." He remembers a nurse mopping his brow with a damp towel and soothing his hair and putting lip salve on his very dry lips.

He recalls that it felt like a regression: "I was utterly dependent on others for everything… I was wiped out by struggle for breath." His illness was so extreme that he faced the prospect of dying: "I have a strong faith and the idea of falling into the arms of a loving God became quite appealing." What pulled him out of this was imagining the impact losing him would have on his family, picturing his sons and his mother: "the idea of her losing her husband of 65 years and her only son in one week was horrific."

He was supported by people around the world who were praying for him and felt he couldn't let them down. He remembers feeling he had something to contribute as a farmer interested in sustainability and conservation work. It was a sense of purpose that seems to have got him through. The day after his situation began to improve and when he was moved out of intensive care after five days, he knew deep down that he'd made it.

He nevertheless experienced survivor's guilt: during his hospital stay, he described the deaths of a 13-year-old boy and an ENT consultation, describing the ordeal in particular of seeing the child struggle in his last hours as "harrowing" (*The Guardian*, 9 April 2020).

The boy he was referring to was Ismail Mohamed Abdulwahab from Brixton, South London who had tested positive for Covid-19 on Friday 27 March. Apparently, he had no underlying health conditions. He died in the early hours of Monday 30 March. "Ismail started showing symptoms and had difficulties breathing and was admitted to King's College hospital," the family said. Dr Simon Clarke from the University of Reading said: "While the old are much more likely to die from coronavirus infection, the young are certainly not immune from it" (*The Guardian*, 31 Mar 2020).

The consultant who died, Amged el-Hawrani, 55, was the first confirmed hospital frontline worker to die after testing positive from coronavirus. His death brought the total number confirmed in hospitals at that time to 1,228. The NHS National Medical Director, Stephen Powis described Amged's passing as "not just an individual human tragedy, but a stark reminder to the whole country that we all must take this crisis seriously" (*The Guardian*, 29 March 2020).[6]

Stress, Sufferings and Survival

Given the administrative constraints it is important to listen with full attention to the experiences of those on the frontline. In an anonymous letter published by *The Guardian*, one reflected with passion and sadness about the everyday realities of his hospital experiences, and the physical and ethical stresses everyone working in the NHS was under. The clinician addressed their "fellow healthcare workers." They described the conflict they felt in turning away patients for intensive care: with the result that many were "sicker for longer" and increasing the likelihood that they "might not survive."

The letter turns to the various groups that the doctor sees as being let down in the dire situation. Addressing their consultant, to whom they frequently turned, they expressed empathy for that impossible situation: "How do you allocate the scarce resources… Often it is a three-person decision." They note that turning to data offers "little ethical guidance." Turning to their colleagues who take on those patients turned away from intensive care, they reflect with sadness of the "grim" odds for patients, and that their chances would not be significantly impacted even if a different decision was made.

The doctor portrayed the chaos their colleagues were left: "waiting on more ventilators, more nurses, more testing, more everything." Addressing the nurses and healthcare assistants: they acknowledged the colossal stress of their caring responsibilities: "I know you are stretched. You are here, you are trying and that's all any of us can do at the moment…"

Reflecting on their own mental health, they described being in tears on their commute home, and seeing fellow passengers move, having "no idea what to say." They described having the "faces of those patients I couldn't accept to intensive care etched in my mind. I replay the conversation I had with parents about their child's prognosis saying they could not visit their daughter." They shared their fears of dying of the virus themselves.

Despite the despairing, exhausted tone of the letter, the clinician ends on a hopeful note, saying: "I'm so grateful for my health. I will be scared at the end of this, but I will survive. We will survive. We have to" (*The Guardian*, 30 April 2020).

Multiple Deaths and Rewriting History

Helen Ward, a professor of public health at Imperial College London, criticised the government's slowness to implement lockdowns, in an op-ed for *The Guardian*, even with pressure and evidence from the scientific community. She relates a colleague telling her that "for the first time in his life he was more concerned than his mother, who had been relatively blasé about the risks of Covid-19."

She used this example to illustrate the gap in concern between scientists and non-scientists, explaining that, "Two months on, that anxiety has not gone, although it has been joined by a sense of sadness." She places the blame for multiple deaths on the fact that "our politicians refused to listen to an act on advice. Scientists like us said lock down earlier; we said test, trace, isolate. But they decided they knew better."

Ward criticised the politicians justifying their decisions on "science" "as if it is a neutral, value-free process resulting in a specific set of instructions," ignoring the processes of revision and response required to follow the evolution of medical understanding of epidemics.

She recorded how the government alarmed many public health experts by abruptly on 12 March abandoning containment and announcing that community case-finding and contract-tracing would stop, in the hope that the spread would slow. When the government announced measures on 12 March that neglected to include social distancing in any significant way, she concluded that "Neither the advice not the science were followed that week" (*The Guardian*, 15 April 2020).

As Nesrine Malik has assessed the history:

> Here's what we already know. The government delayed implementing the lockdown for no clear reason – perhaps it was the prime ministers outsized regard

> for the "freedom-loving instincts of the British people", or a misguided bid to pursue "herd immunity" – and then reversed its position. Weeks were wasted and thousands of lives were lost.
>
> *(The Guardian, 27 April 2020)*

At the time of the pandemic and in its immediate aftermath, it was clear to see that governments across the world were concerned with how their actions were reflected in the media. In the UK it was particularly clear that the government tried to exert as much control as possible over the news cycle. Nevertheless, dissent narratives circulated. Emily Pierskalla, an American nurse, also questions the *distractions* from the lack of preparedness and responsibilities that government authorities carry for the multiple unnecessary deaths by calling health workers "heroes" when many feel they are just doing their jobs in situations made actively more dangerous because of the lack of PPE. She powerfully reflected on this in a piece for the Minnesota Nurses Association:

> If I die, I don't want to be remembered as a hero I want my death to make you angry too. I want you to politicise my death. I want you to use it as fuel to demand change in this industry… to mobilise others. Use my name at the bargaining table.[7]

As journalist Emily Apple reported, UK leaders scrambled to "shift the narrative" on Covid. She criticised their approach as "gaslighting the public by rewriting history to omit their failures," and using the news cycle as a tool to do so. In Apple's words, "daily press briefings are not keeping it accountable; they're allowing it to recycle soundbites." She perceived a lack of "scrutiny" at press conferences for the duration of the crisis."

She noted:

> Everything about this crisis and the way it's unfolded is political. The people who have made the decisions that have cost lives need to be held to account. We must never forget or forgive what those in power have done. We must fight for better wages and conditions for all those who've kept the country functioning during this pandemic. And we mustn't let our politicians get away with rewriting history and erasing their role in the spread of this deadly virus.
>
> *(The Canary, 16 April 2020)*

It did *not* have to be this way and other countries have shown that there were policies that *could* have been followed that would have saved lives and warning people much earlier about the deathly threats they faced with the spread of Covid-19.

Notes

1 Leo Baeck College teaches rabbis for the Reform, Liberal and Masorti movements in Great Britain. For some years I have taught there and originally it was teaching rabbinic students that helped shape my book *Jewish Philosophy and Western Culture* (London: I.B.Taurus 2007). The *Forms of Prayer* for Sabbath and Festivals are published by the Movement for Reform Judaism (London: 2008). The Liberal Movement used *Sidur Lev Chadash* published by the Union of Liberal and Progressive Synagogues (London: 1995).

2 bell hooks the African-American feminist academic writer and activist had vision that broadened over time since her early work *Feminist theory: from Margin to* Centre (Boston: South End Press) to include a materialist understanding of human being as embodied, emotional and spiritual selves. See, for example, *Sisters of the Yam: Black Women and Self-Recovery* (New York and London: Routledge 2015) and *All About Love: New Visions* (New York: William Morrow 2016). She remains an inspiration for a renewal of social theory and philosophy.

3 "Coronavirus: Stories from behind the mask" was a BBC Radio 4 programme for the Series *File on 4*, first broadcast on Sunday 17 May 2020 at 17.00. The broadcast at the time of writing is unavailable, and the quotations here have been transcribed by the author from the original broadcast.

4 For studies that share the experiences that doctors and nurses went through in the early days of the Covid-19 pandemic see, for instance, Dominic Pimenta *Duty of Care: One Doctor's Story of the Covid-19* (London: Welbeck Publishing 2020); *Crisis* Louise Curtis *A Nurses Story: My Life in A&E During the Covid Crisis* (London: Pan 2020); John Wright *Coronavirus Doctor Diaries: Stories from the NHS Frontline* (Independently published 2022).

5 An understanding of the everyday ethics of care and insights into the world of patients and nursing written with the fullness of heart is offered by Christie Watson *The Courage to Care: Nurses, Families and Hope* (London: Vintage 2021). See also her *The Language of Kindness: A Nurse's Story* (London: Vintage 2019).

6 A narrative of a hospital and what it lived through and how it survived the Covid pandemic to secure PPE and completely redesign the hospital is given by Adam Jarrett *In the Time of Covid: One Hospital Struggles and Triumphs* (Independently published 2020).

7 Emily Pierskalla, RN "I want my death to make you angry" (mnnurses.org, 13 April 2020).

11

TRUST, GENDER POLITICS, CARE HOMES AND DISPENSABLE BODIES

Broken Trust, Anxieties and Political Failures

Writing when public trust in the government was breaking down and people were asking questions about the lockdown and why the UK seemed to have one of the highest death rates from Covid-19, journalist Polly Toynbee described politicians as "taking the public for fools," and squandering public goodwill. As scientists expressed significant "differences of opinion" on what counted as "safe" measures, politicians were unwilling to be honest about that uncertainty. As Toynbee points out, "No one knows all the right numbers yet, but trust shrinks when the government missuses them anyway." She sees a cultural correlation between this rejection of doubt and the "absolutist Brexit cast of mind" gripping a large proportion of Tory ministers (*The Guardian*, 18 May 2020).

Toynbee perceived this as politically exposing. She considers, for example, Matt Hancock's dumbfounding claim on Friday 15 May: "Right from the start we've tried to throw a protective ring around care homes…we've made sure care homes have the resources they need." As horrifying accounts emerged from care workers and relatives of the vulnerable occupants of care homes besieged by the virus, Toynbee asks: "What sentient voter doesn't know that to be a flat-out lie. On Tuesday 26 May 2021, during seven hours of evidence to MPs, Cummings accused Hancock of promising ministers that all care residents in England were being tested before being discharged back to their homes and then lying about this.

Politicians in a panic grab for two life rafts, Toynbee explains: internal fall guys and public enemies who are to be blamed and held responsible when the strategy of "following the science" – which often means ducking behind the scientists to let then take the flak – has grown thin as it becomes clear that scientists have different views that the public cannot be trusted to know. Teachers were first to occupy the latter role,

DOI: 10.4324/9781003296874-11

and then came the doctors' turn: and "the most unfit government in living memory" watched as essential workers were pilloried. By not seeming to learn from these mistakes, Toynbee suggested, they were "eroding any trust in the notion that their prime motive might be serving the public's best interest, not saving their own skins."

John Crace in his political sketch has traced how Matt Hancock's "normal Tiggerish enthusiasm and good will" had been dented by criticism. He portrays Hancock as "not just under attack from a country that wonders why the health secretary hasn't done rather more to protect the nation's health" but as a "scapegoat" for his own "cabinet colleagues" preparing for "the inevitable public inquiry" (*The Guardian*, 18 May 2020).

Of his House of Commons performance presenting his coronavirus statement, Hancock seemed aware of the "pure fantasy" he was repeating, but was "not quite ready for the admission of failure," according to Crace. Speaking of the virus like a "mild inconvenience… rather than the worst public health crisis for 100 years" he blithely repeated that, "The government had done brilliantly, hospitals had coped and mental health services were there for anyone who needed them."

Trust is undermined by politicians who cannot admit when they have made mistakes and are incapable of acknowledging when they do not know something, or even when there are doubts about the advice they might be getting. Too often this has been a trait of male politicians shaped by having to compete within a patriarchal culture. Their experiences are formed by having to live up to a dominant masculine imaginary. Whatever happens, they cannot show signs of vulnerability because any sign of weakness is a threat to your male identity.

So it is that in politics, across political parties, men will often find it hard to acknowledge when they are unsure or do not know something. They feel obliged to be in control even when they are not. This helps to shape the language they use and the authoritative voice they learn to assume. Often it does not inspire trust because people eventually stop listening to whatever they have to say. They have learnt not to trust and once trust is broken it can be difficult to repair.[1]

Dis/Trusting Toxic Masculinities

After months of minimising the threat of Covid-19, Donald Trump denied that he ever did such a thing and if he did it is others – the Chinese – who are to be blamed for it. Drawing on the rhetoric of war that dominant masculinities often fall back on to affirm their threatened masculinities, Trump shifted to labelling Covid-19 as an "invisible enemy" and positioned himself as a "wartime president". He described his pandemic responses as "our big war" and he assured Americans that his "aggressive strategy" would end in "victory."

As Trump tweeted on 28 March 2020 10.30: "With the courage of our doctors and nurses, with the skill of our scientists and innovators, with the determination of the American People, and the grace of God, WE WILL WIN THIS WAR. When we achieve this victory, we will emerge stronger and more united than ever before!"

As Lisa Wade and Tristan Bridges write on a blog for *Gender and Society*, Trump "invoke(es) militarized masculinity… adopted by men who see themselves as fighting for a feminised "homeland": a rhetoric long used by US presidents. They add that for many US citizens, masculinity is "strong, fearless, self-assertive" and that it encourages individuals to "face down danger": a tendency that is "deadly" in a pandemic.[2]

Instead, Wade and Bridges speculate that our toolkit for surviving the coronavirus is non-violent: wash your hands, shelter-in-place, wear a mask for essential errands, and quarantine if you've been exposed." They point out: "We need people to hunker down, not 'man up'", but see that this runs "contrary to traditional notions of manliness. This may be why men are substantially less likely than women to wash their hands" (*Gender and Society*, 13 May 2020).

Rosie Frasso, program director of public health at Thomas Jefferson University is quoted by Alyson Krueger in the *New York Times* as saying: "We need to make sure men don't feel too macho to worry about germs." Personal hygiene habits have far-ranging consequences in the Covid-19 pandemic. It seems that men traditionally express less concern for a range of potential threats and so are less concerned with handwashing, face mask use and avoiding crowds. They seem more likely to think that certain risks are worth taking and they can feel that risk-taking is a habitual way in which they affirm and so prove their male identities. As Frasso says, "We need tailored messaging for a lot of things, so it would be logical that this is no difference. For one thing, we know men are less likely to seek health care than women" (*The New York Times*, 17 March 2020).

In relation to Covid-19 this means that men might discount symptoms more easily and also be hostage to early messaging that insisted the virus was little more than the flu and it would be no bad thing it you got it because you would be assured of immunity and could return more easily to work. This messaging proved lethal for many. It has also meant that men have reported to doctors only once the symptoms proved to be really serious, so endangering their lives when they eventually had to go to hospital.[3]

Of course, not all dirty hands can be pinned on men. While Frasso believes women are more hygiene-conscious than men, she recalls in an airport on 8 March, she saw two college-age women coming out of the bathroom without washing their hands. Only after she called them out did they return for a proper 20-second cleanse. Just the fact that both men and women are closely watching their neighbours, also about wearing facemasks, can make a difference. After all, "social norms change behaviour," she said. But with lockdown and the closing down of social spaces, the opportunities to observe others in public are closing down.

Often men across different class, racial and cultural backgrounds learn within Western modernities to be independent and self-sufficient. This can make it difficult to really trust that others – even those in intimate relationships – can really *be there* for them. Often men feel unconsciously, though they might not verbalise it, that when the chips are down, they are on their own. They feel a constant need to prove their worth as men and that they can never really take their masculinities for granted.

Within a neoliberal capitalist culture masculinities are refigured and intensified as time becomes a scarce commodity. Men, across boundaries of class and race, can feel they have to be constantly in control over their lives so that they are constantly planning ahead. Time has to be carefully ordered and not wasted. They constantly have to be active, doing things to prove their worth and affirm their success and achievements in their own eyes. They are fearful of their own existence as vulnerable humans. This can make the inaction, passivity and restrictions of lockdown difficult to bear. It can mean middle-class men, able to work from home, pushing themselves to work harder to prove themselves in the eyes of their line managers. This can bring tensions to home life, where both adults might be working under different neoliberal office regimes.[4]

But the separations from everyday routines and relationships at work can sometimes be difficult for men in particular ways because they can be more externally or other-defined as David Riesman explored in the classic *The Lonely Crowd*. They can feel that the control they feel they need to have over their everyday lives is threated when they cannot leave home, and the demands of children's education and domestic life which they might find hard to balance with the demands of work, causing tension in the gender division of labour at home.[5]

Men can find it hard to acknowledge their own fears and anxieties, as the lockdown goes on and they can take out their frustrations out on their partners and children behind closed doors. They can find it hard to deal with the multiple time demands, especially if they cannot withdraw into a space of their own. With both middle-class parents working from home in restricted spaces, tensions emerge as they are negotiating competing demands.

As Wade and Bridges note, pandemics require primarily cooperation, shared vulnerability and collaboration: leaving little room for individualist and traditionally 'masculine' behaviours. These tendencies towards independence as autonomy and an abiding fear of dependency have moved across the boundaries of gender and they can make things even harder to negotiate within lockdown. Within a neoliberal common-sense it can be difficult across genders and sexualities for people to acknowledge their fears and anxieties because they seem to threaten the autonomy as self-control that they have learnt to identify with so firmly.

Wade and Bridges assess the US are correct in thinking that the effects on the pandemic are long-term, entailing a "survival-mode" mindset. However, in a time of gender fluidity, prescribing gender-based traits like humility, vulnerability and community-mindedness seems problematic and reinforces gender stereotypes. This approach may not be helpful in fostering inclusivity and understanding.

Different generations of men, partly under the challenges of feminisms and ideals of gender equality, have worked to transform attitudes, feelings and relationships in ways that have questioned traditional gender binaries. As they acknowledge, society must evolve beyond associating gender with leadership in these narrow terms.

Gender, Power and Leadership

Robin Dembroff, assistant professor of philosophy at Yale University, wrote that during health crises, "macho leaders are a weakness not a strength." He recalls that "days after California had declared a state of emergency and Seattle schools begun to close, Donald Trump asserted that Covid-19 would simply 'go away.'" Dembroff sees parallels with Ronald Reagan's first term, and his reluctance to take the Aids health crisis seriously: despite the virus killing around 30,000 Americans by 1987, the then-President dismissed it: saying, "it would go away" (*The Guardian*, 13 April 2020).

Shortly before Trump said Covid-19 would "go away" he said it would "disappear…like a miracle." In Brazil his closer admirer, Jair Bolsonaro, had described Covid-19 as a "little flu" that would not want "hysteria" and claimed that Brazil would be protected from the virus by its climate and youthful population. Supposedly it would only kill the old and they were dispensable anyway.

Dr Robert Kirby, a men's health expert suggested that "dominant, aggressive, (and) risk-taking" behaviour that typifies 'toxic masculinity' encourages men to see health problems as "effeminate and weak" choosing "discomfort" over the "emasculation" of getting medical help. When faced with the prospect of contracting the virus, Bolsonaro claimed that his "manly history 'as an athlete' would protect him from the virus." Men brought up within the terms of traditional masculinity can find it hard to acknowledge their own emotional needs. They can have an instrumental relationship with their bodies, as I argue in *Embodying Masculinities*, which can make them less aware of their bodily symptoms, treating tiredness or bodily pain for instance, as a limit they have to transcend and so prove themselves against.

Dembroff saw a need for "traditionally 'feminine' traits such as empathy, solidarity and compassion" in order to appropriately deal with the virus, and a rejection of toxic "political self-interest" (*The Guardian*, 13 April 2020).

As Australian journalist Gay Alcorn has reported, these are qualities that Jacinda Ardern and other female leaders have been able to access in their leaderships. Of Ardern she notes a "combination of steel and compassion." Following an inert start, her address to the nation announcing a four-week shutdown: "Kiwis go home," was "clear and unequivocal," outlining in simple terms the 'four-stage alert system' in New Zealand.

Alcorn recognises that key to this was her "'tone at the lectern." On the restrictions, she was direct: without them, she claimed "tens of thousands of New Zealanders will die. There is no easy way to say that." Concluding her address, she called on citizens to "Be strong and be kind." Alcorn compared her response to that of Scott Morrison in Australia, who gave a statement on the 13 March that despite having effectively banned mass-gatherings, he would still be attending a rugby league game himself. Morrison's government was also hurt by its step-by-step approach, advocating strong measures but not an enforced shutdown, as Ardern had instructed in New Zealand. They were to pay the consequence in higher levels of deaths.

Alcorn cites social researcher Dr Rebecca Huntley's research into crisis management: "What people need are hard and fast rules. When you give people discretion, at a time of panic, then that's difficult for them." She advocated that politicians lead with clarity, and tap into their humanity (*The Guardian*, 25 March 2020).

Clarity, Compassion and Empathy

Ardern had the compacity, so lacking in Boris Johnson and Donald Trump, to really combine clarity and compassion and to speak directly to people's anxieties and concerns and to help them order a time frame, warning people *not* to despair because there would be an upward rise in deaths because of the time-lag between the shut down and its effects. She was able to identify and *show empathy* for the stressful times people were living through while encouraging them to look out for elderly neighbours, asking if they could drop food for them while being careful to maintain social distance.

There was an informality in her video addresses, apologising not being in her work clothes, that people could relate to and stands in contrast to the masculine tones of authority that Johnson assumes in giving people instructions, while being incapable of really expressing *empathy* for the grief so many families around the country were experiencing. He would express regret at the multiple deaths and insist that each death counted, but this was *not* the point. He could *not* emotionally connect with the grief widely felt as Tony Blair had been able to do at the shock of Princess Diana's death. He had found helpful words in calling her "the people's princess" but was also able to express them with feelings.

On 1 April Silveria Jacobs, prime minister of the small island Sint Maarten, addressed her nation's 41,500 people. Amidst the rising coronavirus cases, she was well aware of the peril faced by the island, which annually receives 500,000 tourists but possesses only two ICU beds. While reluctant to enforce a stringent lockdown, she emphasised the necessity of observing physical distancing, as reported by journalists Jon Henley and Eleanor Ainge Roy. She issued the message: "Simply. Stop. Moving… If you don't have the bread you like in your house, eat crackers. Eat cereal. Eat oats. Eat… sardines." She knew how to get through and communicate with feeling and empathy to her people and how to set clear boundaries that they needed at this moment of panic. She did not have the global profile of Merkel or Ardern but was an effective communicator.

Henley and Roy saw a global trend of women leaders, including Germany, Denmark and Taiwan, rising to the challenge of Covid with particularly successful results, nothing that "few (nations) with female leaders have done badly."

They cited the then-Chancellor of Germany, Angela Merkel, as being praised for "uncharacteristically personal public interventions" and striking an empathetic tone that male leaders often cannot find within themselves. Capacities for empathy cannot be willed into existence, whatever efforts are made. Words often sound false, and people see through them.

Thanks to extensive testing from the outset – that was never abandoned as it was with such devastating consequences in the UK on 12 March – and plenty of intensive care beds and Merkel's periodic forthright reminders that Covid-19 was "serious – so take it seriously," Germany has recorded far fewer deaths, in relation to population than the US, the UK and most EU countries. With a doctorate in quantum chemistry, Merkel could get to grips with the different scientific views. She could explain them clearly to the public, without having to defer to the scientists, as Johnson did, seeking protection from criticism while at the same time presenting a false idea of scientific knowledge.

In Denmark the decisive action taken by the prime minister, Mette Frederiksen, who closed the country's borders as early as 13 March going into a firm lockdown a few days later, seems to have spared the country from the worst of the pandemic. There were fewer than 8,000 confirmed cases and 370 deaths. She could draw on the cultural trust people have for their government and their sense of social solidarity, as Danish citizens facing a shared crisis. She also showed a sense of fun, posting a Facebook clip of herself doing the dishes while singing along to the 1980s Dodo and Dodo, during the nation's weekly TV singalong. The effectiveness of her actions is shown in her approval rating and the widespread support she has for a careful opening of primary schools, as part of a gradual softening of lockdown conditions.

Kathleen Gerson, a professor of sociology at NYU recognises that women leaders are more likely to be elected in "a political culture in which there's a relative support and trust in government – and that doesn't make stark distinctions between women and men. So, you've already got a head start." Since the very best leaders are both strong and decisive and capable of displaying feeling, women could, perhaps, "lead the way in showing that these are not competing and conflicting attributes, but complementary – and necessary for good leadership," she said (*The Guardian*, 28 April 2020).

Gender and Sexual Differences

As columnist Arwa Mahdawi insists: "Being a woman doesn't make you better at handling a global pandemic – but women generally have to be better in order to become leaders." We need to be careful not to reinforce "sexist and unhelpful ideas that women are innately more compassionate and cooperative." She recognises – invoking a 'we' as a shared experience amongst women – "we are held to a far higher standard than men… With a few notable exceptions you've got to be overqualified for a top job" (*The Guardian*, 11 April 2020).

Mahdawi sees the dire situation in the USA as a consequence of the fact that "Instead of expertise, Trump's administration has led with ego." She notes Trump's pandemic activities: tweeting, and "lashing out at the press and state leaders." Columnist Simon Tisdall sees globally that, "authoritarian leaders are exploiting, exacerbating or grossly mishandling the response to the pandemic, placing selfish interests ahead of public good."

These toxic masculinities and resulting behaviours that make it harder to listen and learn, cost multiple lives. These leaders share dysfunctional characteristics such as a war fixation and a poverty of imagination. As Tisdall understands, "Lack of empathy (is) a common denominator, even among self-styled "man of the people" populists." He notes of leaders of this ilk who " (personally) believe that they… know best are the worst-behaved, least effective pandemic performers" (*The Guardian*, 26 April 2020).

Turkey's "strongman" president Tayyip Erdoğan was accused, like Trump, of politicising the crisis. His initial response to a growing Covid-19 threat was to put the economy before lives, before imposing a "rushed" set of restrictions that merely added to the sense of panic and prompted food shortages. Tisdall also cites the macho leader of the Philippines, Rodrigo Duterte, who like Erdoğan minimised the Covid-19 threat, then over-reacted. With regard to those who did not comply with the regulations Duterte ordered the police and military to "Shoot them dead."

As pointed out by Tistall, Duterte's assumption of emergency powers resembled "power-grabs" seen in countries with weak "democratic accountability." Hungary's Viktor Orban similarly claimed that indefinite ruling by decree could be "revoked any time", raising concerns about the potential lack of parliamentary oversight to do so. Moreover, Tisdall argues, Xi Jinping exploited the pandemic for political purposes, evident in the "opportunistic" arrest of 15 Hong Kong pro-democracy campaigners. He used the confusion of the pandemic to his advantage, justifying further crackdowns after the previous year's unsuccessful attempts to quell anti-Beijing protests (*The Guardian*, 26 April 2020).

While fully acknowledging that spread and death rates depend on many variables, including population density, wealth and past decades of health care preparedness, as Covid-19 moves across borders in the global South, it can still be helpful to note wider social phenomena. Alice Eagly, a psychologist at Northwestern University, found in her research that in leadership roles, women were generally "more participative and collaborative in leadership" and men more likely to be "authoritarian and top down" (*Politico*, 5 January 2020).

As political journalist Elizabeth Ralph notes, the former approach is particularly "effective" in situations requiring 'buy-ins at all levels – from national governments to local mayors." It can also be helpful that "Women are more communal, the more compassionate sex showing empathy and caring," says Eagly. "That's stereotypically true, but it's also actually true in data." In a situation where people are suffering and dying, where many are fearful, "to emote, to recognise that people are having a hard time," is key.

Cultures of Care and Disposable Bodies

Reflecting upon the status of people with disabilities within the coronavirus pandemic, Rabbi Elliot Kulka introduces themself to Alice Wong in the Disability Visibility Podcast saying, "I am a rabbi as well as personally chronically ill and disabled." They are also a trans activist working for the Bay Area Jewish Healing Centre.

Kulka notes:

> ...from the very beginning of this pandemic... it felt clear that disabled, chronically ill, elder, fat lives, the lives of other marginalised people were being seen as disposable... it was before there was the immediate medical rationing happening in this country. But at that point... the earliest messaging was, "Stay calm. Don't worry. This virus is pretty mild. The only people that might be at the risk of dying are, you know, elders and disabled people. So, it's not that much to worry about," with this very dehumanising way of talking about our lives as disposable.

They recognise how:

> ...the tone of the conversation from the beginning was really alarming to me and really dehumanizing. And the conversation really has continued that way... and that means that on a triage list... you know who has the best chance of surviving and who has the most years left and categories that are not going to benefit us. And those alarms that were raised for me at the beginning just kind of keep ringing and that sense of feeling disposable.

In an article he wrote for *The New York Times*, "My life is more 'disposable' during this pandemic," Kulka opens by pointing out that for them and others also living with health issues and disabilities, "staying at home is not new." What changed rapidly for them was a "gnawing feeling of dread" partly driven by a "pestilence of ableism and ageism" prompted by the pandemic (*The New York Times*, 19 March 2020).

Kulka's saw evidence of this in the choices being made about the elderly, the disabled and the chronically ill Covid-positive patients forgotten by healthcare systems, whose "lives are considered, quite literally, more disposable." This, they point out, indicates the approach of a "perfect storm" of uninsured citizens, workers without appropriate sick-leave protocols and strained healthcare providers.

Feeling "disposable" is, Kukla shares, "not new to me... knitted into my bones and my sinews." They criticise the attitudes of those with power in healthcare, who decide "my transgender, fat, disabled body is simply worth less than other bodies", which is "even more true for my black, brown, poor, disabled and ill friends."

As the child of a Belgian at the mercy of Nazis, they describe a long, embodied memory of a history of violence against disabled bodies: the term "useless eaters" used by Nazis to describe the disabled and chronically ill, who were murdered first. They cite research into trauma at cellular level found in the families of Holocaust survivors, describing how their "father's story lives in my own overactive immune system, and thus my body's response to this pandemic right now." Bodies carry memories, hurts and feelings of abuse, across generations in ways that can take time to emerge, let along name and feel safe and confident enough to express. Sociology has yet to come to terms with these transgenerational emotional legacies.

They share the devastating impact that the phrase "useless eater" continues to have. Kulka shares that his father lives with dementia and Parkinson's in a care home, where pre-pandemic it was "a struggle for people to act as if his life was still worth protecting… The term 'useless eater' hangs just beyond what's said aloud." Kulka concludes that the only way to unspool this cellular, generational trauma, is through others: "to survive illness and trauma, whether individual or communal, we need one another."

Ageism, Disrespect, Care Ethics and Generations

Journalist John Harris recognises the need for a fundamental shift in attitude towards the elderly, the vulnerable and disabled and how much we can learn from different communities. Speaking to Javed Iqbal, a community worker in Alum Rock in Birmingham, an area badly affected by the virus, he shared how he had lost 11 older relatives to Covid-19, a loss not just to him and his family, but to wider society. "These are the pillars of our community: our elders," he said.

As Harris recalls, this was "a stark reminder of what the secularised, divided part of the UK's demographic map lacks, and which we urgently need to recover, as these horrific times put us ever further apart" (*The Guardian*, 26 April 2020).

He recalled a poignant conversation with Richard Kempner, whose 86-year-old mother passed away from Covid-19 in a care home during the lockdown. She couldn't have visitors and died alone, without proper testing and PPE for the caregivers, according to her son. "Covid walked into her room," he said, "Because she couldn't, and didn't walk out of it." Harris noted the UK's collective shame as deaths were underrepresented in official statistics, a crucial aspect of their virus experience, "compound(ing) a sense that such fatalities do not quite count."

As Richard insists, the plight of care home residents needs "to be shouted about, not hidden," speculating that the political silence could be due to their shame of how the pandemic unfolded for the most vulnerable older people. For Harris, the way that the government have neglected and let down older people "long predate(s) the crisis," and draws attention to the phrases "underlying health conditions" frequently used in the same breath as reporting fatalities during the pandemic, as if it is "the natural order of things" for someone with a complex condition not to be spared by the virus. Harris surmises that a charitable reading of this could be "a collective coping mechanism," but nonetheless shows that it "highlights a set of prejudices about older people that have set in the culture for far too long."

Harris recognises how up until a few months before, "residential settings for older people rarely figured in the national conversation," that the "archetypal care home existed in our shared imagination as somewhere distant from everyday life…

still and silent." It existed as a place and time apart if you didn't have relatives there, in a world of its own.

Dr Anna Down, a GP in Ealing, West London shared her deep anger with Robert Booth, *The Guardian*'s social affairs correspondent. She scanned her computer for figures to show how Coronavirus had ravaged her care home patients, sharing that in two homes, "50 per cent of the residents died in the space of 10 days."

As Booth reported:

> Her anger goes beyond grief…early warnings to public health authorities about the risk to care residents have not been acted on. Infected patients continue to be discharged into care homes from hospitals, spreading the virus; and staff shortages are blighting attempts to keep the virus isolated.
>
> *(The Guardian, 22 April 2020)*

If issues of abuse of power ever made it on to our television screens, they would be treated as singular cases that needed to be investigated by regulators and rarely allowed to challenge the everyday relations of power that allow for systematic neglect and abuse by people who often feel devalued and unrecognised themselves, taking it out on those in their power they are supposed to be caring for.

Research published by the Royal Society for Public Health in 2018[6] found that a quarter of people aged 18–24 believed it *was normal* for older people to be unhappy and depressed – across all age groups, nearly a third of people surveyed agreed with the statement "being lonely is just something that happens when people get old." Strikingly also two thirds of the respondents said they had no friends with an age gap of 30 years or more.

They also noted that those from a black ethnic background had an attitude to ageing nearly three times more positive than the average. This shows how much can be learnt about respecting elders as sources of experience and wisdom in a media culture that too readily identifies knowledge with information and has often theoretically learnt to discount experience as a source of knowledge.

"Ageist attitudes about in society and have a major impact on the public's health, and yet they are rarely treated with the seriousness they deserve," said Shirley Cramer, the RSPH chief executive, pointing out that "…often ageist behaviour and language is trivialised, overlooked or even served up as the punchline to a joke – something we would rightly not tolerate with other forms of prejudice" (*The Guardian*, 8 June 2018).

Reporter Amelia Hill reported on research for the Society for Ageing Better entitled "Doddery but Dear?" that shows that older people are widely mocked, patronised and demonised and are mostly seen by the young as incompetent, hostile or a burden to others. The report calls for a "fundamental culture shift… to overturn what it calls an ingrained culture of "pity and dislike" towards older people" (*The Guardian*, 19 March 2020).

Anna Dixon, the group's chief executive says: "The response to the Covid-19 crisis have thrown up serious question about the way we think and talk about older people, and highlighted what an impact those attitudes can have." She goes on to suggest that labelling older people as a "burden" by the media is not only insulting but also perilous during the Covid-19 crisis. It fosters a dangerous belief among the younger generation that their freedoms should not be restricted since only the elderly were truly at risk.

As long as the young were wearing masks, they felt they could walk with ease in the middle of the street, obliging older people to get out of their way since they were already doing their bit. Ageism will fundamentally undermine older people's participation in society and will contribute to greater isolation and loneliness which is already a dangerous feature of the lockdown.

Harris highlights how the generational divide, particularly during Brexit, has led some young people to view older individuals with contempt. The challenges faced by younger generations, coupled with age-based lockdown measures, have seemed to create a society "devoid of older people." It emphasises the cruelties of the virus and its impact on our age-segregated society.

Neglect, Care Homes and Cruelties

If there are cultural traditions which respect the elderly as elders in their own communities there will be different priorities, whatever Johnson's government might claim, and lives would have been saved because the NHS would *not* have been given such a clear priority. It was in care homes where people were *most vulnerable*, yet they were *not* given priority, as Martin Green, CEO of Care England told the Parliamentary Health and Social Care committee on Tuesday 19 May. Social Care had not been a priority for the government during the crisis.

It was clear that priority had been given to the NHS *as* an institution. Professor Martin Green criticised the government's approach to care homes, suggesting that they should have known that they were the "high-risk area", when it was "clear that from the very start of this that people will long-term and underlying health conditions were the most vulnerable." He asks: "why wasn't the response quicker?" (*The Care Home Professional*, 4 May 2020).

According to CareUK's Chair, Mike Paris, the government's lack of planning to protect care homes during the pandemic was evident. In March, the care sector took proactive steps to restrict visitors, but there was no corresponding action from the government. Consequently, the government was always playing catch-up due to its slow response. Unfortunately, the government seemed to accept higher infection rates in care homes as inevitable, despite the possibility of avoiding this outcome with adequate support.

Green highlighted that the government prioritised the NHS, resulting in the withdrawal of medical support from care homes and disruptions in PPE supply chains. Moreover, the policy of discharging infected patients into care homes contradicted practices in other countries where symptomatic individuals were isolated outside care homes. This challenges Health Secretary Matt Hancock's repeated claims that the government had placed a protective ring around care homes from the outset, seemingly attempting to convince the public through repetition.

As the committee heard also from Professor Terry Lum at Hong Kong University, Hong Kong recorded zero deaths in care homes from Covid-19 by employing strict infection control measures that were ignored in the UK. He said that Hong Kong had treated the outbreak like Sars, the killer virus that hit Asia in 2003 while by contrast, the UK's response to coronavirus was at least initially based on planning for a flu pandemic. What was vital was, unlike the UK, they had made it a priority "stopping the transmission from hospital to nursing home."

As he said:

> We do a very good job on isolation. Once we have a person infected, we isolate them in hospital for three months and at the same time we isolate all the close contact people in separate quarantine centre for 14 days for observation. They do tests regularly in that 14 days to make sure they don't have the virus.
>
> *(The Guardian, Tuesday 19 May 2020)*

He also noted that care homes went through a drill simulating an infection outbreak four times a year, so infection control becomes "a well-worn practice."

The MPs also heard from Isabell Halletz, responsible for care homes in Germany, who said there had been fewer than 3,000 Covid-19 deaths in care homes in Germany, partly because no one was allowed in from hospitals without a negative test, or had undergone, quarantine in designated centres or repurposed hotels for at least 14 days. There were a host of other factors and as James Bullion, President of the Association of Adult Social Services, pointed out, the movement of agency staff between locations was "a consequence of the structural model we have got," requiring a radical rethink in terms of financing and hiring practices (*The Guardian*, 19 May 2020).

Grief Upon Grief

Following a conversation with Buckinghamshire care home nurse Julie Roche, correspondent Robert Booth described the horror an outbreak of Covid caused: eight patients lost in the span of three weeks. She describes their relatives saying their goodbyes "by phone or through bedroom windows, the solace of touch made impossible by fear of contagion."

She recalls the only option for the wife of one dying man was to stand close to his window in the care home's car park with her daughter and granddaughter. She passed a bottle of her perfume in the hope of making one final connection with her husband. "I could see it broke his wife's heart."

She says other people handed in cards for carers to real to their dying loves ones before they died. "We do it, we cry," Roche says. Many carers consider the residents as an "extended family," and they have grown very close to them emotionally having cared so closely for them. She also says that funeral directors have been asked to drive coffins past the windows of homes and pause on the way to the crematoria so friends can bid farewell.

> Some of these residents we have lost, we have looked after for years… It will hit us at some point. We are on automatic. We haven't had time to grieve. Once we get through this we will sit and reflect and deal with it.
>
> *(The Guardian, 9 April 2020).*

Some care homes made sure their residents didn't die alone. Julie Raynor, a compliance director, says, "We ensure that families are supported to continue to visit if a resident is at the end of their life, no matter what their cause of death will be… Infectious control risks can be safely managed."

Romaine Lawson at Apple House Care, a learning disability specialist group, said that they made every effort to evaluate cases individually, despite a "general 'no visitors'" policy, and said that they "involved the loved one, their family and the whole multidisciplinary team in any decision we make, which means we take the full responsibility of decisions away from one single person" (*The Guardian*, 15 April 2020).

Maggie Kinloch, chair of the Humanist Society, Scotland, has said the impact on grieving families of also not being able to attend funerals with friends and family supporting them would be profound and last a long time. She noted the "a generalised sense of grief across the world" which was "massively compounded when a family loses someone they love" during the pandemic: "It's grief upon grief. If you are unable to attend their funeral, it's yet another layer of grief" (*The Guardian*, 14 April 2020).

She said, "Families want to give their relatives the best possible celebration of their life, surrounded by people who knew them. The comfort of hugs and handshakes is hugely important. These life rituals are shared acts of community."

Michael Cooper from Durham who was unable to attend his mother's funeral after she died from the virus aged 87 confirms this. The ceremony was livestreamed to him and other close family, but he said he was left with feelings of guilt and shame. "The ceremony was impeccable, except there was no one there who should have been there. I felt my mother was alone."

Hopes for a New Social Order

Half of Europe's Covid-19 deaths were in care homes. Weeks after her 113 birthday Maria Branyas found herself confined to her room in her care home in north-eastern Spain. She fully recovered and is believed to be the world's oldest Covid-19 survivor. She had lived through the 1918 flu epidemic, two world wars and the Spanish Civil War, but "reeled" from the effects of the pandemic, exposing the poor social treatment and ostracisation of elderly people, saying of those left to die of the virus: "They didn't deserve to leave the world in this way."

As correspondent Ashifa Kassam reports from Madrid, she thinks that we need to learn and take action to create a new world order – "It will have to be done all over again and differently" – a social transformation that we owe as a debt to those who died in the pandemic. In her care home in Olot, some 70 miles north of Barcelona that was hit by the virus in late March, at least 17 of the 133 people living there died (*The Guardian*, 16 May 2020).

An estimated 17,500 people have died in care homes in Spain, particularly humbling for a society in which "the reverence shown towards the elderly is a point of pride." As Branyas says, "Governments need to pay attention and provide funding and qualified staff in care homes." As her daughter Rosa Moret says of her: "She says… you have to keep looking forward. I think that's why she's lived so long."

But she was keen to outline the changes she wanted to see for her 13 great-grandchildren in their lives – "A change in values, one that prioritises education, health and research… fewer weapons and far less spending on so many politicians."

Notes

1 For reflections on dominant white heterosexual masculinities and how they are often identified with self- control in ways that identify emotions as signs of signs of weakness see, for instance, Victor J. Seidler *Man Enough: Embodying Masculinities* (London: Sage 1997); *Transforming Masculinities: Men, Cultures, Bodies, Power, Sex and Love* (London and New York: Routledge 2005) and *Young Men and Masculinities: Global Cultures and Intimate Lives* (London: Zed Press 2006)

2 The *Gender and Society* blog that Lisa Wade and Tristan Bridges contributed too was May 13, 2020 at 2.26. For some similar reflections on Trump's masculinity see, James W. Messerschmidt 'Donald Trump, Dominating Masculine Necropolitics' in the Special Symposium: *Masculinity and Covid-19* in the journal *Men and Masculinities 2021, 24(1) 189–194.*

3 Research and reflections on men's relationships with their bodies, emotional life and health which explore links between masculinities and men's health are shared in Donald Sabo and David F. Gordon (eds) *Men's Health and Illness: Gender, Power and the Body* (Thousand Oaks, CA: Sage Publications Inc. 1995); Steven Robertson *Understanding Men and Health: Masculinities, Identity and Well-being* (Milton Keynes: Open University Press 2007); Brendan Gough and Steve Robertson (eds) *Men, Masculinities and Heath: Critical Perspectives* (Basingstoke: Palgrave Macmillan 2009).

4 For some interesting reflections on shifting masculinities within global neoliberal capitalist regimes see, for instance, Andrea Cornwall, Frank G. Karioris and Nancy Lindisfarne (eds) *Masculinities Under Neoliberalism.* (London: Zed Books 2016) and Charlie Walker and Steven Roberts (eds) *Masculinity, Labour and Neoliberalism: Working-Class Men in International Perspective* (London: Palgrave Macmillan 2018) which explores active ways men have deal with forms of economic and symbolic marginalisation and the barriers they've faced in doing so.

5 David Riesman's *The Lonely Crowd: A Study of the Changing American Character* (New Haven CT: Yale University Press 2001) helped to shape a psycho-social engagement with changing work cultures. This influenced studies Richard Sennett has done on the changing nature of work in, for instances, Richard Sennett and Jonathan Cobb *The Hidden Injuries of Class* (London: Verso 2023); *Respect: The Formation of Character in an Age of Inequality* (London: Penguin 2004); *The Corrosion of Character: The Personal Consequences of Work in the New Capitalism* (New York: W.W. Norton and Co. 1998) and *Together: The Rituals, Pleasures and Politics of Cooperation* (London: Penguin 2013).

6 "That Age Old Question": How Attitudes to Aging Affect our Health and Wellbeing 2018.

12

RITUALS, TECHNOLOGIES, GENDER, GRIEF AND POVERTY

Everyday Rituals, Mournings and New Screen Technologies

Thursday 23 July 2020. The shock at witnessing the murder in real time in Minneapolis by a white police officer kneeling on the neck of George Floyd stopped us in our tracks, wherever we were. The demonstrations in the US and Europe mid-pandemic drew the world's attention to the Black Lives Matter movement. The deaths of African Americans and BAME people in the UK through the Covid-19 pandemic were disproportionate. BAME people were also more likely to be working in the health, care and emergency services and less able, because of housing conditions, to isolate safely.

At weekends I went to Brent Park. The religious Jewish school had opened across the road. Though in the early days they took precautions with boys gathering in small bubbles waiting to be taken in by teachers, now they have abandoned these steps. Part of a community that has been hit hard with Covid-19 deaths, they still seem to feel they will somehow be protected. If they say their prayers the plague will pass over them.

The head-teacher said he felt children were safer at school where they played together in large groups. This doesn't assuage my anxieties and I will be happy when the term ends, and the street becomes quiet again. There are more car journeys being made. The world is gearing up to return. People *want to believe* the pandemic is over. They are getting restless about wearing masks and the lockdown. Growing numbers want it all to end and life to "return to normal".

For our daughter's birthday on 4 July 2020 we were able to hug each other for the first time in months. We had a barbecue in the garden carefully organised by Richard, Lily's partner. It felt like a moment of freedom to *be together* as a close family. None of us anticipated that after the summer there would be another

DOI: 10.4324/9781003296874-12

lockdown and another after that, and an even longer lockdown when Christmas was suddenly to be erased and we were to find ourselves back in isolation and unable to leave home. This is a time that people seem very anxious to forget, not wanting to be reminded of the hardships and losses.

It had become a ritual for me to attend the morning Shachrit prayers at the Leo Baeck College on Zoom. Tony's name was mentioned each morning as we said Kaddish – the prayer for the dead. They separate the list according to different stages in the grieving process. The Jewish tradition is helpful in giving *time* set apart *for mourning* when you can depend upon the support of a community, but also recognising – as Freud does in psychoanalysis – that you can sometimes get caught in your grief. It is important to mark a time when it is over. But it's quite misleading to talk of "closure" as if we can ever "move on." As I'm finding out – and had very soon to find again – it *is* a matter of learning *how* to live with grief and live in a different relationship with those who have died.

In Jewish tradition, prayers are said for the year and traditionally you refrain from certain activities. But there is a time when it ends, and you can prepare to return to the joys of everyday life and relationships. Writing is a process that take time and you move through different stages. It is uncanny to become aware that I was re-reading these pages and revising the manuscript exactly a year later – last night being 6 April 2021, marking exactly a year since Tony died. Writing had been part of a practice *of* mourning. Preparing the manuscript to let it go somehow corresponded with exactly the ending of a year since his death.

I'm now revising again in February 2023 preparing to mark a year since my wife Anna also died, but from a sudden heart attack, not from Covid. We cannot anticipate what life will bring. As I'm making final revisions, a year is closing when as a family we have supported each other since Anna's death. I'm aware that across the world people are still suffering from those who died from Covid but also from other tragedies. Yesterday they announced the multiple deaths following the earthquake in Turkey and Syria and the sufferings, yet another natural disaster has wrought.

There are losses that continually remind us of our existence as *vulnerable humans*, even if we are living in very different material and cultural worlds within different networks of interdependence. With new media and global communications, we are often positioned as witnesses of sufferings from across the world in real time, that in previous generations we might have only read about after they were over. We are challenged as ethical humans in different ways.

We need a global ethics that can make living connections between the personal and the structural, the intimate and the communal within a renewed vision of global justice. We might be living through our personal grief, but along with so many grieving their own painful and irreplaceable losses. Covid-19 has been a shocking reminder of our existence as vulnerable humans but also of our responsibilities to others who are living much more unequal lives.

In 2021 I settled into a certain daily ritual feeling the need to give a structure to my life during Covid-19. I planned the different Zoom groups I joined more carefully, so as not to be overwhelmed. I learned to relate differently to Anna and appreciate her different needs for contact, daily time for herself but also for her friendships. We were having to shape our everyday relationship differently since Covid-19 had blocked usual work routines and shifted the terms of intimacy and contact. We would try to walk together in nature, as much as we could.

Around the world, people renegotiated their everyday lives in very different circumstances with very different risks of life and death before the vaccines became generally available. We lived closely from day to day with each other in ways we had not planned or anticipated, but which looking back I now feel very grateful for. We would walk in Big Wood in Finchley a few afternoons a week. We got to know the people and dogs that had also made this part of their routine of survival in threatening times.

Lockdown forced people into very different and unanticipated situations, obliged to make decisions they felt insecure and anxious about There have also been generational *shifts* as families have had to negotiate responsibilities for relatives who might live in isolated areas. Grown up children have been concerned about their elderly parents and whether they have been taking the right precautions. There were different attitudes to the vaccines that to some people could seem experimental and carrying their own risks.

Different generations had different access to medical research on the Internet that could help the family learn about the virus and the shifts in knowledge about it. There could *also* be pressure from a generation who suddenly felt they had to watch over their parents and make sure they did *not* take unnecessary risks. Gradually around the world with access to social media and multiple sources of competing information, there were growing divisions, especially in relation to the vaccines. Through social media people could rely upon very different sources of information and learn to live within oppositional media worlds that accused others of spreading fake news.

People were learning to come together in competing groups on zoom as they promoted sources of scientific research while maintaining social distance. New screen technologies like Zoom enabled people to feel emotionally close in unexpected ways. The Covid pandemic has enabled people across the world to experiment with new modes of communication. Many people have been able to get through the crisis though contact that has been established on Zoom and other social media. Through these new technologies everyday life and contact across the world has been transformed and people have learnt to take them for granted.

Like so many families across the world, we have been locked into our own grief through Covid-19 times. Mourning for Tony would have taken a different shape had we been together in the same space able to grieve together. There is also a strange temporality of grief and loss when you cannot anticipate what you might feel from day to day, week to week. As part of a vulnerable group because of age, you can be locked into taking precautions as part of an elder's group that is clearly at risk. You seem *locked into time* in a different way from younger generations you see walking around more easily and gathering in bars. You seem to be carrying your body in a different way and can feel uneasily locked into yourself, fearful of contact.

Many younger generations in 2020 and 2021 still seemed to think it was *only* a risk for older people and those with pre-existing health conditions. This was reflected in how they walked in the middle of streets. They wondered what all the fuss is about. Now that the virus seems to have ebbed away in the summer months, the government is encouraging people to socialise. The Chancellor Rishi Sunak's Eat Out to Help Out campaign offered 50% off food or non-alcoholic drink up to £10 per person for diners. It was launched with television footage of Sunak serving people their burgers. In March 2023 we have learnt about disagreements in government at the time and how it was a super-spreader initiative they are still to be held responsible for.

People across different age, class and ethnic groups also responded differently. A social researcher, about to turn 40, visited his parents in their garden for the first time in months felt something had changed in him about the *value of life* and how precarious relationships could be. He felt he had taken his parents for granted but now could no longer feel they would always be there. Asked what he wanted as a birthday present, he asked each of them to write the story of their lives for him.

He wanted to live with a different awareness. He thought this would make a difference to how he approached his research project on refugees and asylum seekers. They were people finding ways to make new lives for themselves, often separated from their own families back in Iraq, Afghanistan and Syria. At the same time people could feel locked into more restrictive worlds, tuned into what was happening to family and friends, but their contact with the sufferings in the wider world mediated through their screen lives. As lives were disrupted, so people could feel strangely disconnected from the wider world and locked into an isolation that could sap their self-confidence.

Economic Crisis and Transformations in Work Cultures

On Monday 13 July, nine days after the lockdown was suspended on Saturday 4 July 2021, people returned to the shops in Oxford Street. Newspapers talked of freedom and independence. The *Evening Standard* reported a very different story. People had not gone back to the shops because they still worried about going on public transport and because the instruction was still to work at home if you could. Many of the restaurants and cafes could not make opening up pay for them. The *Standard* front page read: "*REVEALED: True Scale of London Economic Meltdown: Capital Facing a Crisis not seen for Generations*" (*Evening Standard*, 13 July 2020).

Reporting on the impact of the virus on Central London, the report notes that previously "heaving streets from Mayfair in the west to Docklands in the east have been left virtually deserted," with no commuters, and no tourists in sight.

Des Gunewardena of a fine dining group ruminated on a 40% decrease in "Super Saturday" revenue, and even "tougher weekdays with revenues way down because of no corporate business." Compared with France and Germany where 30 to 40% of workers had returned to the office, London presented figures of around 3 or 4%, accounting for this gloomy outlook.[1]

Boris Johnson said employees should "go back to work if you can" deviating from previous advice, and the Cabinet Office minister Michael Gove went further saying: "We want to see more people back at work, on the shop floor, in the office, wherever they can be." Yet, confusingly, the government had not yet removed official advice on its website to "work from home if you can". Many owners of hard-hit restaurants, bars, hotels and shops in "Central London's bustling but fragile economic ecosystem are concerned that the Government's change of heart could have come too late to save them." In the technology sector, Russ Shaw, founder of Tech London Advocates, noted that the "Tech city" had turned into a "ghost city."

When *The Evening Standard* updated its report on Thursday 23 July 2020, they found that many large UK companies "have no immediate plans to return many staff to offices… tens of thousands of staff of will continue to work remotely this summer, with some business giants not expecting staff back at headquarters all year." Even though Johnson ditched the work from home guidance from August 1 and gave companies greater discretion on bringing back staff provided workplaces were Covid-secure, ministers were criticised over pushing responsibility for the office return onto the shoulders of bosses, who feared being sued if an employee contracted the virus at work.[2]

Significant numbers of London employers continued to be apprehensive regarding their staff's commute on public transportation. Josh Hardie, of the Confederation of British Industry, stressed that "safety comes first" and that "changing people's behaviour and confidence will take time". RBS (Royal Bank of Scotland) said about 49,000 of the bank's staff in the UK would continue to work from home into 2021. Property website Rightmove had more than 530 staff who had moved to home-based working in March. Chief Executive Peter Brooks-Johnson said: "We're in no rush to bring everyone back. We see the transition as a gradual one."

In light of the potential impact on cafes, restaurants and shops, the government took measures to enhance people's confidence in returning to work. Despite prior confusion surrounding the policy, the authorities made wearing facemasks mandatory, aiming to instil a sense of security and encourage a safe environment for businesses to operate in.

Sir Martin Sorrell who now runs C4 Capital criticised the government for providing "mixed" policies that offered little guidance to employers, yet claiming that the "ecosystems around the office are crumbling… we have to get back to work". There were new trends being put in place of working from home that would continue after the pandemic, as new technologies made it possible. Concerns about a work-life balance had been re-focused as part of a shift in values, which meant workers were making demands that allowed them to limit days they had to work in the office (*Evening Standard*, 23 July 2020).

Toxic Masculinities, Values and Gender Politics

"Not once did the Chancellor mention childcare in his summer statement, despite the mounting crisis in the sector," pointed out Labour's Tulip Siddiq, the shadow minister for children and champion of working mothers. "You can pump as much money as you like into protecting jobs, but parents won't be able to go out to work without childcare" (*Evening Standard*, 23 July 2020, p. 6).

Despite the headline-grabbing £30 billion plan to prevent unemployment in Chancellor Rishi Sunak's statement, in between the VAT cuts, the restaurant vouchers and a stamp duty holiday, there were no policies directed at women, though women were set to be the losers in the pandemic. "It's like a throwback to the dark ages," Siddiq said. "It feels like I'm banging my head against a brick wall. This is not a cabinet that listens to women" (*The Guardian*, 24 July 2020). As the Inquiry was to learn, there were disagreements with scientists about Sunak's plan "Eat out to help out" in the summer of 2020. Professor Dame Angela McLean, a chief scientific advisor, in a WhatsApp message with John Edmunds, a professor of infectious diseases, referred to "Dr Death the Chancellor" – he thought it played a role in prompting the public to take more risks.

As he said, "I'm still angry about it... 45,000 people had just died. I don't want to blame eat out to help out for the second wave, because that's not the case. But just the optics of it were terrible – this was a scheme to encourage people to take an epidemiological risk." Naomi Fulop of Covid-19 Bereaved Families for Justice said:

> This inquiry has made clear that there was absolutely no consultation with the government's scientific advisers on Eat Out to Help Out, that it contributed to the loss of thousands of lives. It's unbearable to think that if it wasn't for Rishi Sunak's reckless, unscientific and callous approach, my mum might still be with me.
> *(The Guardian, 19 October 2023)*

It was also revealed that opponents of lockdown measures were referred to as the "let it rip brigade" by Patrick Vallance, then chief scientific advisor who kept a diary at the time.

Research showed that women were *more* likely to be working in industries like hospitality that had been affected by the economic downturn. The Institute for Fiscal Studies reported that mothers were combining "paid work with other activities – almost always childcare – in 47 per cent of their work hours, compared with 30 per cent of father's work hours." This insensitivity to women was hardly surprising given that nearly all the government departments were led by men and dominated by men. When Johnson was in intensive care with the virus, the government was run by a "quad" of men to discuss key decisions on the virus response (*Evening Standard*, 27 May 2020).[3]

The men had probably *not* noticed, as Hillary Clinton has appraised across the globe: "Women have been demonstrating the kind of inclusive, empathetic, science-based leadership that we should be trying to promote across the world"

(p. 6). Former Tory Minister Caroline Nokes, chair of the Parliamentary Women and Equalities Select Committee, described the British Government's problem as "institutionalised thoughtlessness… it's about 'he who shouts loudest.' There's a reason why that saying is 'he', it's not she."

As journalist Sophia Sleigh reported in the *Evening Standard*: "The PM's persistent public schoolboy bluster can give the impression that the Chamber is, in fact, the common room of a boarding house at Eton." Observed Nokes: "You see pictures of the Prime Minister doing push-ups, but you can't quite imagine Theresa May ever doing that. I do think it's a macho thing."

Nokes said the failure to put access to childcare at the heart of government policy risked sending women back to the 1970s. "The specific needs of women are not on anyone's agenda right now," she said. "In order to even stand still on gender equality at this moment you would need real drive and ambition, but we are not seeing anyone grasp that."

Sleigh reported one Tory expressing exasperation at the "sheer prevalence of "rugger bugger" public school boys across the party," saying that "They never learnt how to speak to girls until they went to university – and then they were drunk." Baroness Jenkin, a Tory peer who co-founded Women2Win with former Prime Minister Theresa May in 2005 said the trajectory of female candidates was "disappointing." She noted that "Women's lives have been and will in the future be disproportionately affected by Coronavirus and they need to be better understood" (p. 7).

Journalist Heather Stewart in *The Guardian* also reported that Johnson was presiding over an "incredibly blokey" administration with "key decisions in the hands of a tight circle of powerful men," with a male-dominated "inner circle" (*The Guardian*, 11 July 2020). Even if Johnson and Gove had sought to make up and put the past behind them, at some level Johnson must still have had feelings of revenge for the man who betrayed him and allowed Theresa May to become prime minister.

Stewart reported a "shakeup" of cabinet committees resulted in uninspired groupings mainly chaired by Michael Gove. The strategy committees were overwhelmingly male, and entirely so for climate change. She recalled during Johnson's hospitalisation with Covid, key decisions were taken by senior male ministers. On the prime minister's return, and facing trouble with the hospitality sector amid a pause in tourist activity, the group assigned to spearhead the revival of the sector, the "save summer six" was also exclusively male.

As Jill Rutter, a senior research fellow at UK in a Changing Europe said, with the exception of Munira Mirza, the then director of the Number 10 Policy Unit, the senior team leading the Covid response was a "bunch of blokes." She pointed to the daily Covid press conferences, chaired in nearly all cases by a man, as another indication of where the power was, that recalled a "throwback to the 1960s – without Barbara Castle." As Stewart noted: "The junior minister Penny Mordaunt is widely regarded as being on the naughty step after criticising Cummings's trip to Durham during lockdown."

Amber Rudd, former Conservative home secretary, said: "The fact that they have concentrated power into such a small group means it's easier to exclude women and make like it look like a coincidence." It's striking – even laughable if it were not tragic – that when Matt Hancock, the health secretary, was challenged about ethnic diversity in Johnson's cabinet, he said: "It's diversity of thought that's the really important thing when you're taking those big decisions around the cabinet table."

An anonymous woman who worked closely with Johnson doubted that Johnson was aware of the poor optics: "I just think he has a view of the female role and that is never at the top table." It was a legacy of a boy's public school, a vision that when the chips are down or you are up against the wall, women cannot really be trusted. It is your mates that you can rely upon. Tim Montgomerie, who worked for Johnson for a few months in Downing Street, complained in *The New Statesman* of what he called "Dom's frat house," complete with joshing nicknames as a feature of the macho boys' culture they had re-created.[4]

Johnson's chaotic indecisiveness delayed lockdown measures, and in his evidence Cain, his communications director said Johnson has the wrong "skill set" to lead the country through the pandemic. Cummings told the Inquiry that "pretty much everyone" called Johnson "the trolly" due to his constant veering about, while vulnerable people like the poor or victims of domestic abuse were "almost entirely, appallingly neglected" at the start of the crisis. He also criticised Johnson's focus on the media, especially with the *Daily Telegraph*, which pushed against lockdowns (*The Guardian*, 31 October 2023).

As the nastiness, arrogance and misogyny of No 10 was exposed to the Covid Inquiry Cummings, apologising for his abusive sexist language towards Helen MacNamara, deputy to the cabinet secretary, who he would "personally handcuff her and escort her from the building" – "we cannot keep dealing with this horrific meltdown of the British state while dodging stilettos from that cunt" – which was "obviously appalling" while denying it was misogynistic because he was "much ruder about men" (*The Guardian*, 31 October 2023).

In her evidence a day later Helen MacNamara said, "We were looking at harm through a very narrow lens, without realising that, of course, there can be all sorts of other consequences of things you can't see." As late as 15 April she felt compelled to ask if anything was being done about "the fact that most PPE isn't designed for female bodies", despite 77% of NHS staff being female. In her witness statement she talked about the lack of a female perspective" led to "significant negative consequences, including the lack of thought given to childcare in the context of school closures." She also notes, "I am sure there would have been kinder ways of managing pregnancy and birth especially given the differential clinical outcomes for women and their babies who become stressed." She says, "there was a disproportionate amount of attention given to male pursuits" (openDemocracy.net, 1 November 2023).

As Tim Adams reported, "it was McNamara, quietly upstaging her nemesis, who had the last word… [she] was by contrast, self-effacing and human – and among the few clearly determined to speak truth to power". In this spirit, she delivered a devastating assessment of the "macho and heroic" tone of the government response to the pandemic, which clearly contributed to the scale of death and damage. But he also notes, "For all their temperamental differences, it was striking how often Cummings and MacNamara agreed about the nature of the problems that had occurred." They both had heard Hancock promise "again and again" that detailed plans for every eventuality was in place. There was no plan (*The Guardian*, 5 November 2023).

But she recognised, "We need a modern culture of organised collaboration, not a superhero bunfight," she wrote in a draft report in May 2020, where "everything was contaminated by ego." As the crisis deepened women became "invisible overnight" in decision making – mute on zoom calls or silenced sitting at the back of the room. What Cummings and Johnson shared was an active hostility to the existing machinery of state, which was to have terrible consequences when they ignored the existing network of public health directors across the country. As MacNamara said the violent and misogynistic language "was miles away from what is right or proper or decent or what the country deserves." As she noted, "everything was contaminated by ego. It was positively unhelpful when the country needed thoughtful and reflective decision making."

Women, Childcare and Politics

Stewart pointed out in a report that there was hope within No. 10 to hire a woman to lead the new televised daily lobby briefing as part of the government communications radical shakeup. The envisioned role for this individual would have been to inform the public on decisions rather than being involved in their formulation. Sam Smethers, director of the Fawcett Society (the UK's leading charity campaigning for gender equality and women's rights), said Johnson's government had a "gender blind spot," which she argued may have contributed to a string of issues including the reversal on free school meals and the lack of support for childcare.

"They just don't get it," she said. The announcement that beauty salons would be allowed to open followed a backlash from female Conservative MPs who complained on WhatsApp that the industry had been ignored. They didn't seem to understand that childcare played a role in the job losses of almost half the women made redundant since the pandemic hit.

A survey which gathered detailed responses from almost 20,000 working women in 48 hours, was a "cry for help," said Joeli Brearley, founder of the campaign group *Pregnant then Screwed*. In the study, approximately 50% of women surveyed revealed that the lack of childcare negatively influenced how they were regarded or treated at work; 81% of respondents said they needed childcare to sustain their employment, while 72% reported having to reduce their work hours due to the absence of childcare. Additionally, over half of the participants reported facing backlash from their employer regarding childcare challenges.

Brearley expressed exasperation to journalist Alexandra Topping that working mothers had been "ignored during the pandemic," and were now facing job insecurity, saying that "mothers are the sacrificial lambs from the economy contracting."

According to research conducted by the *Early Years Alliance*, about 25% of early years providers worried about potential closure, rising to 33% in disadvantaged regions. Early years childcare seemed to be part of the £1bn "catch-up fund" but was later excluded. A recent survey found 33% of employed mothers and 44% of self-employed mothers had lost childcare spaces due to costs since March.

That put childcare workers, the vast majority of whom are women, at risk of dropping out of the workforce, as Neil Leitch, the chief executive of EYA, warned. He added that the early years workforce, of whom 97% are women, were severely at risk of losing their jobs due to the government's neglect of the sector.

Breaking Trust and Irresponsible Policy-Making

George Osborne, Chancellor of the Exchequer under Prime Minister David Cameron and editor of the *Evening Standard* from 2017 to July 2020, was critical of Johnson's handling of the pandemic, though at the beginning he was generally supportive. He noted the public embraced the advice and followed the rule more than "any behavioural scientist advising the Government imagined," noting the strength of the collaborative spirit of the nation in those initial months, all the more extraordinary after years of division between Brexiteers and Remainers (*Evening Standard*, 13 July 2020, p. 12).

However, this did not last. Osborne noted that this "solidarity" quickly "faded" as the public began to turn away from the "ministerial briefings" they had previously "hung on every word of in the spring." He asked why the British public had withdrawn their support, when other European citizens maintained "high levels of public confidence" in their politicians, even with the uncertainty of a moment when the vaccine was a remote possibility, and all were feeling the economic effects.

"The answer," Osbourne suggests, "lies in part in performance. Britain has not done as well as most in preventing deaths." On Johnson, he said that those who opposed his leadership were "furious", believing that he was "literally getting away with murder." However, Osborne thought not all the blame could be laid at Johnson's door and that people recognised that scientists' advice was contradictory. But the scientists were *agreed* that the lockdown should have come weeks earlier and that the opening up should have been done with more care, as in Scotland and Wales.

Lives were put at risk and even then the government was *not* clear or consistent in the policies it adopted, with weeks of uncertainty about the wearing of facemasks and only clarifying if face coverings were to be mandatory in shops and supermarkets just hours before the regulations were to come into force in July 2020. In his speech to Parliament, on 14 July, Health Secretary Matt Hancock said the death rate from the virus of sales and retail assistants was 75% higher than the general population for male shop workers and 60% higher for women.

As Osborne had realised, people were no longer *really listening* to the government. A catalyst of this was Dominic Cummings' now infamous run-in with Durham constabulary in Barnard Castle, and Osborne suggested that the "slide" continued. Illustrating how much public solidarity had receded, he presented a "challenge… to find two members of the public who agree on what the rules are now on what's permitted and what isn't." The confused and unclear messaging, worsened by politicians asking people to "use your common sense," and therefore abdicating responsibility for those key decisions, led people to a point of deep frustration (*Evening Standard,* 13 July 2020, p. 12).

People were also puzzled as to why so late in the crisis, masks were being made compulsory when this could have happened months earlier. They remembered that in March scientific advisors had said wearing a mask made no difference. They might feel anxious, but they *no longer trusted* what the government was saying and thought it had its own purposes, like persuading people to get back to work in the city even when it might not be safe. People followed their own diverse sources of advice, often from social media.

Osborne recognised the reluctance of politicians and scientists alike to admit to their mistakes. When people saw Johnson maskless in public at a time when wearing them was being valiantly encouraged in public spaces, Osborne suggested, this directly influenced the decisions of the people, saying: "if it was serious, they'd make it a rule." It was a rule in shops and indoor spaces where you could not easily sustain social distance. *The Evening Standard*'s front page headline on Wednesday 22 July stated: "Don't Leave without a Mask" in what it called a "last minute bid to end confusion as law comes into force for shoppers on Friday" (The Evening Standard, 22 July 2020).

Masks had been compulsory on public transport for some time, but the official advice was still to drive if you could, which was bad for congestion, air quality and long-term health. Osborne recognised that: "The Kitchener moment has passed," and that the public were owed explanations for how they had been left to interpret and misinterpret rules, suggestions and clear flouting of guidance by the people meant to give consistent and unambiguous advice. We knew that despite whatever Johnson had mistakenly promised for Christmas 2020, life could not return soon to what used to seem normal.

Lockdown Poverty and Everyday Crisis

The Food Foundation found that food insecurity quadrupled during the lockdown. People were going hungry. There was massive public support for the campaign by Manchester United footballer Marcus Rashford to secure children's food vouchers through the summer holidays. Cafes and chip shops had notices in their windows inviting customers to say: "It's for Marcus" to get a free kid's meal. Johnson said at first the government could not support free food for children – until he realised *how* strongly the nation felt.

There was a wider awareness in the country of growing poverty, largely unrecognised by the mainstream media and the government. Coventry University researcher Alison Brigg's work in Stoke on Trent with a local charity that provided an independent food pantry showed a 104% increase in referrals in the first month of lockdown. It was evident that some of the people who were in most need of government financial support were not receiving it.

Briggs expressed despair that charitable organisations were becoming "increasingly relied upon to plug the gaping holes in the social security safety net" that had worsened during the protracted austerity period, and overwhelmed services during lockdown (Breadline Research, Coventry University, 22 July 2020).[5]

With the suspension of face-to-face research, Briggs had kept contact through text messaging to explore everyday lives and relationships during Covid-19. She explored how many low-income families across Stoke-on-Trent were reliant upon informal networks of family members and friends, as well as foodbanks. She also learnt how indispensable local, grassroots charitable organisations were "in ameliorating the material and psychosocial effects of food insecurity."

From her research, she heard how draining it was to manage food budgets that were stretched to their absolute limit. One of her sources, 65-year-old Maggie, living with her daughter and granddaughter, shared "an intensification of anxiety and worry" due to her regular financial support from extended family members disappearing because they had been furloughed.

Briggs explained that "maternal altruism" saw mothers "regularly skipping meals" in order to feed their children: but I wonder whether this should be thought about as altruism – it is a form of self-sacrifice for children that is a feature of poverty.

These are issues of class entangled with questions of race and everyday racism. They are also central concerns to do with social justice. What levels of inequality *are* acceptable in a society of equal citizenship? How do we justify people having second homes when their fellow citizens have to go hungry in order to feed their children? This is a vision we might identify with the novels of Charles Dickens in the 19th century but hardly with 21st-century Britain.

What does this say about the legacies of a neoliberal capitalism and the inequalities of race and class that have been so brutally *exposed* during the Covid-19 pandemic? How do these inequalities, rendered starkly visible, call for new political imaginations, challenging the idea that people on state benefits or low wages are losers with only themselves to blame? What are the responsibilities of citizenship in a liberal democratic society and what are the *limits* to social and economic inequalities that are morally justifiable?

How are we to think about the economy of energy that is absorbed in tiredness and its health consequences for mothers who are going hungry so that their children can eat? As one mother told Briggs by text, her family were so low on food that she had to make one sandwich last for the whole day. To her enormous credit, she found solace in going out in the sun, and reflecting that this ordeal would increase her "patience," but noted her exhaustion, saying: "I still want to be alone" (Marge, text message, April 2020).

As Emma Revie, CEO of the Trussell Trust said at the ENUF food and poverty conference (Evidence and Network on household food security): "The solution isn't food, the solution is income." Income can be seen as something difficult to change as its focus moves towards central government and their benefit policies, but it has to remain central if we are to work towards a society which no longer has to rely upon foodbanks. Their very existence provides a moral and political challenge to government.

In the aftermath of the pandemic, we know that insecure, precarious and poorly paid work is the root of food poverty, and this will increase over the next few months. This makes it urgent to think about *how* we can provide food assistance in that is empowering, participatory and doesn't stigmatise, an issue raised by Val Barron in her blog (Breadline Research, Coventry University, 24 June 2020).

Reckonings, Fears and Futures

Richard Horton, editor of the medical journal *The Lancet* didn't think an inquiry into the government's handling of the Covid-19 crisis should be delayed. He thought we had to learn lessons immediately for the waves to come. He called for a "reckoning" for the "missed opportunities and appalling misjudgements" here and abroad that had led to "the unavoidable deaths of tens of thousands of citizens."

In his book *The Covid-19 Catastrophe: What's Gone Wrong and How to Stop it Happening Again* he lambasts the management of the virus as "the greatest science policy failure for a generation." He attacks the Scientific Advisory Group for Emergencies (SAGE) for becoming "the public relations wing of a government that had failed its people."

He called out health authorities, including Public Health England, for not reinforcing the WHO public health emergency warning back in February 2020, and damned the UK's response as "slow, complacent and flat-footed" revealing a "glaringly unprepared" government and a "broken system of obsequious politico-scientific complicity." He knows that in the future the government will say that "it is all very well in hindsight" to make judgments, but Horton shows that everything was known back in February 2020 if the government had only been ready to listen, and that they cannot avoid responsibility of the many unnecessary deaths that they failed to plan for.

As he told journalist Andrew Anthony: "I'm not criticising individuals, but the system was a catastrophic failure." As editor of the *Lancet*, he published five papers in late January first describing the new Coronavirus in disturbing detail, but they went unheeded. Several of the papers stressed the importance of personal protective equipment, he reminded Anthony:

> And the importance of testing, the importance of avoiding mass gatherings, the importance of considering school closure, the importance of lockdowns. All of the things that have happened in the last three months here, they're all in those five papers.
>
> *(The Guardian, 14 June 2020)*

He still couldn't understand why the government's scientific advisors didn't consult their counterparts in China.

What he knew, from the published reports of Sage meetings, is that scientists were "trying to be as sensitive to economic issues as they were to health issues." That, he says, "is a dangerous place to be" because it compromises the ability of the advisory group to protect health. As a researcher, he's always been concerned with the social and economic structures that shape health outcomes.

During his treatment for cancer, he gained a new appreciation for health workers and the true significance of the phrase "key worker." In being shielded, as Anthony suggests:

> The experience has made him regard anew not just the hospital staff but also, amid a large cast of previously undervalued workers, the couriers who brought him vital medicine when he ran out. These people, he says, his voice full of emotion: 'They're the ones who are making our society work.'

The experience of living through Covid-19 helped him shape a new political imagination and a different vision of possible futures. He knows that the "moral provocation," as he frames it, of Covid-19 is *not* one we can afford to ignore.

Horton believes this pandemic moment *could be* a watershed moment in history, an event that is much larger than simply a crisis in health. "Covid-19 has held a mirror up to our society," he said:

> ...and forced us to look at who really is vulnerable and who has to literally put their lives on the line while the rest of us are secluded in our houses. We've discovered something about ourselves that we may have been conveniently able to hide before, but we can't hide any more. And so the question is what we do with that knowledge now?

Educating Futures and Shifting Fates

Emma Brockes, writing for *The Guardian* from New York, found respect for teachers was to shift dramatically. Teaching unions were wary about returning to the classroom until track and trace measures could be firmly put in place. Brockes traced how admiration for how teachers do this all day was to turn to impatience. Archly reflecting on her experience of home-schooling, she described it as "a hideous grind" involving "bribery, shouting, chaotic Zoom-calls" that left her feeling that "If the virus didn't kill us, the worksheets surely would" (The Guardian, 23 July 2020).

She watched a backlash against teachers with the US being slightly behind the UK in terms of its willingness to reopen schools. Aware she was writing from a privileged situation, she nonetheless speculated on a "horrifying" possibility that there would be no "full return to school in September," likely to further exhaust and demoralise parents.

In New York, she was facing a "blend of in-person and online learning," where children could expect to be in school half the time. She recalled herself saying more than once: "If McDonald's is open, the schools should be open" though she knows there is no logic to this since no one was permitted to eat in at McDonald's, let alone spend five hours – a school day – breathing on staff.

She was aware of the class divide, with wealthier parents buying themselves out of the situation with "small learning pods" and "private teachers." She also noted that American private schools with the resources to do so intended a full return for pupils.

As Brockes recognises: "None of this… is the fault of state school teachers, many of whom have their own kids at home." Yet she owns up to seeking the "the small endorphin rush" of "trashing" the teachers, concluding that they are being "over-cautious" not because of research, but because parents "have had enough."

She noted her fatigue with the whole lockdown situation, while fully recognising that so many other working-class people had had it so much worse in so many ways. "We are done… we have no more adrenalin left to burn." Instead of a New York Covid-19 propaganda poster with the heading *New York Tough*, most of the people she knows are not feeling tough but exhausted.

Despite her conflicted feelings, she makes it clear that she supports the teachers and the schools, and that they have gone a long way to make the situations "tolerable" with their care and dedication. Reflecting the sudden shifts in mood, a feature of lockdown in the very different class, racial and gender settings people found themselves in, she says: "And so I have flipped once again. If they say no, that should be enough."

Notes

1 To investigate the challenges that the Covid pandemic made to cities and transformed urban life across the world showing how cities can innovate and change profoundly see Miguel A. Montoya ed *Covid-19 and Cities: Responses and Uncertainties* (London: Springer 2021). For a focus on the transformation of urban and transport planning and moves towards more sustainable and green cities that can promote public health see, Mark Nieuwenhuijsen *Covid-19 and the City: The Covid-19 Pandemic and the Transformation of the City* (Independently published 2020).

2 How the way that people work and the spaces they work in have been transformed through the Covid-19 pandemic see, Lori and Barbara Rowlandson *The New Normal: How Covid-19 has Changed the World of Work Forever* (Independently published 2020) and Mark Thomas and Peter Thomson *Never Going Back: How Covid-19 changed Work for good* (Henley-on-Thames: Wisework Books 2021) which explores the challenges and opportunities of the pandemic in creating a new work model based on trust and so changes that can build a greener, healthier and more flexible work culture. See also, Becky Tunstall *Stay Home: Housing and Home in the UK during the Covid-19 Pandemic* (Bristol: Policy Press 2022).

3 Investigations into the changing gender division of labour in different spheres of life are offered by Harriet Bradley *Fractured Identities: Changing Patterns of Inequality* (Cambridge: Polity 2015); Harriett Bradley, Steve Fenton and R. Barot (eds) *Ethnicity, Gender and Social Change* (London: Palgrave Macmillan 1999) and Lisa Adkins

and Maryanne Dever (eds) *The Post-Fordist Sexual Contract: Working and Living in Contingency* (London: Palgrave Macmillan 2015).

4 Tim Montgomerie "Why I broke with Boris Johnson" (*The New Statesman*, 10 June 2020).

5 Research into living with poverty in a society of ever increasing social and wealth inequalities is shared in Ruth Patrick, Maddy Power, Kayleigh Garthwaite et al., *A Year Like No Other: Life on a Low Income during Covid-19* (Bristol: Policy Press 2022); Joseph C. Ewoodzie "Poverty, pandemic and peace of mind" (Princeton: NJ Press 2021).

13

HOPES, VISIONS, ECOLOGIES, PANDEMICS AND FUTURES

Capitalist Ethics, Hopes and Alternative Futures

A YouGov poll in Britain showed only 9% of people wanted to *return* to normal once lockdown was over.[1] Mathew Taylor, then chief executive of the Royal Society of Arts, said in response:

> We must use this time to imagine a better future. This poll shows that the British people are increasingly aware that the health of people and planet are inseparable and it's time for radical environmental, social, political and economic change.
>
> *(Royal Society of Arts, 16 April 2020)*

Professor Tim MacMillan from the Royal Agricultural University perceived a "real appetite for change" and a population "noticing differences, at home, in their work and in communities." He said this was especially apparent when it came to food, farming and the countryside, that "alongside the emergency response" the country must hold on to this determination to make changes "to help shape the kind of country we want to be, including the way we want to feed ourselves, when we recover from this pandemic" (Sky News, 17 April 2020).

As columnist George Monbiot recognised, the pandemic was a "tough lesson in the workings of the natural world," providing evidence of the vitality of ecological understanding. We learnt that threats that originate in one part of the world can spread to others crossing insecure borders. He took heart from a recent survey that 60 per cent of the UK's population wanted more investment in health and wellbeing above growth when we emerged from the pandemic (*The Guardian*, 12 May 2020).[2]

DOI: 10.4324/9781003296874-13

Reporting on this survey in *The Guardian*, journalist Fiona Harvey noted:

> The finding comes as millions of people face economic hardship because of Coronavirus and the lockdown, during which some measures of the quality of life – such as air pollution and the natural environment – are showing signs of improvement.
>
> *(The Guardian, 10 May 2020)*

The campaigning group that commissioned the research, *Positive Money*, said the poll showed that the government should publish statistics on such social indicators: health, the environment and quality of life, to help policymakers better target what the public wants. It would also help people understand changes that *affect* their everyday lives.

Fran Boait, from *Positive Money* emphasises the finding that the public is behind measures to increase funding to health and wellbeing. She warned that the government must resist policies favouring "GDP at the expense of lives" and the environment. Post-Covid-19, she argues, there would be a crucial "need" to shift away from GDP as the primary measure of success, as relying solely on economic growth leads to environmental degradation, deteriorating health and rising poverty, all ignored in the process.[3]

As Monbiot understands immense wealth translates automatically into immense environmental impact, regardless of the intentions of those who possess it. The very wealthy, almost as a matter of definition, are committing *ecocide*. He says we shouldn't be surprised to learn that when Google convened a meeting of the rich and famous at the Verdura resort in Sicily in July 2019 to discuss climate breakdown, its delegates arrived in 114 private jets and a fleet of mega-yachts and drove around the island in supercars. As Monbiot recognises "Even when they mean well, the ultrarich cannot help trashing the living world." He noted: "Income is by far the most important determinant of environmental impact. It doesn't matter how green you think you are; if you have surplus money, you spend it" (*The Guardian*, 19 September 2019).

We need to acknowledge, against what Silicon Valley billionaires might think, as Monbiot says: "Money is not a magic wand that makes all the bad stuff go away. In seeking to prevent climate breakdown, what counts is not what you do but what you stop doing."

We need to question the common-sense presumptions of capitalist ethics which governments and economists use, namely that everyone strives to maximise their wealth. Monbiot stresses that the "continued pursuit of wealth" risks "demolish(ing) our life support systems." For Monbiot it is time to decide what "enough" looks like, and how to know when we've achieved it.[4]

The Belgian philosopher Ingrid Robeyns argued that there should be an upper limit to wealth. Just as we recognise a poverty line, we should recognise a riches line. Surplus money allows inordinate power over others – in the workplace, in politics and the destruction of the planet. It undermines democratic institutions and the equal voice and equal worth that people should be able to feel in democratic society.[5]

What level of wealth inequalities *can* be justified in a liberal democratic society? How can a democracy claim to give equal value to its citizens when so many are led to question democratic institutions that leave them feeling ignored, devalued and taken for granted? What level of poverty and social inequality *are* compatible with a democratic society? What are the ethics that *sustain values* of human equality and social justice? To what extent can be freedom be made compatible with equality?

Green Economies and Eco-Lives

Gaia Vince, author of *Transcendence: How Humans Evolved Through Fire, Language, Beauty and Time*[6] which shows how genetics, the environment and culture all contribute to human evolution, reflected on the "sobering truth" that the pandemic, and the standstill it caused worldwide "has barely dented our carbon emissions." Existing targets show that emissions must decrease by 7.6% annually by 2050, which now feels "alarmingly unachievable." Simon Evans of climate science website Carbon Brief said that the continued rates of emissions when we may have expected a pause evidenced that "avoiding dangerous climate change and getting to zero emissions is unbelievably hard" (*The Guardian*, 17 May 2020).

And yet, as Vince also acknowledged that a "sudden, dramatic shift to a less carbon-intensive lifestyle" showed what could be achieved with greater commitment. Richard Betts, head of Climate Impacts at the Met Office insisted, "huge, lasting changes in energy systems" were needed to have "a substantial impact on long-term CO2 concentrations." Hope lay in the fact that because of the Coronavirus crisis people now had some experience of transformational changes *in* their everyday lives and relationships, so it might be easier for them to *imagine* alternative futures if they could become aware of the dangers to the planet they face.

Evans reflected on the "temporary" nature of the pandemic, speculating on the resumption of "normal" life: "When we drive again, the car still burns petrol." Instead, structural change would mean people *accepting* they need to swap their combustion engines for electric vehicles. More fundamentally, Evans clarified, this would require huge feats of urban re-planning: "a shift towards a low-carbon society can't happen via individual action alone."

The economist Kate Raworth pointed out the interdependent nature of human and planetary health, and suggested that politicians accordingly use "one space" to reflect on health, employment and environment. This means radically *revisioning* relationships between nature and culture. It means appreciating that the fear of being labelled a loser within a competitive culture can make you ill – as you constantly overstep limits as you continually try to prove yourself in the eyes of others.[7]

As Vince reported, the pandemic revealed how deadly pollution is. One study found that a tiny increase in particulates was associated with a 15% increase in the Covid-19 death rate, almost certainly contributing to the terrible death rates seen in cities. In Italy, the high death rates seen in the north of the country correlated with the highest levels of air pollution (*The Guardian*, 17 May 2020).

A momentum for environmental protection predated Covid-19 but possibly the crisis proved a *tipping point* in public consciousness. As Ken Caldeira at the Carnegie Institution for Science, based in Washington DC said:

> Just as we have seen that early action to deter the virus was far more effective than trying to contain the damage after it spread, transforming our energy system now to prevent the expansion of excessive heat over our planet will be more effective than trying to adapt to the consequences later…

Vince noted the strong negotiating position that the government was in to "push a sustainable agenda," overriding pressures from industry, and described it as "vital" that the moment was "not squandered on kneejerk bailouts" in sectors such as oil and food.

Economist Mariana Mazzucoto at University College London claimed that this was about aiding businesses with the "cashflow to survive" and be able to "transform… to be a more functioning part of society." She insisted governments must take the *longer view* and use stimulus packages to actively mould a cleaner economy, something that South Korea had pledged, for instance.

Vince visualised a "post-pandemic economy" that could minimise the possibility of future climate disaster and contagion, because having "experienced a cleaner, quieter and kinder alternative," people were rejecting a return to how things were.

Globalised Capitalism, Resistance, Visions and Possible Futures

A "crossroads" moment confronted politicians in the summer of the pandemic, according to *Guardian* columnist John Harris, writing that July. Boris Johnson was hoping for a restoration of "significant normality" by Christmas, but his optimism seemed at odds with the "inescapable" gloom and "feeling of dread" that was pervasive during a "strange, uneasy summer."

Even Johnson said a few days later that the virus was still with us and going to be with us for a while to come. The second wave that came to pass was attended with a "gathering avalanche of numbers" of debt and risk of mass unemployment, that anticipated an "economic disaster" (*The Guardian*, 19 July 2020).

"Politics is failing us," Harris concluded, perceiving a "spectacle of absurd displacement activity" with civil service restructuring and threats to do the same to the NHS, and ongoing coverage of Brexit movements. Meanwhile, the opposition was facing a challenge to win back potential voters and reconcile the party after the fallouts of the Corbyn leadership, and were strangely quiet on the potential for "social and economic disaster."

Anthony Barnett, the founder of openDemocracy, the independent, international media platform, wrote an online essay "Out of the Belly of Hell".[8] It assessed the crisis of Covid-19 and what it meant for the way countries had been run for the past few decades. He said the gift of Coronavirus was that it: "Makes clear that the future of humanity is a matter of our choice." Globalisation, as Barnett sees it, has two increasingly irreconcilable aspects. It embeds a neoliberal "profit maximisation and marketisation," and insists that human values can be identified exclusively with market values. It's the market alone that can determine value and we have to be ready to submit to its demands.[9]

But at the same time, according to Barnett, it has produced a generalised capacity for people to *become* citizens, with expectations of human rights and state protections. Millions of us might be exploited, but we also have a deep awareness that "we share the same planet – at the same time as each other". At some level we share the same fate and in a cosmopolitan world we realise that we exist beyond the terms of the nation state. The pandemic, Barnett argues, "initiated a new era." The economy was forced to take a backseat whilst life-saving measures took centre stage, ultimately "precipitat(ing) an ideological breakdown."

This new era is manifested not just in the politics of the virus itself and what it has exposed about structures of racial, class and gender inequalities, but also what this helped precipitate in the Black Lives Matter upsurge. Movements of resistance in lockdown have had the time to reflect upon their *values* and what really matters in life: their families, their friends and their communities. They have helped create alternative ethical imaginations that acknowledge the importance of self-care, love and emotional and spiritual integrity. They have created new visions of solidarity, alliances and co-operation across differences.

But we also experienced polarisation in communities across the world with powerful anti-vax movements identifying with Trump, Bolsonaro and other populist leaders. While some had found *how* they are dependent upon each other, so challenging in everyday life a neoliberal common-sense, others have been affirmed *in* libertarian and populist convictions. Living in states which have imposed restrictions on public health, they have insisted that it is *only* your individual freedom *as* an autonomous and independent agent, able to decide whether or not to wear a mask, that could really matter to you. Populist politics and accusations of fake truth on social media have helped to polarise societies, but the realities of multiple deaths can also bring a sense of ethical realism, especially when people close to you, who refused to wear masks, died.

As Barnett recognised, breakdowns are *not* the same as revolutions, where there is a choice to return to how things were: "The outcome is decided afterwards and has to be achieved, it is never inherent in the crisis." We were now faced, in the terms Barnett frames, with a central "incompatibility": "economic market dogma" and "an expectation of the right to life."

I think we need a broader vision of the right to life that, as he would agree, connects to the *equal worth* and *equal voice* of citizens promised within a democratic society. This goes beyond electoral visions of representative democracy and raises questions, at least in Britain, about the importance of health, free at the point of delivery within the NHS. This raises questions about fundamental *values* and visions of human equality that shape our visions *as* ethical humans who acknowledge vulnerability and responsibilities to others living in very different material conditions of injustice and oppression.

According to Barnett, the two key questions of our time are "whether a more human, collectivist way of thinking *can* finally be pushed to the fore, and what a different kind of economy and society might look like." But we need to be careful *not* to reproduce an unhelpful binary between liberal individualism and a socialist collectivism – while we learn to *value* the freedoms that individuals have claimed as they shape their ethnic, gender and sexual identities. We need to challenge structural inequalities and the growing inequalities between the 1% and the 99% per cent. ("We are the 99 per cent" was the slogan used by the Occupy movement, referring to wealth inequality in the United States.) It means facing the issues framed by the Occupy initiative and opposing the culture of white supremacy radically challenged by the Black Lives Matter movement.

Harris suggests that despite the absence of major themes in the Coronavirus conversation, we should discuss and address them on a crisis-appropriate scale. This might involve adopting a "partially directed economy," implementing a green new deal and reallocating resources for sustainability. Furthermore, a substantial public housing programme should revitalise town and city centres, while blurring the line between paid work and voluntary care with a basic income.

Harris joined his voice to Barnett's, adding that the way we collectively deliver public services should be *reshaped* by what Barnett calls an explosion of empathy, social awareness and networking, recently seen in spontaneous community action across different countries during the pandemic.

As Harris insists, we need to rethink the *kind of state* we want, having all witnessed England's tragic handling of the pandemic, making radical changes to the creaking, centralised system of government currently reliant on "ossified practices and institutionalised prejudices." This directly contrasts with the Boris Johnson-Dominic Cummings model (when Cummings was chief advisor to Johnson as prime minister) which saw regeneration dropped on places from on high and firmly controlled by the centre.

Harris's investigation revealed the pandemic's exposure of flaws in Britain's centralised state. He cited the Health Secretary's approach to Covid testing, favouring a centralised model with "drive-through testing centres" outsourced to private firms like Deloitte, Sodexo and Boots. He contrasted this with Germany's successful "devolved, pluralistic" approach.

He notes how the development of a "system of contact tracing" was also contracted out to private companies such as Serco, "staffed by new recruits… given the most cursory training" (*The Guardian*, 25 May 2020).

Local authorities, who *had* the forensic local knowledge and experience any successful tracing operation would depend on were left in the dark till the last moment. Less than three weeks before the system was meant to be in place, local councils who had their own public health experts had *no idea* of what they were going to be asked to do. The announcement came "at one minute to midnight" as one city leader told Harris. The government announced that councils would be working with Whitehall to support test and trace services in their own communities and develop tailored outbreak control plans.

As Harris recognised:

> Just about everything in our current national impasse proves that the old, centralised game is up, and that England needs a new constitutional settlement… Power needs to be taken from the centre and dispersed. The future needs to be found in a huge boost to councils' share of tax take, the devolution of everything from health to transport, and fully localised response to any future emergencies.

Lockdown Inequalities and Precarious Futures

The beginning of the end of lockdown, as journalist Nesrine Malik noted, was marked by a "new fear" and "sharpened" sense of our own "grossly unequal society." She traced a vital moment that revealed the masculine disdain in the government as like a "boys' club" (*The Guardian*, 31 May 2020).

What started out as a firm but restrained refusal to admit any wrongdoing on the part of Dominic Cummings had descended into menace and mockery. (Cummings had driven his wife and child from London to the north of England during the lockdown when other people had been fined for walking a dog in the remote countryside.) Malik described Boris Johnson as increasingly "aggressive and ratty" in public briefings, senior figures such as Matt Hancock and Michael Gove "laugh(ing) and scoff(ing) in interviews," urging people to "move on," portraying a government no longer committed to a show of resilience or support.

Malik suggested that the country would *not* forget or forgive the attitude of the "tight-knit group of arrogant and talentless entitles" steering the government. They showed "no interest in our safety – or our respect" (*The Guardian*, 31 May 2020).

As she knows, the labour force was divided between those who could work from home and those who had to go out and be on the frontline; between those who could continue to protect themselves at home and those who could not afford it. As the predicted recession bites and unemployment rises, the power that employers have over zero-hours workers grateful to have any income will produce more and more abuses, especially for undocumented workers.[10]

Malik highlights the plight of a group of these vulnerable migrants whose legal status does not protect them from the pandemic's impact. Despite paying extortionate rates for "visas, residence permits and access to the NHS," they remain excluded from accessing public funds. While some individuals received support during the universal lockdown phase from friends, family or furlough schemes, these lifelines were temporary. As the furlough scheme wound down, "non-shielding helpers" would resume their regular lives and jobs, leaving the vulnerable migrants without a safety net.

She wrote: "The pandemic quickly thrived in society's cracks, claiming lives and livelihoods according to race, access to healthcare, work risk profile and economic status." She anticipated that these "fissures" would deepen in the "unforgiving new landscape of sharpened inequalities."

Malik had already written earlier in May to speculate on the possibility of a recession following the pandemic. She envisioned major sectors, including hospitality and retail, on their knees, small businesses "operating on the thinnest of margins… dying out" (*The Guardian*, 18 May 2020).

Remembering the aftermath of the 2008 global financial crisis, Malik learnt that the first thing that happens in a recession tends *not* to be a radical re-engineering of the economy. The first impulse is to make a quick calculation: *who* should be saved and who *is* dispensable. In the US after the 2008 crash, the banks were recapitalised and the economy stabilised, and 10 million Americans lost their homes. As she notes "The only factor that mattered was how many people could be lost without disrupting the economy for everyone else."

Analysing the "deliberate" language of "a resilient infrastructure doing its best," Malik warns vigilance against the complacency that comes from reframing "failures" as "challenges," and in the case of the NHS, characterising their response as successful as they are no longer described as "overwhelmed."

In the final stages, Malik traces policies to help the vulnerable launched at the start of the pandemic that would soon be quietly dropped. A pledge to review the NHS surcharge for foreign doctors has come to nothing. A popular programme to house homeless people in England in hotels was quietly scrapped. The homeless returning to the streets will be joined by others sent there by the economic downturn. Malik fears the "scapegoat(ing)" that may occur when this happens. We must learn, she concludes, not to buy in to the cover-ups that may follow in the "shattered aftermath" of the crisis.

Disruptions, Nation-States and Liberal Moral Theory

Philosopher and author John Gray wrote in *The New Statesman* that the crisis of Covid-19 was a turning point in history because the era of peak globalisation was over. "This is not a temporary rupture in an otherwise stable equilibrium," Gray noted. He anticipated the end of "unceasing mobility", claiming that people would live more "physically constrained and more virtual" lives, perhaps leading to a "more fragmented" but "more resilient" world" (*The New Statesman*, 1 April 2020).

This shows, as I also argued in *Ethical Humans: Life, Love, Labour, Learning and Loss,* the significance of sociology *as* an art of living. It is *not* just a matter of beliefs, values and norms, but of everyday embodied ethical practices and relationships. It's a matter of *how* we treat each other, and how we learn to live together with our differences that can be valued and respected. Many had now experienced different relationships with space and time that have been confining and often dangerous. They sought alternative ways of living and relating as *vulnerable* humans on a precarious planet. Some moved towards a vegan diet determined to live and relate differently.

Liberalism with all its talk of freedom and choice was, Gray argued: "In practice the experiment of dissolving traditional sources of social cohesion and political legitimacy and replacing them with the promise of rising material living standards. This experiment has now run its course."

The global financial crisis of 2008 revealed *growing inequalities* between the 1% and the 99% which years of austerity only served to deepen. It showed that structural inequalities of class, race and gender had proved enduring. Discrimination is not just a matter of individual prejudices that can be challenged, but also of institutional relationships of power that need to be named within an alternative radical vision that can focus upon the lessons we learnt through the pandemic and the grief so many are living with, rather than being forgotten within a technological vision of "returning to normal." With a global climate emergency already well underway, we need to shape new moral and political imaginations that illuminate the stark realities we are living with and narratives that explain why those who created the 2008 financial crisis were never held accountable.

There has been a need to question a postmodern ethic that can too easily foster myths of living in societies that are post-racial and post-gender – as if individuals have somehow been freed to create their own individual realities so they only have themselves to blame if they fail to achieve individual success and happiness. The return to Marx and an awareness of structural inequalities of class, race, disability, gender and sexuality needs to learn from social movements that have raised concerns about democratic accountability and the equal worth of citizens. We need to challenge an environment that has often been hostile to immigrants who are seeking refuge from war zones and are often obliged to survive as undocumented migrants in precarious conditions.

Post-pandemic, and on the restarting of the economy, Gray argued: "it will be in a world where governments act to curb the global market." He speculated that governments would move to decentralise supply chains to avoid a situation, such as "the world's essential medical supplies originat(ing) in China – or in any single country". Gray notes that "The notion that a country such as Britain could phase out farming and depend on imports of food will be dismissed as the nonsense it always has been." He also speculated that "harder borders are going to be an enduring feature of the global landscape. A narrow goal of economic efficiency will no longer be practicable for governments."

He recognised that the most successful responses to the epidemic were in Taiwan, South Korea and Singapore, saying:

> It is hard to believe their cultural traditions, which focus on collective well-being more than personal autonomy, have not played a role in their success.

> They have also resisted the cult of the minimal state. It will not be surprising if they adjust to de-globalisation better than many western countries.

In relation to China, however, he noted: "The virus has provided a rationale for expanding the surveillance state and introducing even stronger political control. Instead of wasting the crisis, Xi Jinping's regime is using it to expand the country's influence."

The strength of Gray's thinking is his questioning of the idea that "pandemics are blips rather than an integral part of history." Covid-19 is telling us permanent changes in how we live will have to be made if we are to be less vulnerable in future.[11] In Gray's vision this is where the protective state comes in because he says at its core, the British state has always been Hobbesian. Peace and strong government have been the overriding priorities. At the same time this Hobbesian state has mostly rested on consent, particularly in times of national emergency. Being shielded from danger *has* trumped freedom from interference by government.

This inclines him to think that as a result of the Covid-19 global pandemic, people would lean in to "bio-surveillance for the sake of better protection of their health," despite these measures being deeply "intrusive", and inviting more "pervasive" state influence.

But it's a strength of his conservatism, at some level echoing Simone Weil's later work, to recognise: "Those who believe personal autonomy is the innermost human need betray an ignorance of psychology, not least their own. He characterises Liberalism as a "systematic denial" of the importance of "security and belonging" and furthermore, "a denial of (the individual's) dependency on families, friends, and communities." Gray says that as a response to lockdown, many have "re-evaluate(d) their lives and relationships with nature… revisioning their sense of what it means to be ethical humans and what really matters to them."

As William H. McNeill wrote in *Plagues and People,* the idea that we can return to normal is questioned when we have also learnt that an "obscure parasitic organism can escape its niche and expose dense human populations to some fresh and devastating morality." As globalisation advanced, so had the risk of pandemics spreading. Commenting on how some plagues have been understood by historians, McNeil notes: "For them as for others, occasional disastrous outbreaks of infectious diseases remain sudden and unpredictable interruptions of the norm, essentially beyond historical explanation."[12]

As Guiseppe Conte, then Prime Minister of Italy, said in March 2020 when Italy was at the centre of the global pandemic, neglecting to "rise to the unprecedented challenge" risked the "whole European structure loses its raison d'être for the people" But for Gray it was the non-EU Serbian president Aleksandar Vucic who was blunter and more realistic, saying: "European solidarity does not exist. That was a fairy tale. The only country that can help us in this hard situation is the People's Republic of China. To the rest of them, thanks for nothing."

Anticipating Impossible Futures and Alternative Imaginations

In an interview in his apartment in Rio de Janeiro with *Agência Pública*, in 2019, the Brazilian anthropologist Eduardo Viveiros de Castro, said he felt as perplexed *as* everyone else, saying "We can't tell the difference between truth and lies anymore." He felt the truth had become unbelievable, claiming "We're witnessing a final offensive against Brazil's Indigenous people" (*Agência Pública*, 10 October 2019).

Recalling the words of the social anthropologist Claude Levi-Strauss, de Castro saw this as evidence of "western civilisation (destroying) substance of its own existence." He shared Levi-Strauss' conviction that "humanity is complicit in its own extinction, given that the representatives of the species who consider themselves most advanced are precisely those who are contributing most radically to the deterioration of the material conditions humanity needs for its survival."

He comments on the "surreal" circumstances orchestrated by Bolsonaro's administration in Brazil. Even before Covid-19, he saw its "big push" to destroy indigenous ways of life, noting that if "they're not buying them out, they're sending in missionaries to break them, prohibiting *pajelanca*" (traditional medical and religious systems). He notes that the Amazon is the last piece of Brazil "yet to be destroyed, 'civilised', 'conquered'", and portrays the Bolsonaro government as a return to 16th-century colonial values.

He notes that Brazilian "big business and agribusiness" whose interests are aggressively pursued by the government regard indigenous people as a threat as they live "outside the land market," which goes against the privatising agenda of the political class.

Asked why Bolsonaro had identified the Amazon and the indigenous peoples as enemies, his answer is a "belief that Brazil is essentially a European country… There's hatred towards non-whites in Brazil. There's anti-Black racism, and a double-racism with a territorial element towards the Indians." He sadly reflects that Brazil is "a colony of others and a colony of itself."

Viveiros de Castro thought that in a time of Covid-19 and the ongoing climate emergency, we have to shape alternative imaginations *if* we are to survive. We could learn from the Indians about the end of the world, since their world has been ending since 1500. In contrast to western culture's visions of human superiority, Indigenous people regard themselves as "part of a universe," and reject anthropocentric ideas of hierarchy.

As he remarked, humans have an arrogant belief that "we're gifted with something that will save us from any problem, that other species will become extinct, but not ours," a dangerous delusion.

Viveiros de Castro recognised that what we call developed countries are really super-developed – "in the sense that they consume far more than necessary, far more than is reasonable, and far more than is possible given the material conditions of the planet."

As ethical humans, how can industrialised societies morally justify super-developed large cars that populate our cities and consume disproportionate amounts of fuel? As de Castro recognises: "These countries have to *underdevelop* so that other countries, other peoples, can develop a little more, so we can have more equality in our conditions of existence. Because if this doesn't happen, the planet will explode."

Covid-19, Big Tech and Polarised Societies

The divisions created within nations *as* populist supporters of Trump in the United States and Bolsonaro in Brazil refused to take the *threats* of the virus seriously, as Johnson also initially refused to do in the UK, deepened over time. Significant minorities, across age groups, identified themselves *against* state regulation and the avoidable harms that they saw as consequences of lockdowns, for example to children's education.

There were demonstrations in cities across the world against lockdowns and then against vaccines being made compulsory in certain lines of work. There was agitation on social media. Different sources of information challenged claims made for the vaccinations. These were not straightforward left-right distinctions, though there was considerable alignment between Trump supporters in the United States and those insisting that it was a matter of individual freedom to refuse mask wearing and the vaccine.

In the US, Naomi Wolf in *Bodies of Others: The New Authoritarians, Covid-19 and The War Against the Human*[13] said the state was using the Covid pandemic to realise other long term authoritarian goals. As she argued, the threats directly posed to human life by the pandemic needed to be understood in relation to the aims of major corporations to undermine the freedoms of democratic citizens.

In writing *The End of America: Letters of Warning to a Young Patriot*[14] she was already aware how the terror threat post 9/11 was being used by the Bush administration: "To hype fear and strip us of our civil liberties." She said: "There are 10 steps to fascism that leaders who want to crush democracy will always take. You start with invoking a terrifying internal and external threat. It can be a real threat, but its hyped. You go on to surveil citizens."[15]

You can sense the appeal to conspiracy when Wolf moves quickly to say:

> You create militia groups unaccountable to the rule of law. You create a Gulag. You start to demonise whistle blowers and critics. You start to call dissent, treason or espionage or subversion. And then you get to step 10, which is martial law, declaring emergency law.

For Wolf: "Well, here we are at step 10" and the evidence was when in July 2020, when still under lockdown in New York, governor Andrew Cuomo: "Stated that we couldn't have more than six people in our homes, which is a massive violation of the Fourth Amendment and the First Amendment, right to assembly, the right to privacy."

For Wolf:

> This had nothing to do with a public health emergency. What we were seeing was step 10. We were seeing a wholesale race to exploit what was messaged as a global pandemic in such a way as to strip us of our remaining liberties and to terraform America conceptually into being ready to accept a CCP-style (Chinese Communist Party) World Economic Forum (WEF) guided post-humane and post-constitutional world. And that's only escalated.

She noted that:

> Big Tech companies massaged pandemic policy in various ways to suit their ends. Millions (of dollars) are flowing to Big Tech companies as a result of completely medically unnecessary pandemic policies. What the tech companies are driven by is that human beings in human space, having human conversations with human smiles are a competition that they cannot compete with. So, a lot of the policies rolled out as a public health emergency really serve to kill off that human advantage and transfer assets to Big Tech. (Big) Pharma isn't even the main driver as powerful and scary as it is.

The conspiracy was clear for Wolf:

> It's a pretty, fully-fleshed out methodology that involves Big Tech, involves CCP, involves World Economic Forum, and now the WHO as a delivery method to create a One World matrix in which nation states are meaningless, parliaments and congresses are meaningless and all of us are surveilled and tracked and regularly injected or forced to take whatever pill or treatment or intervention they want us to take in such a way as to make freedom a thing of the past. And also in such a way as to harvest all our data continually, which is gold for tech companies.

Threats, Bio-Security and Social Divisions

Giorgio Agamben, the veteran Italian philosopher, born in 1942, author of *Homo Sacer: Sovereign Power and Bare Life,* lost support in Italy because of his criticism of the "techno-medical despotism" of quarantines and lockdowns. In a society that respects science, expertise confers power. In 2004, at the height of the so-called "war on terror" – a term later put aside – Agamben refused to be fingerprinted and declined a post at New York University rather than submit to it.

He warned that such data collection was passing itself off as an emergency measure but, if we weren't vigilant, would inevitably become part of normal everyday life. With Covid he was concerned that the emergency declared by public-health experts was a *pretext* for withdrawing rights and privacy from citizens.

"Biosecurity" now serves as a reason for governments to rule in terms of "worst-case" scenarios, the American journalist Christopher Caldwell expounded. Caldwell noted: "Many European governments, including Italy's, have developed national contact tracing apps that allow them to track their citizens using cell phones" (*The New York Times*, 21 August 2020).

Wars have bequeathed to peacetime a "series of fateful technologies," Agamben reminded us, from barbed wire to nuclear power plants. Such innovations tend to be ones that elites were already agitating for, or that align with their interests. Epidemics, he suggests, are no different. "For fear of getting sick," Agamben writes: "Italians are ready to sacrifice practically everything."

The politics of the pandemic seemed to expose a deeper ethical and metaphysical erosion where people came to see their neighbours not as fellow human beings but as spreaders of pestilence, as portrayed in Allesandro Manzoni's *The Betrothed* which describes how human relations degenerated in Milan during the plague of 1630.[16] With Covid-19 also, for Agamben: "The threshold that separates humanity from barbarism has been crossed," as shown in the treatment of the dead.[17]

> How could we have accepted, in the name of a risk that we couldn't even quantify, that not only the people who are dear to us, and human beings more generally, should have had to die alone but also – and this is something that had never happened before in all of history from Antigone to today – that their corpses should be burned without a funeral?
>
> *(The New York Times, 21 August 2020)*

In a blog "The Invention of an Epidemic" in February 2020, so in the early days, Agamben called the reaction to the virus "frenetic, irrational and entirely unfounded." He accused state authorities of misleading the public about the threat of Covid-19 which he, along with Trump, Bolsonaro and Johnson dismissed as no more dangerous than the flu. He was quick to argue: "the invention of an epidemic offered the ideal pretext for scaling (exceptional measures) up beyond any limitation."

I don't know if he was later to regret his words when the reality of the deaths from Covid-19 became evident, but he decried people's willingness to accept a disruption of every aspect of their lives, as conveyed to us by his translator Adam Kotsko (*Slate*, 20 February 2020).

Kotsko first learnt of Agamben's Covid scepticism when he was asked to translate some of his blog posts. As the months passed and the pandemic took hold, Agamben maintained his critique of the pandemic emergency measures. Far right politicians have invoked his considerable intellectual authority to advance conspiracy theories and decry the supposed persecution of anti-vaxxers.

Agamben's paranoia led Kotsko to question the philosopher's previous work. He noted that In *Homo Sacer* (Latin for "The Sacred Man") Agamben argues: in the West "Political power… is founded on the decision to include some people within the protections of the law and exclude others… to a state he designates as 'bare life'."

Agamben's primary example of "bare life" is the Nazi Shoah where Jews were not only expelled from society but included in it as a subhuman class. According to Kotsko, this led Agamben to consider Nazi Germany as "paradigmatic for modern politics" rather than an "exceptional deviation."

Kotsko gave the "expansive emergency powers" of George W. Bush's administration during the "war on terror" as an example of this: making Agamben's observation "alarmingly plausible." Agamben reminds of the legality of the actions of the Nazis, following the "state of emergency" declaration made by Hitler in order "to suspend civil rights and normal legal processes."

The fact that western nations have increasingly declined to govern by means of normal constitutional processes with the rise of authoritarian populist leaders, like Trump and Bolsonaro, means that, according to Agamben: "the state of exception has become the norm".

But it *is* important to remember that both these leaders, even if they maintain considerable support, were defeated in elections. Johnson's attempts to suspend the British Parliament in the Brexit divisions were rejected by the Supreme Court. There are still disturbing authoritarian populist trends that Agamben *can* help us understand, but we also need to evaluate *how* Covid-19 has been experienced and dealt with in different ways, if you contrast Denmark with Sweden and contrast both with the United States, Brazil, India and the UK.

Anti-vaxxers and anti-lockdown protesters, Adam Kotsko notes, inspired by Agamben himself: "have repeatedly abused the memory of the Holocaust by comparing their own situation to that of European Jews in the middle of the 20th century." Pandemic measures, according to Agamben produced the start of "bare life" in the population: and was even welcomed by the people. But Kotsko adds: "Most puzzling to me was Agamben's failure to see the obvious difference between the Nazi regime, which aimed to exterminate life, and the pandemic measures that were aimed at saving it."

There are different grounds to be sceptical about science and medicine and the difficulties they have in engaging with the whole person – in ways that complimentary traditions seek to do through the link the between the physical, emotional, mental and spiritual. These critiques can move across traditional political divisions, and it has often been the libertarian protests, against regulation, that has tended to monopolise public discourse.

Readers of *Homo Sacer* and *State of Exception*, Kotsko notes, could be led to assume that to solve the problem of the "overuse of emergency powers", we must "return to 'normal' political structures." However, as Agamben posits, this comes with risk. "A more radical solution…is needed: a dissolution of the entire structure of law and power – a possibility that he usually evokes using literary or theological imagery, rather than concrete actionable plans."

But this points to dangers in Agamben's philosophy. Simone Weil also engaged with *how* Roman notions of power and greatness have continued to shape western notions of masculine heroism, freedom and self-determination. But she also framed alternative histories of France and institutional reforms that would offer equal respect, dignity and human worth through a balance between hierarchy and different forms of authority. In her move towards Christianity, she did not lose connection with political insights into human suffering from her early factory work.[18]

We are so deeply formed by our culture's power structure that, according to Kotkso: "A radical alternative is bound to sound vague and paradoxical to us – but if we want to escape we must make the effort." He thinks that Agamben's "excessive distrust of any state authority" has "blinded" the philosopher, leading him to "individualistic approaches (that have) reinforced corporate power while exacerbating the pandemic." Kotkso concludes that "essential workers, along with so many others, have been reduced to disposable bare life, not by direct state intervention but by policies that claim to set them free."

Social Media, Politics, Divisions and Anti-Vaxxers

Writing about the relationship between Covid and politics, Robert Reich, author of *The System: Who Rigged it, How we Fix it*[19] notes that as of October 2021, Covid mortality rates in counties where Donald Trump had significant support (winning by wide margins or at least 60% of the vote) were alarming. Trump-won counties had a death rate of 25 per 100,000, over three times higher than heavily Biden counties with 7.8 per 100,000. Moreover, areas where Trump secured at least 70% of the vote experienced an even higher average Covid death toll. Reich recognised that "Trump counties also have the highest unvaccinated rates in the US. Almost every reliably blue state now has a higher vaccination rate than almost every reliably red state" (*The Guardian*, 28 November 2021).

Trump voters were more hesitant to get vaccinated also because he had *politicised* the issue making it a hallmark of his right-wing populism suggesting that *if* you value your freedom, you won't obey government regulations to get the vaccination. Along with Fox news, he spread false rumours and conspiracy theories about the vaccine. By the time Trump eventually called on people to get vaccinated, the damage had already been done.

There were Democrat voters, well-informed and well-educated, who were equally opposed to getting vaccinated so there are alliances *across* traditional political boundaries. Some felt the vaccine would undermine their immune system and that the most helpful thing to do would be to focus upon strengthening it. They didn't want anything to go into their bodies that they couldn't control and were wary of a vaccination that had been rushed through. They didn't trust big pharma, regarded as greedy global corporations who are focussed upon maximising their profits and were refusing to share the knowledge that would allow other countries to produce their own vaccines.

As Reich, a former Secretary of State for Labour under President Bill Clinton, commented there was widespread distrust of the government, with a belief that it had been "so corrupted by big money that (people) don't trust agencies charged with protecting the public." He suggested in one interview that their concerns, however valid, had to be weighed against the public's overall interest in defeating the epidemic but that people didn't seem to care. He described a "narcissism" that is focused upon individual wellbeing, and a longstanding American "stubborn, selfish, me-first individualism."

Noting a long history of New Age and Far Right ideologies becoming unlikely bedfellows, author Jules Evans reported anti-lockdown rallies in major global cities "attract(ing) both New Agers and far-right groups." He noted that QAnon was an increasingly influential example of this and was disturbed by echoes of Germany in the 1920s and 1930s, when an overlap of this nature emerged with disastrous consequences.

We need to be careful in our own calls for a paradigm shift in the relationships between human beings and nature to recall that the Nazis, like many other Germans, were fascinated by an early environmental holism. As Evans notes: "They passed legislation to protect forests and rivers and moved to ban experiments on animals (while authorising experiments on camp prisoners)." He quotes Ernst Lehmann, a Nazi professor of botany, writing: "This striving toward connectedness with the totality of life, with nature itself, a nature into which we are born, this is the deepest meaning and the true essence of National Socialist thought."

Evans notes how Hitler delivered a conspiracy theory of "a hidden global elite of monsters/vampires/demons – that is, the Jews," that could be fought by "magical light-warriors of the Nazi party" in "cosmic battle, ushering in a golden age of peace and love." These fantasies were based on dubious sources, including *The Protocols of Zion*, a piece of Russian intelligence originating in the early 20th century designed to encourage anti-Semitism.

"Doesn't this sound like QAnon to you?" Evans asks. He points out the parallels: the "hidden Satanic elite, a secret cabal made of up demonic liberals from Hollywood, the Democratic Party and the deep state," performing "monstrous blood rituals on children." They perceive the conspiracy in the mainstream media too: "Any anti-Trump information is planted by the 'lying press' (a favourite Nazi term)" (*Medium*, 4 September 2020).

Journalist David Smith in *The Guardian* (20 August 2020) reported how Donald Trump tacitly *endorsed* QAnon claiming its followers "love our country" and "like me very much". When asked about the theory at a White House press briefing, the US president failed to condemn it. When pressed about the beliefs of QAnon supporters, Trump flippantly denied knowledge of it, but said: "If I can save the world from problems, I'm willing to do it… We're saving the world from a radical left philosophy."

Tommy Vietor, a former spokesman for Barack Obama's national security council, condemned Trump's comments, pointing out that the FBI had identified the movement as a "violent domestic terrorism threat." This played out in the attack on Congress on 6 January 2021. Joan Donovan, research director at the Shorenstein Centre, said that people should be vigilant on the dangers of QAnon, that it was not just an "outlandish conspiracy theory about child-trafficking and Satanism" but a hateful movement "driven by tropes about Jewish people and the one world government narrative" (*The Guardian*, 20 August 2020).

We should be aware of how histories *can* echo in the present without indulging what historian Simon Schama calls the "obscene syllogism": the idea that, as Monbiot recognised, "because the Nazis promoted new age beliefs, alternative medicine and ecological protection, anyone who does so is a Nazi." At the same time, we need to think about *what* has made the most unlikely people become susceptible to right wing extremism. We need to acknowledge how the anti-vaccine movement is a highly effective channel for the penetration of far-right ideas into left wing counterculture.

This gains momentum, Monbiot noted, with the rise of social media "directing vaccine hesitant people towards far-right conspiracy groups,' helping to revive connections between "antisemitic paranoia" and "wellness." As he argues, "the notion of the sovereign body, untainted by chemical contamination, has begun to fuse with the fear that a shadowy cabal is trying to deprive us of autonomy."

According to Monbiot, when the left allied themselves with big business, "the right seized the language they had abandoned… repurpos(ing)… themes of resisting elite power and regaining control of our lives" (*The Guardian*, 22 September 2021).

But Monbiot notes the strange bedfellows:

> A justified suspicion about the self-interest of big pharma clashes with the need for mass vaccination. The lockdowns and other measures required to prevent Covid-19 are policies, which in other circumstances, would rightly be seen as coercive political control. Curtailing the pandemic, climate breakdown and the collapse of biodiversity means powerful agreements struck between governments – which can be hard to swallow for movements that have long fought multilateral power while emphasising the local and the homespun.
>
> *(The Guardian, 7 April 2022)*

Neoliberal Capitalism, Ecologies and Fearful Futures

Attending to how our planet and its peoples have been transformed by neoliberal capitalism, Naomi Klein in *The Shock Doctrine: The Rise of Disaster Capitalism* in 2008[20] focussed on how, in conditions of socioeconomic turmoil, elites can implement far reaching plans that seem to be responses to crisis, but in fact work to secure their own narrow interests. Engaging issues of the climate emergency more directly in *This Changes Everything: Capitalism versus the Climate*[21] she shows *how* a neoliberal order was in effect "now at war with many forms of life on earth, including human life."

Wittgenstein in his later philosophy talks about "forms of life" but this is a way of extending the term more directly into social and political life within shifting historical contexts. This is a theme also developed in Pope Francis's encyclical, *Laudato Si. (Praise be to you my Lord).* Klein also recognised that if we are to break free from the reigning socioeconomic paradigm, we also need to shape a positive vision of the world we might create.[22]

As Klein explained in an interview with *Syndemic Magazine* (syndemic.ca, 8 March 2022) "I try to follow my research where it leads me." She describes her "arrogant idea" expressed by *The Shock Doctrine*, that "if we understand that the very unpopular policies get smuggled in under the cover of crisis – then just knowing that would be armour against this cynical tactic." But when the 2008 global financial crisis came, a lot of people already understood that the crisis was being exploited to enrich elites through pushing through privatisation and deregulation. As she noted: "The slogan on the streets of Europe was, 'We will not pay for your crisis.' But – they *did* pay for the crisis of the bankers."

She learnt that it wasn't enough to say no to their bad ideas and we need our own solutions to the crisis, which led her to write *This Changes Everything.* Recognising that we need solutions on the scale of the disaster, she argued that a Green New Deal could be a systemic response to the climate crisis.

She said: "You can't believe in privatisation and deregulation and growth at all costs, and also acknowledge what is happening with our planet's life-support systems." She writes about the radical steps we need to take in a time of climate emergency.

Klein thinks that the pandemic has been grasped by corporations as a "living laboratory for the permanent and highly profitable no-touch future" which she ironically terms "the screen new deal." When New York Governor Andrew Cuomo was in office during the pandemic he was giving speeches at the time, arguing: "Why do we even need classrooms? Why do we even need teachers?"

Though she believes that governments are exploiting the Covid-19 pandemic she is also concerned that: "We are at a time of peak conspiracy theory and misinformation" and that her ideas are "being used and abused" to justify positions such as those of anti-vaxxers. She is critical of Bill Gates for interfering to protect the patents of drug companies. She thinks he's played a terrible role, but she recognises it is misinformation to suggest that he "is doing all this because he wants to depopulate the earth and the vaccines have tracking devices." As she noted: "It's a new ball game. Conspiracies are always part of disaster ecosystems."

With new technologies and social media landscapes it's so much easier for conspiracies to go viral. The suspicion of mainstream media that was encouraged by Trump led many people to rely on their own sources of information. As Klein recognised: "Steve Bannon's strategy… is 'flood the zone with shit.' The strategy is to make people doubt any kind of fact, so, you don't believe anything at all… It creates a very malleable political moment for people to exploit."

It is paradoxical, since it gives many dispossessed people who feel on the margins a chance to affirm a sense of self-worth through being able to question what the mainstream media is telling them and not telling them. There is a sense of empowerment that *can* come from disbelieving what the authorities supposedly want you to believe.

Klein also noted an interesting US trend in the "anti-mask and anti-vaxx crowd" that they "provided incredible cover to the people who want to privatise the school system... so if their kids don't have to go to schools that are either doing remote learning or requiring vaccines or masks, they can spend that money in private schools." She concluded that the pandemic was being used as an excuse to "wage war on public education."

Klein calls for: "The real investments that make a society able to weather shocks. You can't put everything on a vaccine mandate. You need to invest in the infrastructure of care." As she *recalls* in her conversation with historian Ian McKay: "In the early days (of Covid)... We didn't make the big infrastructure investments that would have made it easier for people to gather more safely in schools or make our hospitals more resilient."

As she noted:

> It's just been the vaccine, the vaccine, the vaccine. This has created an atmosphere that is very ripe for conspiracy theories, because people are seeing the huge profits that are being won by a small group of people. It doesn't feel right, so they're looking for explanations.

Ian McKay wondered about her prognostications for the decade to come, noting: "People are just exhausted- they're so sick of this. Many are bereaved and mourning loved ones. It doesn't strike me as a likely time for an energetic movement of resistance."[23] Klein responded saying:

> I think we have a right to a pandemic dividend, and I think we need ambitious movement leaders who demand it and inspire us. And I think we need artists to help revive our spirits after this period of trying to weather these shocks on our own. We're in the uncharted territories.

At the same time, she thought:

> The technology-enabled isolation of Covid is quite unique: to be two years as separate from one another as possible. So, my hope is that the thrill of being able to be together because we are social beings will be such that we will be overcome with energy. We will be energised by being in each other's company.

But she also saw the risks of eco-fascism saying: "I see a risk of the climate crisis being folded into a narrative around 'great replacement' fears" (a racist conspiracy that European people being replaced by non-Europeans) "and white supremacy, creating an even more toxic cocktail than climate change denial." She is also concerned about a convergence between the wellness worlds and the conspiracy and far-right worlds:

> You will hear things like: 'Well I have a great immune system' and 'I take care of myself – so why should I have to sacrifice for all these people who aren't taking care of themselves? Maybe they should die.' This is a fascist world view.

Politics, Power and Resistance

Long-haul truckers who descended on Ottawa, gathering round the parliament building, protesting at compulsory vaccination to cross the Canadian American border (agreed by both countries), managed to shut down the Canadian capital for days. Judy Rebick and Corvin Russell, while challenging the failure of the left to really engage the well-funded anti-vaxxers and anti-maskers, noted that the lorry drivers had substantial support among Conservatives and Greens. "More importantly, this mobilisation provides one of the few outlets for many people to express anger and frustration around legitimate grievances with government failures during the pandemic."

As they recorded in ways that echo governments beyond Canada: "These failures have been real. While China adopted airborne precautions as early as January 20, 2020, authorities in Canada and other western countries at first denied the usefulness of masks." They point out that former chief advisor to President Trump, Anthony Fauci came clean later that this narrative was pushed due to concerns that demand would outstrip supply for masks. "By the time they'd reversed course, the damage had been done."

They noted:

> What's needed to manage the pandemic sustainably is clear and doable – N95 masks and rapid tests for all, vaccines for the world, ventilation and filtration upgrades in shared indoor air, and support for people and workers isolating. Yet governments and businesses have taken a penny-wise, pound-foolish approach and invested in an implausible vaccine-only exit strategy, hoping that the short-term expense of needed structural fixes including permanent ventilation improvements could be avoided.
>
> *(Rabble, 4 February 2022)*

Richard Horton, editor of *The Lancet*, opened an analysis of systematic Covid failures by quoting Laurie Garrett's *The Coming Plague*: "While the human race battles itself, fighting over even more crowded turf and scarcer resources, the advantage moves to the microbes' court. They are our predators."[24]

The US Institute of Medicine in its evaluation of the 2003 Sars outbreak, came to a similar conclusion, noting that "The rapid containment of Sars is a success in public health, but also a warning. If Sars recurs, health systems worldwide will be put under extreme pressure. Continued vigilance is vital" (*The Guardian*, 9 April 2020).

However, "The world ignored these warnings and Austerity blunted the ambition and commitment of government to protect its people... The result was to leave the country fatally weakened." Horton explains that governments should have been prepared for a new epidemic given the history of HIV's emergence in the 1980s, infecting 75 million and claiming 32 million lives. Though not as rapid as Sars-CoV-2, HIV's impact should have served as a warning to be ready for future viral outbreaks.

He further acknowledged that the Anthropocene entailed a high degree of human influence on the environment: but that the pandemic revealed an "astonishing fragility" at the heart of our societies. He contemplates the very real possibility of societies learning nothing from Covid, and leaning further into dangerous "complacent exceptionalism."

If people cannot mourn the many who have died and so learn the lessons from their deaths, it will be as if these terrors we lived through never really happened. We will fool ourselves that nothing really needs to be learnt and the transformation in our understanding and relationship with nature, which is so vital for the world in the face of the climate emergency too, will just not happen. This is why we need to join the young activists who have in so many ways led the struggle for climate justice, as part of a much wider movement. As Klein notes: "It really does take everyone" (syndemic.ca).

Grief, Memories and Vulnerable Futures

How are we to remember the Covid-19 dead and honour their memories? *The New York Times* filled its front page with names while Germans made shrines out of burning candles. India created a memorial website while in the UK people created their own memorial wall on the Thames Embankment and an online book of remembrance at St Paul's Cathedral.

Laura Spinney, author of *Pale Rider: The Spanish Flu of 1918 and How it Changed the World* highlighted the "paradoxical" nature of pandemics: forcing us to reckon with huge numbers of fatalities that we are naturally unable to, that quickly "shades into meaninglessness." However, "because pandemics destroy people but not infrastructure – unlike wars, which destroy both – humanity tends to recover from them relatively quickly."

She reflects on their cyclical nature: "They are both ephemeral *and* perennial. Whenever we think we've beaten the invisible enemy, we've really just entered a new round." She is impressed with the idea of Martin Gomez Platero, the architect of a new memorial in Montevideo. It's a shallow bowl in concrete and steel suspended over the South Atlantic. It wants to express – "humankind is not the centre of the ecosystem in which we live, as we will always be subordinate to nature." The beauty of this world memorial is that it will commemorate *all* pandemics, as

Spinney notes: "The one we're living through, the ones we've forgotten and the ones still to come" (*The Guardian*, 18 March 2021).[25]

Already in 2020, Spinney was warning that:

> Letting the virus that caused Covid-19 circulate more or less freely is dangerous not only because it risks overwhelming hospitals, but also because it could delay the evolution of the virus to a more benign form and potentially even make it more lethal.

She talks about "the biological arms race between a pathogen and its host." In November 2020, she was struck by the differences in death rates between Sweden – which took a relaxed approach to containment until much later into the pandemic – and Norway, whose measures were much stricter. Sweden had more than three times as many deaths per 100 cases as its neighbour. She noted: "If the conditions are right, the slightly more virulent viruses will begin to predominate and cause more damage. In Sweden conditions have allowed those slightly more virulent variants to flourish."

"Protecting people through public health measures," she argues, "buys us time" by delaying contagion, which in turn "could make a huge difference to all those people in the world who don't have access to adequate healthcare." The influenza epidemic of 1918 spread around the world largely because of the unprecedented mingling of people on the Western Front in the First World War showing the *active* role humans can play, sometimes unwittingly. Something similar happened with global air travel in the case of Covid-19 (*The Guardian*, 19 November 2020).

In an interview with Ian McKay for *Syndemic Magazine* (syndemic.ca, 23 March 2022) Spinney explained:

> We talk about spill-over events, zoonotic diseases that come from animals into humans. Yet we shape the whole ecosystem that makes that possible through our use of the environment, through farming, through wildlife and trade. Once the pandemic is upon us, we shape the virus in terms of how it mutates, how it evolves, how infectious it is, and how severe the infection is. Vaccines put enormous selective pressure on the virus. The uneven rollout of the vaccines across the world that we're seeing at the moment, is another way in which we're shaping its evolution, because the pressure will be on it to escape.

McKay questioned her talking about a "biological arms race" between a pathogen and a host and wondered how helpful it was to use war metaphors in talking about the pandemic. He said:

> Martial language encourages us to think still that we're at war with a virus, when in fact we have co-evolved with the virus. It's really a question of managing our metabolism with nature in a more rational way, rather than being at war with it.

Spinney acknowledged that she was guilty of using these metaphors, saying her thinking has been evolving. She thinks Biden used this language to help people get over a kind of natural passivity. He wanted to persuade them to act. She also thinks that it *can* reflect a changing understanding of pandemics: "There's a certain justification for talking about it as an enemy which is trying to outwit us. There is a sense in which we need to outwit it." For her, it's probably not too damaging for us to use this kind of warlike language if we understand that the enemy is a virus.

As Spinney said about the writing of *Pale Rider:*

> I was trying to explain to myself, as much as to anyone else, why our memory for pandemics is less good than our memory for war. We forgot this terrible catastrophe (The 1918 flu) that killed more than any disaster in the 20th century. There's a very different way in which we document these kinds of disasters and then, because of that, in the way that we remember them.

McKay's reading of her book is that she's saying: "Well, one of the problems of public memory here is that the pandemic didn't have the right shape. It doesn't conform to the beginning, middle and end, of a classic narrative structure." He notes, "It's very hard to tell when a pandemic is over and also the heroes and villains are going to be hard to discern in this one."

With shifts in technology, it is possible to remember in different ways and as Spinney suggests:

> Anyone in the world who has access to the internet, could have, if they wanted, from the beginning of this pandemic, tracked infection rates and mortality rates in (almost) real time. They could have had a general overview of the whole global phenomenon. This wasn't the case in 1918. It took a very long time for people in the world to realise they were looking at one pandemic, rather than lots of local outbreaks of disease.

The naming reflects that. It was given several different names to begin with. But she asks: "If we are better at documenting this one, does it mean we'll remember it better?"

Global Inequalities and Threatened Democracies

In *The Covid Consensus: The New Politics of Global Inequality*, Toby Green critically examines the emergence of the scientific consensus surrounding the Covid-19 lockdowns, suggesting that it has worked to *amplify* global inequalities. Even if these policies were not intended to do so, this has effectively been a consequence and it has also blocked countries that might have followed a different course given their locations and contexts in the global south. Green views lockdowns as the most intrusive public health measure which resulted from the politicisation of the public health crisis and the difficulty of alternative views getting a hearing on mainstream media.[26]

He asserts that while tech companies, pharmaceutical corporations and remote workers were able to benefit from lockdowns, front line essential workers, the hospitality sector, those engaged in art and culture, women and children and many in the global south were adversely impacted. These beneficiaries helped to *shape* the consensus through the media, even if they were being questioned on social media outlets. Green argues that following a blanket approach meant that different socio-economic realities were being ignored *at* the cost of many, particularly in the global south.

Green draws on wartime comparisons to argue that unlike in the Second World War, citizens were instructed to sacrifice the future *for* the present rather than left to decide the risks they were willing to take with their own lives. He raises the question about the proportionality of benefit to loss during the first lockdown. One set of risks was *not* weighed against another, for example issues of children's education, mental health of individuals and sexual violence. He exposes the reasons why authorities did not acknowledge the initial failure to evaluate these risks.

Challenging the myth that the Covid-19 was a great leveller because we were equally exposed to the virus that would not discriminate, means questioning the moral foundations of a culture of deliberate ignorance. This neoliberal commonsense, framed in individualist terms about health risks, ignores the *devastating* socio-economic and health impact of the international response to the pandemic in the global south.

Borders were suddenly imposed, and people were encouraged to forget the world that existed beyond their own national boundaries. The global poor were to be abandoned by policy makers. Ethical considerations for vulnerable populations were put aside. This meant countries in the global south had to use their reserves for immediate relief, which Green argues could have been invested later in health and education. This worked to *increase* the inequality gap within countries as well as the inequality gap between the global north and south.

Green traces the quick shaping of the consensus and how fear was mobilised to ensure compliance and close down discussion of different options so that it took time for "all in this together" idea to dissolve and for class, race, and gender inequalities to be exposed through the numbers who were dying. He was surprised at how easily people willingly ceded their rights to fight a disease within liberal democratic societies where freedom is fundamental.

He argues that the estrangement of people from democratic capitalism has paved the way for authoritarian capitalism where a capitalist market economy exists alongside an authoritarian government that is ready to sacrifice constitutional freedoms for its own short-term policy agendas. He is concerned that freedoms will be permanently abandoned in post-pandemic times because people will accommodate themselves to new realities.

Possibly people were more accommodating of the early lockdowns because it was in the context of a public health emergency. People were rightly fearful before the vaccines became available, even if this fear was to be manipulated by authorities who did *not* seem to be obeying the laws that they had legislated. There were anti-lockdown protests and people across the world questioned them for a whole range of different reasons. A thoughtful review by Chinmayee Mishra (LSE Blogs, 17 February 2022) suggests Green's book devotes "less space to the benefits of lockdown in places in the global south where the number of public health facilities is disproportionately small relative to the size of the population."

The Covid-19 response has *had* devastating consequences for democratic rights and the poor worldwide. Whatever we might think about the wisdom of the lockdowns at different stages in the pandemic and in different places, Green shows that as the fortunes of the richest soared, nationwide shutdowns devastated small businesses, the working-classes and the global south's informal economies. He shows how gender-based violence soared and the education and mental health of young people was severely compromised.

Toby Green and journalist Thomas Fazi confront the refusal of the global political class and mainstream media to report the true extent of the erosion of democratic rights and the socioeconomic assault on the poor. Whether you are persuaded by their arguments against lockdown, it is undeniable that such restrictions have disproportionately affected the young and the poor. Even in the face of viruses and death, some humans are still "more equal" than others.

Taking Liberties and Threatening Democracy

Tracing the attacks on democratic rights in the UK, Adam Wagner's *Emergency State: How we lost our Freedoms in the Pandemic and Why it Matters*, will resonate in different ways in countries across the world. He shows how on 26 March 2020 a new law appeared which in 11 pages restricted our freedoms more than any other law in history, justified by the rapid spread of a new deadly virus. Even though you might have expected it to be fiercely debated in parliament, it wasn't debated at all.[27]

A state of emergency was declared, meaning the law came into force the moment it was passed. Though the emergency was supposed to be short, it lasted for 736 days allowing ministers to bring in by decree over 100 new laws. These were almost never debated though they severely restricted freedoms people had learnt to take for granted. In this way "our democracy was put under threat during the pandemic," as Lady Brenda Hale, former President of the Supreme Court who had to deal with Johnson's illegal prorogation of parliament, acknowledged saying: "We must never let the Emergency State – all powerful but ignorant and corrupt – take over again."

In an article for *Prospect Magazine* called "Taking liberties: Covid-19 and the anatomy of a constitutional catastrophe" Adam Wagner opened with a question: "How quickly does freedom die?" and suggested that though we might get many of our personal freedoms back: "Such have been the abuses of Parliament, police and the law that we may never recover our standing as free citizens." He acknowledged that this question was a strange one to ask "in a country that thinks of itself as blessed with venerable and supremely liberal constitutional arrangements" (Prospect Magazine, 26 March 2021).

Wagner noted that "visceral evidence of our loss of liberty" was coverage of the Metropolitan Police "manhandling peaceful participants in a vigil for the murdered Londoner Sarah Everard," which was swiftly followed by the government "push(ing) through measures that gave police powers to permanently limit such assemblies." As he acknowledged: "The question is fast becoming: how quickly can you resurrect freedom? Or is that impossible when the authorities have grown too comfortable with the public living without it."

He questions a seductive argument we often hear throughout history, that democracy, and the civil liberties that underpin it, are "peacetime niceties." He says history teaches us that the opposite *is* true: that these things are even more essential during times of upheaval.

> Cuts to our democracy leave scars, and once normality returns, the deepest cuts may never heal. Many emergency powers have ended up remaining in place. Look at the post-9/11 anti-terrorism laws and associated intrusive state surveillance, which have become permanent even as that threat has receded.

The lockdown was justified but the law ultimately put in place, as Wagner remarks: "Was radically different to any other in English legal history assuming that people would be forbidden from doing anything unless the legislation said, in terms, that they could." He appreciates that:

> The easier it is for freedoms to be taken away, the greater the temptations to limit them in the future. A government which, had, only months before, unlawfully prorogued (closed) the legislature was not going to be held back by such niceties as debates and primary legislation.

Instead of amending the Coronavirus Act 2020 that included parts relating to restrictions on gatherings and school closures, the government decided to impose lockdown through secondary legislation – regulations made by ministerial decree – under the Public Health (Control of Disease) Act 1984.

It would be possible for there to be *no* Parliamentary scrutiny or approval for 28 days after the law had come into effect. Last minute legislating became a habit to cut down liberties people had long taken for granted. As Wagner notes: "No matter how grave the breach of civil liberties, there was no presumption of scrutiny. The government's systematic bypassing of Parliament seemed designed instead to stymie scrutiny and remove the opportunity for MPS to examine the all-important detail." Interviews with police officers showed him that some despaired that the "too wide" rules had become a "farce and pretty much unenforceable." Morale had sunk, they said because "everyone hates us." One worried about "the need for public support, now and in the future."

Wagner recognises: "Pandemic law-making will have left an indelible stain on the rule of law and on the relationship between citizen and state." He laments the "radical contempt" shown for democracy by Parliament. He points out how far down the agenda keeping the public informed became: "As the government endlessly iterated and experimented, it has shown a worrying lack of concern for explaining exactly what it is doing and why."

Concluding his powerful assessment, Wagner stated that the "so-called unwritten constitution is simply too weak to protect our basic liberties." He saw that moment as an "opportunity to rethink and codify the ground rules of our freedoms… with the clear-eyed understanding that while freedoms may occasionally need to be checked and balanced, this must always be temporary, proportionate, and – just as much – argued for and explained."

These are questions about the *rule of law* and *everyday justice* that concern liberal democracies around the world in the global north, as much as in the global south, where populist and authoritarian rulers, even if they have an electoral mandate, have been able to use Covid-19 to strengthen the authority of the state to undermine democratic accountability. *If* we are to learn the lessons of the pandemic, they have to do with recreating forms of democratic accountability within societies where economies and societies have been built back differently, as was promised, less marked by structural inequalities of class, race, disability, ethnicities and genders.

As ethical humans threatened by a climate emergency, we need to learn that we are *part of* the natural world that we depend upon. We need to challenge the terms of a globalised neoliberal capitalism that has fuelled increasing inequalities through the pandemic and treated nature as a means of exploitation and extraction. We need to shape moral imaginations that uphold the equal dignity and worth of human beings as part of the natural world and new visions of equality and global justice. The terrifying earthquake in Turkey and Syria in February 2023 reminded us of the need for global communities of support that can learn from their different traditions and values.

Notes

1 This was a report by YouGov that was reported on Sky News, Friday 17 April 2020 also reporting that 'More than half (54%) of 4,343 people who took part in the YouGov poll hope they will make some changes in their own lives and for the country as a whole to learn from the crisis. The survey was commissioned by the Food, Farming and Countryside Commission (FFCC).

2 To engage with developments in George Monbiot's thinking around ecology and planetary development see, for instance, *Manifesto For a New World Order* (New York: New Press 2004) that emphasises not only that things ought to change, but how to change them; and *Regenesis: Feeding the Earth without Devouring the Planet* (London: Penguin Books 2023) which weaves the poetry of soil into the politics of farming and offers a hopeful vision of techno-ethical equilibrium between humanity and nature.

3 For challenges to traditional economics that is organised around notions of economic growth and fails to engage with questions of political economy and growing social and economic inequalities see, for instance, Tim Jackson *Prosperity without Growth: Foundations for the Economy of Tomorrow* (London: Routledge 2016). He argues for a new

economics which works for people, planet and prosperity, providing an alternative to passivity, selfishness and cynicism. See also his *Post Growth: Life After Capitalism* (Cambridge: Polity 2021) where he argues that the relentless pursuit of more has delivered climate catastrophe, social inequality and left us unprepared for a global pandemic. A world beyond capitalism is a world where relationship and meaning take precedence over profit and power.

4 For some reflections on living in ways that question a capitalist ethics that always wants more see, for instance, John Naish *Breaking Free from the World of Excess* (London: Hodder Paperbacks, 2009) who argues we need to develop a sense of enough and from a Christian theological vision; Will Davis *Enough: Finding More by Living with Less* (Grand Rapids, MI: Revell 2012) who challenges us to discover the peace through contentment with what we have and compassion for those in need.

5 An interview with Ingrid Robeyns with David Maclean "Can Limitarianism Save the World?" (iai.tv, 13 December 2017). See also Ingrid Robeyns, "Why Limitarianism?" *Journal of Political Philosophy 30*(2), pp. 249–270) (Hoboken, NJ: Wiley) and "What, if Anything, is Wrong with Extreme Wealth?" *Journal of Human Development and Capacities 20*(3), 2019. She basically argues that eliminating excess wealth prevents the super-rich from undermining political equality and there will be more resources available to address any urgent unmet needs in society.

6 Gaia Vince *Transcendence: How Humans Evolved Through Fire, Language, Beauty and Time* (London: Penguin Books 2019).

7 Kate Raworth is a renegade economist, creator of the Doughnut of social and planetary boundaries and author of *Doughnut Economics: Seven Ways to think like a 21st century economist* (London and New York: Random House Business 2017). This means to meet the needs of all within the means of the planet and so to ensure the dignity and prosperity for all people. See also Jason Hickel *Less is More: How Degrowth Will Save the World* (London: Windmill Books 2021) who offers a radically possible vision of a post-growth future through showing how the insatiable drive to increase GDP has caused the ecological crisis. He reveals the historical and colonial roots of capitalism also in *The Divide: A Brief Guide to Global Inequality and its Solutions* (London: Windmill Books 2018).

8 "Out of the Belly of Hell: Covid-19 and the humanisation of globalisation" (opendemocracy.net, 21 May 2020).

9 Anthony Barnett's investigation into whether Biden and the liberal centre can ally with progressives under the banner of humanity to renew our democracy and save our ecosystem in post-Covid times is *Taking Control: Humanity and America after Trump and the Pandemic* (London: Repeater Books 2022).

10 To grasp changes in the neoliberal capitalist economy and the experiences of zero-hours and undocumented labour that reveals the everyday lives of undocumented migrants and how they navigate the pressures they are under see, Alice Bloch and Sonia McKay *Living on the Margins: Undocumented migrants in a Global City* (Bristol: Policy Press 2017); A. Bloch, N. Sigona and R. Zetter *Sans Papiers: the Social and Economic Lives of young, undocumented migrants* (London: Pluto Press 2014) and Alice Bloch and Giorgia Dona *Forced Migration: Current Issues and Debates* (London: Routledge 2019).

11 For a sense of the development of John Gray's writings, see for example, *Heresies* (London: Granta Books 2004); *Straw Dogs* (London: Granta Books 2003) and *The Silence of Animals: On Progress and Other Modern Myths* (London: Penguin 2014).

12 William McNeill *Plagues and People* (New York: Bantam Doubleday Dell 1977) gives an interpretation of world history seen through the impacts, political, ecological and demographic of diseases on culture.

13 Naomi Wolf *Bodies of Others: The New Authoritarians, Covid-19 and The War Against the Human* (Livermore, CA: All Seasons Press 2022).

14 Naomi Wolf *The End of America: Letters of Warning to a Young Patriot* (White River Junction VT: Chelsea Green Publishing Inc 2007).

15 This is taken from an interview with Dr Joseph Mercola https://freedom-school.com/freedomThe-Bodies-of-Others-An-Assault-of-Our-Liberties-by-the-Technocrats.pdf.
16 Allesandro Manzoni *The Betrothed* (London: Penguin Classics 1983).
17 For a sense of Giorgio Agamben's philosophical work see, for example, *Homo Sacer: Sovereign Power and Bare Life* (Palo Alto: Stanford University Press 1998) where he shows how throughout the history of Western political theory notions of sovereignty have implicitly invoked notions of power over "life". See also his *State of Exception* (Chicago: University of Chicago Press 2005); His more recent writings on the Covid-19 pandemic are presented in *Where Are We Now: The Epidemic as Politics* (London: Eris 2021).
18 Simone Weil frames an alternative vision of post war France in *The Need for Roots* (London: Routledge 1978). For a discussion of the development of Weil's work and how certain themes about inequality, power, oppression and suffering endure see Lawrence Blum and Vic Seidler *A Truer Liberty*: *Simone Weil and Marxism* (New York: Routledge 1989). See also, Peter Winch *Simone Weil: The Just Balance* (Cambridge: Cambridge University Press,1989) and Mary Dietz *Between the Human and the Divine: The Political Thought of Simone Weil* (Lanham, Maryland: Rowman and Littlefield 1988).
19 Robert Reich *The System: Who Rigged it, How we Fix it* (New York: Alfred Knopf 2020).
20 Naomi Klein *The Shock Doctrine: The Rise of Disaster Capitalism* (London: Penguin 2008).
21 Naomi Klein *This Changes Everything: Capitalism versus the Climate* (London: Penguin 2015).
22 Naomi Klein's writings developing a critique of neoliberal corporate capitalism and its relationship with Covid-19 and the climate emergency include *The Shock Doctrine: The Rise of Disaster Capitalism: The Rise of Disaster Capitalism* (London: Penguin 2008); *This Changes Everything: Capitalism vs. the Climate* (London: Penguin 2015) and *How to Change Everything* (London: Penguin 2022).
23 An Interview with Naomi Klein by *Syndemic Magazine*, 8 March 2022 – a project L.R Wilson Institute for Canadian History, McMaster University.
24 Laurie Garrett investigates the worldwide conditions that have culminated in newly discovered diseases and epidemics of diseases migrating to new areas in *The Coming Plague: Newly Emerging Diseases in a World out of Balance* (London: Penguin Books 1995) This frightening vision of a microbial catastrophes in a global ecology also questions Enlightenment beliefs in progress through science and technology.
25 Laura Spinney writes a devastating story of the Spanish flu with a death toll between 50 and 100 million, showing how the pandemic was shaped by the interaction between the virus and the humans it encountered in *Pale Rider: The Spanish Flu of 1918 and How it Changed the World* (New York and London: Vintage 2018). Its impacts were as devastating as the two world wars but in popular conception it exists largely as a footnote to the First World War.
26 Toby Green was sceptical about government policies in relation to lockdown and develops a critique from the left in *The Covid Consensus: The Global Assault on Democracy and the Poor.* (London: C. Hurst and Co. 2021).
27 Adam Wagner traces how the government in the UK was ready to put aside constitutional freedoms to consolidate its power during the Covid-19 pandemic in *Emergency State: How We Lost Our Freedoms in the Pandemic and Why it Matters* (London: Bodley Head 2022).

COVID-19: AFTERTHOUGHTS

How Different the World Needs to Be

Renewing Democratic Politics and Ethical Imaginations

We will never know how the Covid-19 global epidemic is going to end or whether in 2023, at the time of writing, three years after its beginning, we are still waiting for new strains to arrive. We don't know when a new pandemic might strike. We might anticipate that in time, Covid-19, like influenza before it, is going to weaken, even if each year it is going to take many lives, especially of the elderly and the frail during the winter months. Will we eventually just accustom ourselves to getting an annual Covid-19 vaccination along with a flu jab? Will we build resistance to the virus as our immune systems learn more?

But if it is hard to anticipate an ending, it is clear that many people across the world are determined that it *is* over, even before the threat of new infections is not. They don't want to be reminded of their lives as vulnerable humans living in isolation, the loneliness in lockdown and the pain of grief. They *want* to put the fraught and frightening last few years behind them, as if they never really happened at all. Many prefer denial than facing difficult truths and coming to terms with global inequalities as vulnerable humans.

But philosophy and sociology as disciplines that are still learning how to listen and learn from each other are both concerned with *making sense* of experiences in difficult social and historical contexts. Ethnography helps us learn from different voices as they are making sense in uncertain times and listening to diverse voices has helped to shape this project that has always been shared and collective at its heart.

In a piece for *The Asean Post* on 3 June 2022 entitled "Why Did We Forget COVID So Quickly?", Brigid Delaney cited coverage in *The Washington Post* that

DOI: 10.4324/9781003296874-14

week that even though high infection rates persisted and were five times higher than the same period in the previous year, people's behaviour did not reflect this:

> People know but don't want to know at the same time. Parents of children too young to be vaccinated are making cross-country travel plans. Octogenarians are venturing into to bars. Families are celebrating graduations and weddings with throngs of mostly unmasked revellers.

There were echoes of the ending of the Second World War. Child survivors from Auschwitz, like Kitty Hart, were warned by their families in Britain *not* to talk about the terrible experiences they had lived through. The attitude was that people just didn't want to hear it. They wanted to put the war firmly in the past. They didn't want to be reminded of the horrors they had lived through and they didn't want a young refugee to ask questions. Kitty was told that if she wanted to be accepted, she would have to put her traumatic history behind her and learn to live as if it hadn't happened at all.[1]

It's hard to anticipate and prepare for pandemics to come if we insist on moving on with the present, feeling intolerant, even abusive, to those who insist on wearing masks to keep safe.

Delaney, this time writing in *The Guardian*, noted that in June 2022, partly encouraged by the government insisting that the vaccine was the answer to everything, people felt Covid was over. She describes this phenomenon as the "pandemic's social death," noting that people's wish to cease dwelling on Covid is consistent with the "mass forgetting" that follows "mass trauma." She speculates that the severity and insidiousness of the "disruption" caused by the virus was felt so deeply, that individuals simply feel "(they) cannot incorporate it into (their) present and future narratives" (*The Guardian*, 2 June 2022).

She turned her attention to the attitudes displayed in Australia, at that time dealing with new cases surging to up to 35,000 per day. She suggests with high vaccination rates, individuals have forgotten to act and modified their behaviours to prevent the spread in the first place. As she points out at that time, just a year on from the lockdowns:

> …the daily press conferences and "the numbers" – police fining people, seems like they are from another era, one we've tacitly all just agreed not to talk about, or remember, or dwell on… (with) a taint of embarrassment about it.

Delaney perceives that this shaped a "collective consciousness" that the pandemic had ended, although the figures clearly contradicted this. People yearned for the end of the pandemic: so, judged the "*medical* ending" of the pandemic to be when mass fatalities were no longer reported: perhaps around the point when the Covid zero policy was discarded. The "*psychological* death," Delaney explained, could only come about when people no longer felt afraid, and felt able to carry on, "business as usual," which she noted was "fascinating to watch from a sociological perspective – or horrifying, if you are vulnerable or immunocompromised."

She concludes the article with the declaration: "An era has ended, and maybe one day we'll wonder if it ever happened."

Vulnerable Humans and Hopeful Selves

To forget it had happened was not possible for the millions around the world who are suffering from Long Covid and felt pushed to the side lines. George Monbiot reflected on what we now knew about Long Covid:

> We know how the virus attacks our cells, "traumatic brain injury" looks less like an analogy than a description. The outcomes can be devastating, ranging from extreme fatigue and breathlessness to brain fog, psychotic disorders, memory loss, epilepsy and dementia. We are all playing Covid roulette.
>
> *(The Guardian, 26 January 2023)*

As cholera was stopped by providing clean water, the spread of Covid would be halted by clean air, Monbiot suggested, citing a study that found that mechanical ventilation systems in classrooms reduced the infection rate by 74%. He additionally pointed out that parliament, and government buildings where ministers work, had these systems. At the World Economic Forum in Davos in 2023 they were in every room.

Writing in the *British Medical Journal* without sharing her name (10 February 2023, p. 337), a doctor with Long Covid said she felt abandoned by the NHS. Her account imparts difficult truths that many would want to forget, or at least ignore. She expressed her dismay at the "collective silence and the lack of protections and support mechanisms in place" that followed the crisis, which caused thousands of healthcare workers like her to develop this debilitating chronic health condition, whilst trying to protect and care for others.

She described *how* medics neglected their own health, becoming too ill to work, and were then confronted with the possibility of a hit to their salary, or even unemployment: thus feeling that they had little choice but to carry on. She describes her experience, shortly after despairing over the discrepancy between shows of public support, and "troubling attitudes" to staff safety, of falling ill herself: "Within a few weeks of working during the first wave of the pandemic, I was sick and stuck in bed, my oxygen levels dropping whenever I stood or walked."

Even then, she was working when she was physically able to: as she and her colleagues "pushed through" the punishing first stages of Long Covid, due to what she describes as the "martyr complex instilled by medical culture." She reflects on how deeply her sense of self is influenced by her profession, and her sorrow that she could not do her job: being "in constant pain… (struggling) to sit, walk, or play with my children." She starkly describes how her disability made her feel "left behind" and "thrown away."

The pandemic may have been "declared 'over,' " but for her and thousands of others like her, she was living day to day with its consequences, and as she points out, people were still becoming ill. Damningly, she states the "shameful" discarding of workers has been justified by institutions, "because they can no longer provide the same level of productivity."

Michael Rosen, the children's author was so severely ill with Covid that he spent six weeks on a ventilator. He said:

> It feels like a pre-death, because it's a nothingness." He didn't have a clue what kind of man would emerge. He told Simon Hattenstone of *The Guardian*: "I couldn't stand up, so I thought: 'Oh I'm the kind of person who can't stand up,' and there was a bit of me that resigned myself to the fact that I would be in a wheelchair."
>
> *(The Guardian, 30 September 2020)*[2]

Rosen said:

> I'm the kind of person who is pathologically certain. Now, suddenly, all that certainty has gone. "What will I do, what will I be, how will I cope with the fact that I can't see out of this eye or hear in this ear? And, of course, what can I do if I can't work? We're not very good at accepting that people come out of a big crisis damaged, because we go: 'Oh well, at least he's alive; at least she's still with us.' So, I guess people have transferred that response from people who survived being bombed in the war: 'You survived… great, well shut up, then'."

Philosophy, Sociology and Vulnerable Humans

The Covid-19 pandemic was often described as an "unprecedented" disaster, which required completely *new ways of living* in the world that is at the same time threatened by climate emergencies. What are the new ways of organising economic and social life now that the pandemic has so clearly disrupted existing social orders? Now it has rendered visible the depth of global inequalities and social injustices, not only within countries and also between the global North and global South?

The conviction that there has to be a different world, a more equal and just world that emerges from the years of Covid pandemic, is *shared* by many but we are still to learn whether this hopeful vision can be realised. This calls for a renewed vision of ourselves as ethical humans inspired by an eco-human imagination that puts an ethics of care, extending across different species, at the heart of a re-imagined politics.

At the heart of this is the concept of vulnerability: a notion that has coming into cultural prominence over the past few years, dovetailing with the sense of human fragility that many reckoned with during the pandemic. The songwriter and singer Nick Cave published a series of conversations in 2022 under the title *Faith, Hope and Carnage*[3] in the wake of the crisis, and mused extensively on the power of vulnerability (*The Marginalian*, 12 February 2023).

Cave poignantly suggests that in the course of a life: "You somehow grow into the fullness of your humanity, form your own character, become a proper person, someone who has become part of things, not someone separated from or at odds with the world." He explicitly states his feelings on the importance of vulnerability, or this embracing of being a cog in the machine: "It is in our vulnerability that we find our deepest freedom. My experience in creating music and writing songs is finding enormous strength through vulnerability. You're being open to whatever happens, including failure and shame." Another great songwriter of our time, Bob Dylan, in an interview with Jonathan Cott observes that vulnerability is absolutely key to being "sensitive to reality… being vulnerable is just another way of saying that one has nothing more to lose."[4]

Erich Fromm framed a similar awareness, uniting vulnerability and hope in the sense of the individual being part of a wider whole, in *The Revolution of Hope: Toward a Humanised Technology,* writing: "Hope is a decisive element in any attempt to bring about social change in the direction of greater aliveness, awareness, and reason."[5] He argued that our capacity *to hope* is rooted in our vulnerable self-consciousness, aware that human beings lack animal instincts (or certainties):

> Humans do not "know" infallibly, as the salmon knows where to return to the river to spawn its young and birds know where to go south in the winter. Humans have to make their own decisions and there is a risk of failure in every decision made. The price that humans pay for consciousness is insecurity. The only certain prediction a person can make is: "I shall die."

Fromm's "appealing to the love for life that still exists in many of us" affirms:

> Only through full awareness of the danger to life can this potential be mobilised for action capable of bringing about drastic changes in our ways of organising society. One cannot think in terms of percentages or probabilities as long as there is a real possibility – even a slight one – that life will prevail.

As he also recognises:

> Hope is neither a passive waiting nor is it an unrealistic forcing of circumstances that cannot occur. It is like the crouched tiger, which will jump when the moment for jumping has come. To hope means to be ready at every moment for that which is not yet born, and yet not become desperate if there is no birth in our lifetime.

Rebirths, Hopes, Ecologies and Global Futures

Thinking through Kafka's story *Metamorphosis,* French philosopher, Bruno Latour entitled his response to Covid, *After Lockdown: A Metamorphosis* suggesting a possibility that suffering had led humans to go through a transformation, like Gregor in Kafka's story. This had led to the possibility of a better understanding of our connections with other living beings, in ways that could be conducive to confronting our climate crisis.

His sequel was called *Down to Earth: Politics in the New Climate Regime.* During lockdown we were unable to be sustained in our taken-for-granted identities through our everyday routines. We were encouraged to explore existential questions, for example: Where am I? Isolation provided a crucial answer that, as humans. we are terrestrials living on earth.[6]

This matters to Latour because a vital idea that emerged with Galileo was that people were not just on earth. We live in the Universe. Science allows us to observe our planet from space and so encourages us to see ourselves and the world from the outside. This gives secular terms to a Christian notion that separated Christianity from its Jewish sources and so also from the Jewishness of Jesus. The earth was to be disdained as a place of sin and suffering, and it was only through *transcending* our animal natures that we could exist as spiritual selves. Bodies were to be identified with sexuality and the sins of the flesh. Human beings were to be imagined as disembodied spiritual selves that had radically separated from earthly lives.

Latour's insight breaks with rationalist traditions of social constructionism, that when we see the earth externally as an object of scientific knowledge, we *misunderstand* our planet and fail to appreciate the "engendering concerns" on earth. This is a term he invokes to refer to the connections, overlaps and interactions between diverse human and natural beings. We lose a sense of the concerns shared among humans, termites, bumblebees, rocks, rivers and air that all become buried.

Empowered by assumed objective knowledge, humans have had the "secularised religious emotion" (p. 57) that they can escape from this world and don't need to be held accountable for their expansions, as Latour frames it. As we learn within Cartesian traditions to identify ourselves with our minds and learn to guide our lives through reason alone, so we often abandon our bodies and what they are telling us. We don't learn to *listen* to our bodies, but we learnt to *control* and *silence* them. This is often at the cost of our own physical and mental wellbeing. Born of the universe, moderns always want to *deny* their issues as they learn to blame others and learn to withhold what is going on for them and escape elsewhere.

Sharing his own experience and change of heart and mind during lockdown, Latour wrote:

> I began to position myself as a terrestrial among other terrestrials once the surprise had worn off and I realise that terrestrials never move around "freely" everywhere in some undifferentiated space. They construct that space step by step. It's feeling confined that gives us this freedom finally to move freely. Turning into a termite assures us that we can't survive for a minute without constructing, by means of saliva and mud, a tiny tunnel that allows us to crawl in complete safety a few millimetres further along. No tunnel, no movement.
>
> *(p. 27)*

In a review, of *After Lockdown*, Dr Rong A, a visiting fellow in the Department of Sociology at the London School of Economics, affirmed: "Lockdown experiences are empowering as lockdown shook off the secularised religions that preach escape from this world" (p. 57). On Earth, confinements have always been terrestrials' direct experiences. Becoming an insect, as Gregor experienced in Kafka's *Metamorphosis*, 'is empowering as we free ourselves of the infinite. In lockdowns, "people know perfectly well that there is no infinite exterior anymore" (p. 55), and "everyone started to live at home but in a different way" (p. 53).

Seclusion grounded people somewhere at last where previously they had *not* lived anywhere in particular, dreaming about freedom and assuming life goes on forever. This is part of the metamorphosis: people replaced the approach of "living in a globalised world,' with "let's try and situate ourselves in a spot we will need to try to describe in tandem with others" (p. 70). In lockdown, people had to cook for themselves and take care of their children. They had to rely upon poorly paid essential workers to ensure the continuity of everyday lives.

As Latour noted:

> We are no longer living in "the Nature invented by the economists so as to have their sums circulating freely in it". We are opening each discussion that the economy aimed to close. Stillness gave people a chance to free their minds from the laws of economics in which they were rotting away.
>
> *(p. 63)*

Rather than shouting about restarting on the path of progress, many people were thinking: "What on earth are we really going to be able to live on, my dependents and I?" Humans were radically shifting their sense of themselves *as* ethical humans as they *realised* the significance of an ethics of care and the ties of interdependence among neighbours, insects and land.

On 24 December 2021 during lockdown, Latour wrote a short piece on the transformation of the pandemic into a "permanent condition" or a "way of life" that he concludes the article with calling "the new climatic regime" and detailing the ways in which the individual and society could learn to exist differently. One key way of doing this is to be mindful of how we coexist with "other living beings that react to our actions," at micro and macro-levels, and being aware that "…if they mutate, we have to mutate as well" (*The Guardian*).

Latour details the importance of learning how "our social relations will be moulded forever by the quick reaction of ecosystems that are rapidly modified by our actions" from how quickly our environments were altered by the virus "at the local as well as the global level."

Ultimately, Latour warns against complacency. The article calls for an attitudinal shift in those "used to the industrialised way of life" of constant expansion, who were suddenly forced to reckon with confinement with entities they had been able to ignore previously: in his examples, "other people of course, but also viruses, soils, coal, oil, water… this damned, constantly shifting climate."

As he wrote in an essay for the AOC cultural online newspaper:

> The first lesson the Coronavirus has taught us is also the most outstanding. We have actually proven that it is possible, in a few weeks, to put an economic system on hold everywhere in the world. This encourages us to think across the world to actively imagine how different the world could be if we learn from this experience.
>
> *(quoted in The Guardian, 24 December 2021)*

In a wide-ranging interview with journalist Jonathan Watts of *The Guardian*, the thinker elaborated on this work towards reimaging the world through the lens of the lessons of the pandemic. He explained a belief that it *isn't* helpful to think about the revenge of nature because anyone who has studied the history of medicine:

> …knows how a virus can make a society feel completely different. We are on a great learning curve… This is a global catastrophe which has come not from the outside like a war or an earthquake, but from within. Viruses are completely inside us. We cannot completely eject them. We must learn to live with them.
>
> *(The Guardian, 6 June 2020)*

When asked about the futures he would imagine, Latour responded ambitiously: suggesting "not only to modify the system of production but to get out of it altogether", and away from a relatively new tendency to "(frame) everything in terms of the economy." He acknowledged that nature is such a wide and all-embracing notion that it is difficult to *think* with: but highlighted that we must reckon with the reality that Earth's critical zone is "finite, it's local, it's at risk and it's the object of conflict", and that "It is not just about physics and energy. It is life."

> It is life which acts to maintain habitable conditions for itself. It reveals something vital about our existence as ethical humans who are part of the natural world and the therapeutic work we need to grow into ourselves and face the traumatic family legacies we carry.

As we learn to challenge the objective, God's-eye view, of science and recognise that humanity *cannot* be so detached, we need to bring the sciences and the humanities into a radically different relationship with each other, as Simone Weil suggested in her critiques of how the Nazis used science in their projects of mass murder. They encouraged scientists to be neutral in their design of mobile gas death trucks, as if there were *no* ethical issues in the movement of dead bodies. These could be considered just as shifting weights.

In an interview with journalist Hettie O'Brien in *The New Statesman*, Latour made clear his intention was never to undermine public trust in science. "The more we show how science is made, the more we can talk with credibility about what it achieves." As O'Brien wrote:

> If anything, our post-truth politics affirms Latour's ideas. In an era of conspiracy-thinking, the fragility of facts and forms of expertise we once exalted is being shown. As Latour writes in *Down to Earth:* "Facts remain robust only when they are supported by institutions that can be trusted."
>
> *(The New Statesman, 6 February 2019)*

Latour says for people *to believe* in a shared set of facts, they have to inhabit a shared world. This is something that mounting inequalities and the erosion of social safety nets have thwarted. The retrenchment of the welfare state and the spread of climate denial are all to be understood as part of a ruling elite seeking *to escape* the climate crisis while at the same time denying its existence by refusing to take the global actions necessary to meet it. "On the other hand," Latour told O'Brien irreverently: "If you read the scientific literature and see how big the problem of changing the world is, the idea of escaping makes a lot of sense – if you're rich that is."

Another giant of public discourse on the environment whose work spanned the twentieth and twenty-first centuries, scientist James Lovelock agreed that the moment of the pandemic was a moment of climate-reckoning, writing in 2021: "I don't know if it is too late for humanity to avert a climate catastrophe, but I am sure there is no chance if we continue to treat global heating and the destruction of nature as separate problems" (*The Guardian*, 2 November 2021).

He further warned:

> My fellow humans must learn to live in partnership with the Earth, otherwise the rest of creation will unconsciously move the Earth to a new state in which humans may no longer be welcome. Covid-19, may well have been one negative feedback. Gaia will try harder next time with something even nastier.

As we learn to challenge the objective, God's-eye view, of science and recognise that humanity cannot be so detached, we need to bring the sciences and the humanities into a radically different relationship with each other. As Simone Weil suggested in her critiques of how the Nazis used science in their projects of mass murder.

Groundings, Philosophy and Everyday Ethics

Lucy Easthope is one of the UK's leading authorities on emergency planning, who professionally assesses the scale of a disaster. Her memoir *When the Dust Settles: Stories of Love, Loss and Hope from an Expert in Disaster* (2022) was reviewed by Fiona Sturges, who noted how her deep understanding of the power of preserving memories to aid in the mourning process. After Easthope lost her first baby to a miscarriage, she kept everything, from the pregnancy test and her first scan to the hospital appointment slips, in a brightly coloured shoebox. She went from making memory boxes to memorialise others, to "doing it for herself. Her shoebox of memories of her baby was, for her 'proof that she had been. That she had existed'" (*The Guardian*, 30 March 2022).

Easthope had been involved in the operations around the 2004 tsunami, the 7/7 bombings, the Grenfell fire and recently around the British response to Covid-19, of which she noted: "We are all disaster survivors now." Sturges noted the "instinctive empathy and compassion" driving Easthope's work: "High up on her agenda" she noted "are the needs of those left behind: the displaced, the traumatised, the bereaved."[7]

Sturges recognised that Easthope's responses to disaster may have come from an innate ability to care for people at the most difficult points of their lives, but also a resigned conviction that these moments of crises are "perpetual, chronic, with a pain that ebbs and flows like tides."

As Lucy Easthope writes:

> The word disaster is formed from the Latin *dis* and a*stro*, meaning bad star. It refers to an ancient belief that when the stars are in a poor position, unfortunate events are going to occur. A misaligning of the astronomical bodies sends the world off kilter.

She acknowledges that most of us don't expect or anticipate major disasters "until they are on the news, after they have already happened" (*The Guardian*, 20 March 2022).

Writing in March 2022, she recognised:

> We will feel the effects of Covid-19 for many years to come. The government's response to Covid-19 has included hefty doses of fear in the messaging. People are afraid of the virus but worse, of each other. We have never been on more of a knife-edge. Fear is a dark genie that is not easy to put back into the bottle. Its effects will linger long after things feel more under control.

She acknowledged:

> Errors made in the response can change the course of the recovery and undermine the longer-term psycho-social health of whole communities. I thought I knew what trauma was and what causes it. But in the course of my work, I have discovered a new enduring loss brought about by the loss of everything-something the people of Ukraine now face.
>
> My soul hopes for the best. My professional experience has taught me the value of a horizon to swim towards. The importance of trying to build something afterwards. But to stay living, breathing, there has to be a purpose, a future, a bluer sky.

Three years after the new Coronavirus began to spread through Wuhan and at least 6.6 million deaths later, we are just beginning to understand its impact and the need to shape a different kind of world. The pandemic is not over, with Covid still moving through China, where it originated, after the lifting of strict controls. Even in the UK, the number of cases rose above 1 million in mid-December 2022.

The pandemic is far from over, even if many people *want* to believe that it is. They are living in denial and refusing to recognise that an estimated two million people are living with Long Covid. We can insist on forgetting but this can only make it harder to "build back better" as we were promised and to learn the lessons as we shape a different, more equal and just world.

For many, however, the intensity of frustration and even anger and despair come from the realisation that there can be *no* simple return to pre-Covid life. It has become clear that Covid-19 has dealt a lasting adverse hit to the NHS. Young people have been specially affected. The full impact may only become evident years or decades into the future.

Cultural Memories, Fearful Bodies and Uncertain Futures

An editorial in *The Guardian* on pandemic recovery (28 December 2022) noted:

> Families of the tens of thousands who died in the UK are still grieving for lost loved ones and want answers about their treatment. Many people lost jobs or businesses. Months of juggling work with childcare, being cut off from friends, worrying about an isolated parent – these too take their toll. The soaring cost of living, or a broader sense of economic, political and social permacrisis, is proving the final straw. The emotional strain of living with ongoing uncertainty and threat is telling.

The pandemic made inequalities much more visible with the poor and black and minority ethnic people much more likely to die while the wealthy were piling up savings. We have become aware of social polarisations and the fragmentation of populations across the world as people dealt with the fear of the virus in different ways, some refusing to acknowledge its harms and then dying in hospitals. The disproportionate burden of caring responsibilities carried by women but also the high levels of sexual abuse and violence reported across the world, have made gender and sexual inequalities more visible challenging ideas of gender and racial equality.

The personal, social, health and economic effects of the pandemic are *not* separate but *interrelated*. Across the world people are coming to terms with the grief they have suffered, and this is *harder* to do when societies are polarised in response to the pandemic. It takes time for people to come together and rebuild social times as they shape new imaginations that help them talk honestly and openly about the fears and terrors, they have lived through during Covid-19.

We need to learn the hard lessons, as the Covid-19 Inquiry is exposing the catastrophic government macho culture in the UK and slowly learning how the experiences of the bereaved provide vital *evidence* through their experiences of loss, rather than personal accounts that can be listened too and set aside. Across the world we have to learn vital lessons to shape different relationships, also with nature, in a time of global emergency.

Rather than forget and put these painful years behind us, we need to be determined *to learn* from them in conversations that share experiences across different nation states and between the global north and the global south. This has to be an integral part of understanding the interrelations between the Covid pandemic and the terrible realities we were already living with in the global climate and biodiversity crisis, that cannot be separated from each other.

We need to listen and to learn as ethical and vulnerable humans who are facing a philosophical need to rethink the terms of European modernities that have undermined our lived relationships as part of the natural world. We need to shape new social and political imaginations that can engage with the inequalities created through globalised neoliberal capitalisms. If humans are to have a future on this planet, it is only going to be *if* they learn to listen to each other as they decolonise their philosophies and social theories and hear the voices of indigenous peoples who have lived their own end of days.

This involves re-visioning conceptions of social justice and being prepared to fundamentally question notions of historical progress that depend upon taken for granted notions of white supremacy and the control and domination of nature. We are still to come to terms with the lessons of the Holocaust and the mass murders of the 20th century that were firmly based on ideas of racial superiority and the hatred of the other. It means a willingness to remember, rather than wilfully forget, the traumatic memories of the global pandemic and experiences as vulnerable humans.

Notes

1 Kitty Hart-Moxon shares her memories of Auschwitz as a child and what it was like for her growing up as a Jewish refugee in post-war Britain in *Return to Auschwitz* (London: Harper Collins 1983).

2 Reflecting on his life and his near-death experiences of Covid-19 Michael Rosen, the children's author has written *Getting Better: Life lessons on going under, getting over it, and getting through it* (London: Ebury Pres 2023); Michael Rosen's *Sad Book* (London: Walker Books 2011) and his *Many Different Kinds of Love: A Story of Life, Death and the NHS* (London: Ebury Press 2022).

3 Nick Cave and Seán O'Hagan *Faith, Hope and Carnage* (New York: Farrar, Straus and Giroux 2022).

4 Jonathan Cott (ed. Bob Dylan) *The Essential Interviews* (New York: Simon and Schuster, Reissue edition 2017).

5 Written in 1968, the year of international student revolts, Erich Fromm writes *Revolution of Hope: Towards a Humanised Technology* (Banbury: Lantern Book 2011) contrasting an increasingly mechanised society bent on mass destruction with a path of humanism and hope. See also his *To Have or to Be* (London: Bloomsbury Academic 2013) and *The Art of Listening* (London: Constable 2001).

6 For a sense of the shifts in Bruno Latour's thinking, partly as a consequence of his engagement with the climate crisis, see *Down to Earth: Politics in the New Climate Regime* (Cambridge: Polity Press 2018) in which he is learning new ways to inhabit the earth while engaging with exploding inequalities, massive deregulation and the conversion of the dream of globalisation into a nightmare for most people; *After Lockdown: A Metamorphosis* (Cambridge: Polity Press 2021) and *Facing Gaia: Eight Lectures on the New Climatic Regime* (Cambridge: Polity Press 2017).

7 Lucy Easthope as a world-leading authority on recovery from disasters who holds governments to account, supports survivors and helps communities to rebuilt has written *When the Dust Settles* (London: Hodder Paperbacks 2023). She has also written *Recovery Myth: The Plans and Situated Realities of Post-Disaster Response* (London: Palgrave Macmillan 2018).

INDEX

Note: page numbers followed by "n" denote endnotes.